INTRODUCING RESEARCH IN NURSING

SECOND EDITION

HOLLY SKODOL WILSON

RN, PhD, FAAN

ADDISON-WESLEY NURSING

A Division of The Benjamin/Cummings Publishing Company, Inc.

Redwood City, California ■ Menlo Park, California

Reading, Massachusetts ■ New York ■ Don Mills, Ontario

Wokingham, U.K. ■ Amsterdam ■ Bonn ■ Sydney ■ Tokyo ■ Madrid ■ San Juan

Sponsoring Editor: Mark McCormick
Production Editors: Gail Carrigan, Cathy Lewis
Cover Designer: Yvo Riezebos
Editorial Assistant: Bob Bledsoe
Compositor: G&S Typesetters, Inc.

Library of Congress Cataloging-in-Publication Data

Wilson, Holly Skodol.
    Introducing research in nursing / Holly Skodol Wilson.—2nd ed.
        p.   cm.
    Includes bibliographical references and index.
    ISBN 0-8053-9405-2
    1. Nursing—Research—Evaluation.   2. Nursing—Research—
Methodology.   I. Title.
    [DNLM: 1. Nursing Research—methods.   WY 20.5 W748i]
RT81.5.W54   1992
610.73′072—dc20
DNLM/DLC
for Library of Congress   92-22043
                                                                 CIP

ISBN 0-8053-9405-2
3 4 5 6 7 8 9 10 -FG- 95 94 93

Addison-Wesley Nursing
A Division of the Benjamin/Cummings Publishing
Company, Inc.
390 Bridge Parkway, Redwood City, CA 94065

For my three daughters, Molly, Emily, and Hillary, as they pursue their own advanced education.

CONTENTS

PREFACE

Introducing Research in Nursing was written for nursing students and nurses who realize that we are in the midst of an information revolution. Coping with the growing body of research literature in our field requires the ability to understand and judge the usefulness of scientific findings. Our commitment to excellence in nursing care demands that we develop the skills of intelligent research consumership. This book has been thoroughly updated and revised in keeping with the spirit and the style of the first edition, with some important new information and improvements. (1) Examples, references, and facts have been updated. (2) All glossary terms appear in easy-to-identify boldface type in the text. (3) Annotated research examples appear in each chapter to illustrate the critique process. (4) Chapter 11, Qualitative Research Methods, now includes uses of the *phenomenologic-interpretive* method in nursing research. And (5) an appendix on statistics has been added.

Research skills can become an integral part of every nurse's role in a variety of ways. Here are some examples:

- A nurse may be asked to comment on the accuracy of a health-related article in the popular press by his or her clinic clients;

- A nurse may need to evaluate the rationale for procedural change on a hospital unit;

- A nurse may need to interpret the meaning of the research reported in a nursing journal.

Introducing Research in Nursing 2e will guide nurses in their first steps on the journey to competence as informed consumers of nursing research. Based on the award-winning *Research in Nursing 2e* (1989), this introductory text conveys the same message: Nursing science and research can become as valuable and interesting to nurse clinicians as they are to nurse scientists. If nursing is to build a body of scientific knowledge, and if nursing practice is to be shaped by that knowledge rather than by tradition, intuition, authority, or habit, then research consumership skills must be as basic to every nurse's repertoire as are communication skills and sterile technique. *Introducing Research in Nursing 2e* offers a clear and practical presentation of these skills.

AUDIENCE

This book is appropriate as the primary text for nursing research courses in all undergraduate curricula, including those aimed at returning RNs. Experienced clinicians who wish to sharpen their research critique skills will also find it a useful addition to their agency or personal reference shelf. An *Instructor's Guide* is keyed to the text chapter by chapter and includes lecture outlines, small group and large class learning activities, and test questions.

CONTENT

The organization and coverage of this text address the needs of the reader who wishes to understand nursing studies. It begins with the basics, which are often taken for granted in introductory texts but which are crucial for all nurses who engage in the research process as consumers. Key questions addressed throughout the text are

- Where do I find reports of nursing research?

- How can I begin to penetrate the unfamiliar, technical language of nursing research?

- What are the ethical issues involved in nursing research with human subjects?

- What is my role in identifying researchable clinical problems?

- How can research findings influence clinical practice?

- What are the criteria for judging the truth of published findings?

The book presents the phases of the research process by emphasizing the information that is important to intelligent consumership. An informal, lively writing style contributes to its readability. Illustrations from current nursing research literature help to bridge the "research-practice gap."

FEATURES

Several design elements enhance this text's utility as a learning tool, including

- chapter outlines

- chapter objectives

- annotated examples

- guidelines for critique

- summaries of key ideas and terms

- a glossary

- an index

In addition, appendixes provide information and guidance on writing proposals, ethical issues and a quick summary of important statistical information. The first of these is particularly useful to students for whom a research proposal is the required term project, while the second and third are essential continuing resources to all nurses involved in clinical research projects, whether in supporting or principal roles.

Holly Skodol Wilson

ABOUT THE AUTHORS

Dr. Holly Skodol Wilson, RN, PhD, FAAN, is a professor in the Department of Mental Health, Community and Administrative Nursing at the University of California, San Francisco. She teaches the required introductory research course for nursing students in the masters of science program. Her other honors include Distinguished Alumni, Duke University, School of Nursing; Distinguished Dissertation of the Year, University of California, Berkeley; the American Nurses' Foundation Scholar Citation; membership in Sigma Theta Tau; a Kellog National Leadership Fellowship, and she is a fellow in the American Academy of Nursing. Dr. Wilson is the author of over 60 scientific and scholarly journal articles and the author or co-author of 15 books. She is a sought after national and international consultant and lecturer who has worked in Colombia, Argentina, Australia, New Zealand, The Philippines, the People's Republic of China, Japan, Africa, Israel, Sweden, Norway, Denmark, England, Canada, and throughout the United States. She is also the single mother of three daughters.

Dr. Sally Hutchinson, RN, PhD, FAAN, is a professor in the College of Nursing at the University of Florida. She teaches research courses with an emphasis on qualitative methodology to masters and doctoral students. Her research focuses on nurses and their work, psychogerontology and bipolar disorders. Dr. Hutchinson is the author and co-author of two books and many scholarly articles. She is a national and international speaker and consultant.

Brandy Britton is a doctoral candidate in the Department of Social and Behavioral Sciences at the University of California, San Francisco. She has a BA in sociology and a BS in biology, with a minor in women's studies. Her areas of specialization include research design and methodological techniques, medical sociology, and women's health. Britton is a Project Director for a National Institute on Drug Abuse grant project that investigates drug abuse among pregnant women.

ACKNOWLEDGMENTS

Introducing Research in Nursing Second Edition was

- inspired by the nursing students enrolled in my research course at the University of California, San Francisco;

- encouraged by the energy and efforts of nursing editor Mark McCormick;

- enriched by the previous contributions of my colleagues, who contributed to *Research in Nursing* (1985) and *Research In Nursing 2e* (1989): Dr. Sandra Ferketich, Dr. Sally Hutchinson, Dr. Diane LaRochelle, Dr. Ada Lindsey, Dr. Linda Moody, Dr. Jane Norbeck, Dr. Sandra Scheetz, Dr. Nancy Stotts, and Dr. Joyce Verran;

- updated and improved through the revisions made by Brandy Britton, doctoral candidate in sociology at the University of California, San Francisco.

INTRODUCING RESEARCH IN NURSING

SECOND EDITION

WHAT IS NURSING RESEARCH?

HOLLY SKODOL WILSON

CHAPTER OUTLINE

In This Chapter . . .

- Why Do Research?
- Ways of Knowing
- What Is the Scientific Approach?
- Types of Nursing Research
    - The Pure-Applied Continuum
    - Classification by Purpose and Design
- Steps in the Research Process
    - Step 1—Stating a Researchable Problem
    - Step 2—Defining the Purpose of the Research
    - Step 3—Reviewing Related Literature and Linking It
        to a Theoretical Context
    - Step 4—Formulating Hypotheses and Defining Variables
    - Step 5—Selecting the Research Design
    - Step 6—Selecting the Population and Sample
    - Step 7—Conducting a Pilot Study
    - Step 8—Collecting the Data Step
    - Step 9—Analyzing the Data
    - Step 10—Communicating Conclusions
- Nursing Research and the Nursing Profession
    - Nursing Research from the 1950s to the 1980s
    - The National Nursing Research Agenda for the 1990s

After reading this chapter, you should be able to:

- Appreciate the meaning and usefulness of the scientific method of problem solving and decision making in nursing practice

- Compare the scientific approach with (1) trial and error and common sense, (2) authority and tradition, (3) inspiration and intuition, and (4) logical reasoning

- Identify the assumptions, characteristics, and aims of the scientific approach

- Locate a nursing study on a continuum based on its relevance to nursing practice

- Recognize types of nursing studies through identification of study purpose and design

- Explain ten typical steps in the research process

- Interpret the implications of past trends for the future nursing research agenda

1

IN THIS CHAPTER . . .

> Expert Nurse: *We had a woman who came in with a diagnosis of diverti-culosis. She had had bilateral mastectomies, and on her laparotomy they found her belly full of cancer. Her surgery was open-and-close. The attend-ing physician told her husband and instructed him not to tell his wife until she had recovered from her surgery. Her prognosis was grave, probably only a few weeks. The day I remember is when she was very close to death and we were all waiting for her son to arrive from Texas. He hadn't seen his mother in several years, but his mother very much wanted to see him be-fore she died. She was delirious and her husband was frantic with anxiety that his son wouldn't arrive in time. I spent much of that time with him in her room talking to them both and bathing her. She was incontinent and bleeding from many orifices. We then heard that the plane her son was on was two hours late, which heightened everyone's anxiety. He [the son] finally arrived and I told him what to expect when he entered the room. They spent 15 minutes together, the three of them, before she died. She was alert and talking the whole time. We all cried that day, amazed and reaffirmed by this example of human strength. [Benner 1984, pp. 57–58]*

The realities of human suffering and joy challenge and enrich the practice of the scientific, professional discipline of nursing. Each day you may carry out tasks that are viewed by others as rewarding, frightening, or even distasteful. You will often have to rely on your own judgment in the absence of complete information. Your work may arouse in you feelings of compassion, outrage, guilt, pity, anxiety, confusion, or curiosity. These experiences may seem far removed from the world of scientific research. Indeed, there seems to be an enormous abyss separating the daily practice of nursing and the seemingly abstract science of nursing.

Voices in the vanguard of leadership in nursing call for bridging the gap between research and practice. This involves a two-way process: making nurs-ing practice (rather than education or administration) a more frequent focus for research, and increasing the application of research findings to practice. Editorials in nursing journals, officers in professional associations, and proba-bly your own teachers all assert that without an empirically grounded body of scientific knowledge on which to base clinical practice, nursing's stance as a profession is weak. Everybody seems to agree that it is critical that nursing develop a scientific base and that research is the way to get it.

One of the aims of this book is to show that research is more than the meticulous application of given procedures to relatively obscure questions. By penetrating the mystique of research methods you will come to know

- what to look for in research studies

- what meanings to assign their findings

- how to put findings into practice

- how to use your curiosity, imagination, and reasoning to adapt the technology of science to acquiring fresh knowledge and solutions to practical problems

The aim of chapter 1 is to define the meaning of science and research for nurses who will be applying study findings in their clinical practice. In this chapter you will learn about the scientific way of knowing as contrasted with the alternatives of common sense, tradition, intuition, and logical reasoning. You will also be introduced to several types of nursing research, the typical steps in the research process, past trends in nursing research, and nursing's research agenda for the future. Finally, you will discover how nursing research can foster your own intellectual development, advance the nursing profession, and improve the quality of care given to patients.

Chapter 1 opens the door to a rich adventure in the world of discovery and scientific competence. Take a stand when you read it. Argue about the ideas. Be opinionated. Later, soften your attitude to one, in Kerlinger's (1966) terms, of "intelligent conviction and emotional commitment." Technical competence is empty without a basic understanding of the nature and promise of research in nursing.

WHY DO RESEARCH?

A mother-to-be was admitted to a California hospital at 3:40 A.M. in active labor. An external monitor was applied, and her membranes broke about 20 minutes later. When her physician's associate checked in at 5 A.M., the obstetrical nurse expressed concern about the monitor tracing and asked him to check it. After he did so and did a pelvic exam on the laboring mother, he suggested that the nurse call the patient's primary obstetrician. Unknown to him, however, was the fact that the obstetrician had left standing orders not to be disturbed between 10 P.M. and 7 A.M., "except in an emergency." Because the associate did not declare this case to be an emergency, the nurse followed the standing orders. By 7:30 the monitor was exhibiting a marked late deceleration, and by 10 the obstetrician had come to the hospital and performed an emergency Caesarean section. The newborn exhibited signs of brain damage. Now, at 3¹/₂ years of age, he is a spastic quadriplegic with mental retardation. [Snyder 1983]

How does a nurse decide what to do in such a situation? Should he or she follow the standing instruction of an authority and abide by the institution's traditions? Or is there an independent accountability to the patient that requires the nurse to recognize the seriousness of the situation from the monitor tracings and make judgments on some other basis?

If you are inclined to favor the latter alternative, consider another situation. Imagine that you have taught prenatal classes to expectant parents for five years. One of your patients has been complaining of severe nausea and vomiting and is taking Bendectin (a combination of doxylamine and pyridoxin). She reads in the local paper that the drug's manufacturer is no longer making and distributing the drug but that it has not been withdrawn from the market and will continue to be available until supplies in the hands of drug distributors, wholesalers, and pharmacies are exhausted. She asks *you* whether it is true that taking this drug will cause pyloric stenosis in her infant. Or will nausea and vomiting, without treatment, themselves increase the same risk? Would she be better off taking a different drug, even though it has not been so well studied as Bendectin? The mother-to-be seeks your counsel. On what basis do you respond?

Or, suppose you are planning a prevention program targeted to the reports that older women get osteoporosis three to five times more often than men and therefore have more bone fractures in later life. Would you recommend calcium supplements, high-protein diets, exercise, or supplemental estrogen? On what bases would you decide? What is the risk to young children of electrically powered beds with automatic bed-lowering controls, or "walk-away switches"? The scientific approach as reflected in nursing research offers you important resources for answering such difficult clinical and health-related questions.

WAYS OF KNOWING

Although this text advocates the scientific method as the way to address the questions posed in the last section, there are alternative ways of knowing:

- *You can use trial and error combined with common sense.* If the other patients in your prenatal class who took Bendectin did not have babies with pyloric stenosis, your common sense might compel you to say that the drug was safe.

- *You can use authority and tradition.* If following the stated rules in procedure books and standing orders is your choice, you will not feel obligated to make an independent interpretation of the fetal monitor's tracings for evidence of an emergency.

- *You can use inspiration and intuition.* If your engaged style of knowing compels you to predict that elderly women are disadvantaged by the level of care they receive, you will be inspired to become an advocate for better care for the aged, minorities, and other disadvantaged groups and support teaching them self-care.

- *You can use logical reasoning.* If your own sense of logic alerts you to the ideas that (1) children and some adults are particularly curious about how mechanical beds operate, (2) the metal underparts of such beds can have a scissors or guillotine action, and (3) being caught between the stationary portion of the bed and its moving frame could crush a child to death, you will conclude that removing or deactivating the "walk-away" down switches on these beds, at least in pediatric and psychiatric wards, is definitely indicated.

WHAT IS THE SCIENTIFIC APPROACH?

The way of knowing developed in this book is that of scientific research blended with what Diers (1983) has defined as "clinical scholarship"—a stretching of one's mind for new insights. Let's begin with some basic *assumptions* that underpin the scientific approach:

1. It is better to be knowledgeable about the world than to be ignorant of it.

2. Scientists can use their senses to apprehend an external reality.

3. Observers of the world are able to relate observations conceptually and make meaning out of them.

4. It is possible to discern an underlying order in the psychosocial as well as the physical world.

5. Cause-and-effect relationships exist in the social *and* physical orders.

Given these assumptions, we can define **scientific inquiry** as a process in which observable, verifiable data are systematically collected from the world we know through our senses to describe, explain, or predict events. The scientific approach has two *characteristics* that the other ways of knowing do not: (1) **self-correction,** or **objectivity,** and (2) *the use of* **empirical data.** The quality of objectivity is the attempt to distance the research process as much as possible from the scientist's personal beliefs, values, and attitudes.

The empirical data, or evidence gathered by the senses, are examined in a systematic way.

The basic *aims* of scientific inquiry are (1) to develop explanations of the world (these explanations are called **theories**—see chapter 5) and (2) to find solutions to problems. Although these two aims in nursing science are related, some research studies emphasize the development of our general understanding of human beings in interacting with their environment, whereas others emphasize the determination of effectiveness of specific nursing interventions in practice situations. Table 1–1 summarizes the assumptions, characteristics, and aims of the scientific approach.

Table 1–1 *Summary of Basic Points about the Scientific Approach to Knowing*

Assumptions	*Characteristics*	*Aims*
Knowledge is more valuable than ignorance	Built-in self-correction or objectivity	To build a body of theories that describe,
Empirical evidence is used	Reliance on empirical evidence	explain, and predict
Conceptualizations are based on observation		To solve practical problems
An underlying order exists in the universe		
Causal relationships exist		

In sum, if as a clinician you began to wonder why some myocardial infarction patients were allowed to drink ice water and others were not, you could draw on books of procedure, your past experiences, trial and error, and common sense to arrive at an explanation. *Or* you could try to use the tools of science to answer your question. Table 1–2 provides a comparison of the scientific approach with the common-sense approach.

TYPES OF NURSING RESEARCH

There are two main types of research, related to the two chief aims of scientific inquiry. Research conducted to develop theories is often called **basic, or pure, research.** It is often compared to building blocks, on which increments in knowledge and further research are based. Research directed toward solving practical problems is usually called **applied research.** It includes not only studies designed to solve problems or make decisions but also **clinical trials** aimed at developing and evaluating a new program, product, method, or procedure.

This distinction between basic and applied research becomes a bit fuzzy when it is used to categorize research conducted in a practice discipline such as nursing. Suppose a nurse were to do a study of the health care needs of elderly Hispanic-American women. The study's purpose and design might be limited to building a data base and thereby contributing to a body of knowledge in an area where there has been little research. In this sense, by the standard definition the research would be basic—knowledge for knowledge's sake. Someone else, how-ever, might subsequently use the findings to alter aspects of nursing care for this population of patients, thus transforming a basic study into an applied study by using the findings to reform the ills of practice.

Table 1–2   *Scientific Knowing versus Common-Sense Knowing*

Scientific Approach	*Common Sense*
Uses conceptual schemes that have been empirically tested	May accept fanciful explanations
Acquires evidence to test theories according to systematic methods	Selects evidence on the basis of personal experiences or preferences, usually to verify a personal position
Uses a controlled method for ruling out other variables that might explain a phenomenon	Makes little or no attempt to control variables
Tends not to deal with explanations that cannot be empirically tested	May be highly metaphysical or spiritual
Has a built-in mechanism for self-correction	Allows explanations to persist even if incorrect

Diers (1979) equates virtually *all* nursing research with applied research when she enumerates three distinguishing properties of research problems in nursing:

1. The potential nursing research problem must involve "a difference that matters" in terms of its consequences for improving patient care.

2. A nursing research problem has a relationship to conceptual issues and therefore has the potential for contributing to theory development and the body of scientific nursing knowledge.

3. A research problem is a *nursing* research problem when nurses have access to and control over the phenomenon being studied.

According to these criteria, all nursing research is a blend of pure and applied research, and the critical point is its *clinical relevance* for nursing practice and our knowledge about that practice.

In sum, according to Diers and many other researchers, knowledge in practice professions is *for something;* specifically, in nursing it is for improving the care given to the consumers of nursing services. If a nurse were to study how baccalaureate nursing students learn to care for terminally ill patients in the context of routine clinical instruction, the nurse would be conducting a study in the field of education, not nursing. But if a nurse were to study the effects of rate of intramuscular injection on intensity and duration of first and second pain, she or he would be conducting a nursing research study.

The Pure-Applied Continuum

An alternative to the old basic-applied distinction that is probably more useful in classifying types of nursing studies is a **pure-applied continuum** based on *how relevant* (1) the subjects, (2) the content, and (3) the conditions are to real-world nursing problems and decisions (Cooperative Graduate Education in Nursing 1975). This continuum can be divided into six stages (see Figure 1–1).

Stage 1—Not Directly Relevant   A nurse physiologist interested in the mechanisms of skin healing and studying the optimum time and temperature of wet soaks on guinea pigs' wounds in a laboratory would be conducting pure research. This research would be identified as a stage 1 study on the pure-applied continuum in Figure 1–1. It would not be directly relevant to the practice of nursing.

Pure Research					**Applied Research**
Not directly relevant	Relevant topic *or* subjects	Relevant topic *and* subjects	Relevant topic, subjects, and trial conditions	Normal field conditions	Advocacy and adoption
Stage 1	Stage 2	Stage 3	Stage 4	Stage 5	Stage 6

Figure 1–1   *Pure-applied continuum based on relevance to nursing practice*

Stage 2—Relevant Topic *or* Subjects   A nurse interested in the concept of hunger might conduct a laboratory study in which college students drink Metrecal through a tube from behind a screen with no visual cues to how much they have consumed. Such a study, designed to determine whether there is a natural factor that influences feeling satisfied, would be located at stage 2 because it is conducted with people instead of animals. However, the topic of hunger and satiation is not specifically related to a nursing activity.

Stage 3—Relevant Topic *and* Subjects   A researcher wanting to know whether premature infants placed in different body positions consume different amounts of energy would be working at stage 3 of the continuum, because the study involves people as subjects *and* compares positioning choices, a topic of direct concern to nursing practice.

Stage 4—Relevant Topic, Subjects, and Trial Conditions   A study to determine whether it makes a difference to the recovery rate of hospitalized children when a nursing care plan also takes into account the needs of the parents would be testing nursing intervention under special conditions, a stage 4 study. (Of course, one of the problems with a study under special conditions is that the conditions themselves may account for the results.)

Stage 5—Normal Field Conditions   Studying the quality of nursing care for chronically ill patients with differing staffing patterns under normal hospital conditions would qualify as a stage 5 study.

Stage 6—Advocacy and Adoption   Research that demonstrated the applicability of primary nursing—in which one nurse is totally responsible for a case load of patients—to a diverse array of practice settings would be at the extreme applied end of the continuum, or stage 6.

Classification by Purpose and Design

Nursing research can also be classified by its purposes and related study designs. Table 1–3 summarizes four of the major purposes of research—to describe, to explain, to experiment, and to test a method—and cites illustrative contemporary nursing studies for each. Study designs are described in detail in chapter 7.

STEPS IN THE RESEARCH PROCESS

The purpose of research is to discover solutions to problems and generate general principles and theory by applying scientific procedures designed to increase the chances that data collected will be reliable, relevant, and unbiased. To increase the chance that any particular study meets these criteria, researchers customarily follow a sequence of actions when conducting the study. Whether the actions in the sequence are called steps, phases, or elements, they are likely to be expressed in different forms and numbers depending on the level of inquiry and the type of

Table 1–3   *Types of Nursing Study According to Purpose or Design*

Type	Purpose	Methods	Examples
Exploratory	To obtain a richer familiarity with a phenomenon and clarify concepts as a basis for further research	Interviews, participant observation, document analysis, case studies	The lived experience of recovering from addiction (Banonis 1989)
Descriptive	To obtain complete and accurate information about a phenomenon	Interviews, questionnaires, direct observation, analysis of records	Nutritional support in HIV infection (Bradley-Springer 1991) Diagnosis of Alzheimer's disease from the spouse's perspective (Morgan & Laing 1991)
Explanatory	To provide conceptual analyses grounded in observation of human behavior	Interviews, participant observation, constant comparative analysis	Cultural diversity as a variable of crisis precipitating factors of individuals seeking intervention (Coler & Hafner 1991) Prediction of maternal depressive symptoms in single-parent families (Hall et al 1991)
Experimental and quasi-experimental	To test hypotheses about relationships	Experiments, quasi-experiments	Effect of lung hyperventilation and endotracheal suctioning on cardiopulmonary hemodynamics (Stone et al 1991) Neurobehavioral assessment ratings for infants with intraventricular hemorrhage correlated with one measure of brain metabolism (Medhoff-Cooper et al 1991)
Methodological	To develop or refine a new research technique or procedure	Validity tests, reliability tests	Psychometric assessment of a new measure of nursing intensity (Prescott 1991) Alternative approach to the multitrait-multimethod matrix approach (Ferketich et al 1991)

study. This section is intended not to present a set of steps set in concrete but rather to use the metaphor of steps to describe the general line of thinking that most investigators consider when planning a study. My list, for the purpose of clarity and comprehensiveness, has ten modular, mobile, and flexible steps:

1. stating a researchable problem

2. defining the purpose of the research

3. reviewing related literature and linking it to a theoretical context

4. formulating hypotheses and defining variables

5. selecting the research design

6. selecting the population and sample

7. conducting a pilot study

8. collecting the data

9. analyzing the data

10. communicating conclusions

Each of these steps is taken up in comprehensive detail in the remainder of this text. To give you a sense of the whole picture, however, each step will be described briefly here.

Step 1—Stating a Researchable Problem

An investigator's task initially involves moving from a broad area of interest to a more circumscribed problem that specifies exactly what he or she intends to study. Most investigators try to define their research problems as precisely as possible. A problem is often stated in the form of a question. Here are some examples from published nursing research studies:

- How many different treatments for pressure sores are advocated by nurses, and what rationales are given for their use?

- Do mothers who are not given a prepartum enema have higher rates of contamination than mothers who are given an enema?

- Do different postoperative activity schedules affect the recovery of physical fitness among athletes?

- Is there a relationship between types of care of indwelling urethral catheters and the incidence of urinary tract infection?

- What is the optimal length of time needed to obtain an accurate oral temperature with a glass thermometer?

- What is the effect of low-frequency auditory and kinesthetic stimulation on neurological functioning of the premature infant?

If a study problem is too broad or is vague, proceeding to subsequent stages of the process becomes very confusing. This is true even in the instance of field research and qualitative analysis, where the study problem per se may "emerge" from the data after a researcher enters the field (see chapter 11). A research question, according to Brink and Wood (1988 p. 2), "is an explicit query about a problem or issue that can be challenged, examined, analyzed, and will yield useful new information."

Step 2—Defining the Purpose of the Research

The second step is sometimes called defining the *rationale* of the study. It is the researcher's statement of *why* the question is important and what use the answer will serve. It lets the reader or funding agency know what to expect from the study. The purpose of a study also influences its review by an institutional review board (see chapter 12). Many nursing studies are challenged on the basis that they seem to be exercises in methodology with no conceivable benefit to anyone. A trivial purpose will influence judgments about the risk-benefit ratio if human subjects are involved.

An excellent example of a purpose statement is found in the report of Kathryn Barnard's (1973) classic research on the effects of environmental stimulation on the sleep of premature infants:

> Previous work with full term neonates and older infants supports the general notion that particular kinds of stimulation assist in the regulation of sleep and arousal status. Given this evidence and the increasing evidence that quiet sleep in the immature infant can improve neurological development . . . *the purpose of the current investigation was to study the effect of regular, controlled stimulation on the neurological functioning in the infant born prematurely.* [p. 15]

Step 3—Reviewing Related Literature and Linking It to a Theoretical Context

If researchers want their study to build on, confirm, or even transcend the existing knowledge in a discipline and thereby qualify as a real contribution to science, they must know what has already been done. A review of the literature provides the researcher with ideas for defining concepts and for creating a study design (see chapter 4).

A **theoretical framework** is an essay in which the investigator summarizes the existing concepts, theories, research methods, and findings and relates them to his or her study question and purpose (Brink and Wood 1988). At the least, constructing such a framework provides relevant concepts for the research; at best, it can give the researcher a full awareness of facts, issues, prior findings, theories, and instruments that might be relevant to the study question.

Step 4—Formulating Hypotheses and Defining Variables

Hypotheses are statements of the relationship between two or more concepts, or variables (see chapter 6). Some studies are intended to *develop* hypotheses (exploratory, descriptive, and grounded theory designs), while others are intended to *test* hypotheses (experimental and quasi-experimental designs). Stating hypotheses requires not only sufficient knowledge of a topic to make a prediction about the outcome of a study but also the ability to specify definitions for the variables under investigation in measurable terms. Hypotheses can be explicitly stated, as Sitzman and her colleagues (1983) did in their study of biofeedback training:

> HYPOTHESIS (H_1): *Emphysema and chronic bronchitic patients who receive a biofeedback training program to decrease their respiratory rate will have a significantly decreased respiratory rate at the end of the training program and one-month follow-up. [p. 219]*

Hypotheses may also be stated as **null hypotheses,** which essentially test the idea that *there are no significant differences* in what is called the criterion, dependent, or outcome variable other than *what can be attributed to chance.*

Because stating hypotheses requires the investigator to specify the concepts being studied, it is also important at this point to determine how these variables are going to be defined for the purpose of measuring them. For example, social support might be defined as a score on a written self-report scale or inventory. This step is called **operationally defining** the variables.

Step 5—Selecting the Research Design

A **research design** is a well-thought-out, systematic, and even controlled plan for finding answers to study questions. It offers a road map or blueprint for organizing a study, from methods of data collection through methods of data analysis. Chapter 7 covers the array of possibilities that are available for structuring the research plan.

Step 6—Selecting the Population and Sample

Once researchers have reduced a general idea of interest to a specific study question, have reviewed the related literature, and have decided on a plan for designing their study, they must choose a study population and select a sample. A **population** refers to the group to be studied. To whom should the study's findings apply? Populations that have been the focus of recent nursing studies include divorced fathers, older persons, hospitalized children, disadvantaged minorities, depressed women, nursing mothers, patients with cancer, persons with AIDS, patients who have had surgery, and nursing students. The **sample** refers to those elements of a population from whom data will actually be collected and from whom generalizations to the population will be made. The various kinds of samples and procedures for selecting them are spelled out in chapter 8.

Step 7—Conducting a Pilot Study

A researcher can learn a lot about the strengths and weaknesses of a large project's intended design, sample size, and data-collection instruments by doing a **pilot study,** or small-scale practice run. Pilot studies have been so helpful in strengthening nursing studies by weeding out problems in advance that many funding agencies are not inclined to approve study proposals unless a pilot study has been conducted.

Step 8—Collecting the Data

Any study that goes beyond "armchair speculation" eventually requires the researcher to collect data. Data sources may be people, documents, or laboratory materials, and data-collection instruments may include interviews, questionnaires, physiological tests, and psychological tests. All of these possibilities are covered in depth in chapters 9 and 11. Data relevant to the variables being studied are collected using the researcher's senses and measurement tools. The amounts of time and energy required for this step vary according to the research design. Field studies, historical research, surveys, and most experiments demand a lot of both during this phase.

Step 9—Analyzing the Data

The next step in the research process involves taking apart the data that have been collected and reorganizing them so that the researcher can make some sense of them in relation to the study question, research objectives, or stated hypotheses. Analyses of numerical data can be accomplished using the statistical procedures discussed in chapter 10. Qualitative data such as open-ended questionnaire responses, observational field notes, interview transcripts, case studies, documents, and the like can be analyzed according to a variety of approaches explained in chapter 11. The most important part about this step is to *have a plan in mind, the requisite skills for doing it, and the realization that this work is the source of answers to the original research questions.*

Step 10—Communicating Conclusions

The researcher's challenge at the final stage is to explain the results of the investigation and link them with the existing body of knowledge in the discipline. The study's real contribution cannot be judged unless the conclusions are communicated to colleagues and critics. As Polit and Hungler (1987) put it, "Even the most compelling hypothesis, the most careful and thorough study, and the most dramatic results are of no value to the scientific community if they are unknown" (p. 41). Communicating the conclusions, interpreting the real meaning and implications of the findings, recognizing the study's possible limitations, and suggesting directions for future lines of inquiry culminate the research process.

Most researchers acknowledge these research steps as conventions, or recipes, and then, with creativity, imagination, and pragmatism, vary and adapt them to the unique situation they are addressing.

NURSING RESEARCH AND THE NURSING PROFESSION

Nursing Research from the 1950s to the 1980s

Beginning at least in the early 1950s, nursing research received increased federal funding and professional support. Centers for research developed, the number of doctorally prepared nurses engaged in scientific enterprise increased, and avenues for communicating research reports (journals, conferences, and meetings) expanded. Nursing research became viewed as a legitimate field of interest not only for students at the entry level but also for *all nurses.* Spruck's 1980 National League for Nursing (NLN) survey of 286 accredited baccalaureate nursing programs revealed that research content was included as required course work in 83% of the schools, and the remainder of the schools were moving toward incorporating a research component. A second survey, by Thomas and Price (1980), obtained usable responses from 205 of the 291 NLN-accredited baccalaureate nursing programs in the United States. Of them, 198 reported explicit provision for teaching nursing research in their programs; the remaining 7 were in the process of developing research content. Our profession had reached a consensus that some involvement in research at all levels of educational preparation was necessary for the advancement of the nursing profession and the welfare of patients. In sum, the question "Should nursing research be taught at all levels of nursing education?" was replaced with the contemporary question "What should be taught about nursing research, at what level, and how?"

In 1983 two history-making announcements were made. The first was the creation of the Center for Research for Nursing by the American Nurses' Association (ANA). It was responsible for developing a distinct and coordinated research program to serve as the source of national data for the profession. It encompassed the former ANA Department of Research and Policy Analysis, American Academy of Nursing, and American Nurses' Foundation. The principal function of the Center was to conduct studies and surveys to:

- support the work of policy bodies

- provide for administration of extramurally funded projects

- prepare grant applications to secure funding for research

- coordinate external fund-raising activities

The second announcement was that legislation to create a national institute of nursing had been introduced in Congress. This move was prompted by recommendations in a 1983 Institute of Medicine report that called for a federally established entity *to place nursing research in the mainstream of scien-*

tific investigation. In 1986 **The National Center for Nursing Research** (**NCNR**) was established as part of the National Institutes of Health (NIH) by congressional mandate. The mandate for the NCNR is to fund nursing research and research training related to:

- patient care
- promotion of health
- prevention of disease
- mitigation of effects of acute and chronic illness and disabilities

The NCNR initially made $19 million available in 1986, and that total increased to more than $33 million in 1990. The number of grant applications rose from 160 in 1987 to 280 in 1989. Establishment of the NCNR placed nursing research in the mainstream of scientific investigation focused on our nation's health.

The **National Nursing Research Agenda** (**NNRA**) of The National Center for Nursing Research is a concentrated effort to set priorities for nursing research. When the NCNR was created in 1986, the newly appointed director, Dr. Ada Sue Hinshaw, proposed a number of initiatives to develop programs of the center. One of these was the five-year plan to provide directions for nursing research within the discipline. The process began with a review of the literature of past priority-setting by nursing organizations. This early work led to two working papers which provided the background for a national conference on research priorities convened in January 1989 and involving more than 50 scientists. The priorities selected, published as a 1988 editorial in the *Journal of Professional Nursing,* consisted of the following:

- low-birth-weight mothers and infants
- HIV infection prevention and care
- long-term care for older adults
- symptom management
- information systems
- health promotion
- technology dependency across the life span

Promising Directions

The research agenda for nursing in the 1990s emphasizes linking research to practice. Experts agree that nursing research should focus on health problems and disease-prevention techniques, such as obesity reduction, smoking cessation, prevention of cancer and heart disease, prevention of complications, and improvement of patient care for problems like wounds and decubitis ulcers. Research on clinical therapies and interventions, such as non-nutritive sucking—which encourages premature infants to use bottles sooner and be discharged from the hospital earlier, thus substantially cutting costs for their care—will also be prominent in the next decade.

The federal **Agency for Health Care Policy Research (AHCPR)**, created in 1990 with a first-year budget of $126 million, is responsible primarily for implementing a program to improve the effectiveness and appropriateness of health services nationwide. It particularly emphasizes treatment effectiveness, or "outcome research." The agency's allotted $166 million in 1991 and $221 million in 1992 include funds for studies of nursing clinical practice.

The National Nursing Research Agenda for the 1990s

The approach to science and research expounded in this text involves closing the gap between research and practice. Research does not become nursing research merely because it is done by a nurse. Many authors have distinguished between what they call nursing research and research in nursing. **Nursing research,** on the one hand, is research into the process and outcomes of care and the clinical problems encountered in the practice of nursing. **Research in nursing,** on the other hand, is the broader study of people and the nursing profession, including historical, ethical, and policy studies. If we agree that the business of nursing is *practice* and also agree that the business of nursing research is answering questions and solving problems about that practice, then nursing practice and nursing research share the common goal of *improving nursing care.*

Research does not have to be complicated to be good and useful. We must be wary of trying at all cost to adhere rigidly to methods that were developed in the natural, or "hard," sciences. They may well be inappropriate for studying nursing phenomena in a natural setting. Emerging alternative methods are increasingly interesting to nurses involved in clinical research.

The shift in recent years toward describing nursing phenomena, evaluating outcomes of nursing intervention, and building empirically based theories that will be the cornerstones of a nursing science does not preclude the value of what Diers (1983) has called "clinical scholarship":

> Scholarship is different from research. It implies . . . contemplation [and] the stretching of the mind for new insights. . . . Good research reporting may well fall into the definition of scholarship; mechanical reports, which provide data but not insight, do not. [p. 3]

Tomorrow's nursing research will continue to emphasize studies of the interaction of physiological and psychosocial mechanisms in human experiences of stress and coping, evaluations of nursing interventions, the transfer of research findings into textbooks and practice, a focus on high-risk and underserved groups such as the elderly, vulnerable families, and minorities, and the creation of a body of scientific nursing knowledge. And today's student of research in nursing will be involved in its conduct and application.

RESEARCH EXAMPLE

Study Problem

applied research

The variables of achievement motivation of pregnant women and of their level of information about breast-feeding are suggested as positive predictors of <u>success in breast-feeding</u>. Success is defined as breast-feeding for at least six weeks postpartum.

Methods

stage 4 on pure-applied continuum, relevant topic, subjects, and trial conditions

Initially, <u>the volunteers</u> for the study, sought through prepared childbirth classes, completed the Personal Data Inventory, the Questionnaire Measure of Individual Differences in Achieving Tendency, and the Information on Breastfeeding Questionnaire. The Breastfeeding Experience Questionnaire was mailed to each participant at six weeks postpartum with a request to return the completed form. Participants numbered 150.

Findings

The hypothesis was supported, with 107 participants successful in breast-feeding. Of those who were unsuccessful, more than 50% weaned their infants within the first three weeks postpartum. The two reasons most cited for early weaning were (1) lack of milk, and (2) sore nipples. The unsuccessful mothers in the study were generally less knowledgeable about breast-feeding than the successful mothers. <u>The need for accurate information about breast-feeding</u> has been recognized and <u>supported by the findings.</u>

explanatory research

Implications

Based on this study's findings, it is suggested that the <u>maternal-child nurse provide</u> basic information about feeding choices early <u>in the pregnancy and encourage</u> the woman to make a commitment. After the woman has given birth, the nurse should be available to reinforce information, answer questions, and provide support.

this is nursing research (vs. research in nursing) on the patient care priority of NCNR; maternal-child issues

Source: Rentschler, DD 1991.

Guidelines for Critique

Is the research basic, or is it applied?

How relevant is the research to nursing practice? Determine at what stage it would fall on the pure-applied continuum.

What type of research is it?
    exploratory
    descriptive

    explanatory
    experimental or quasi-experimental
    methodological

Is it nursing research, or is it research in nursing?

Does the study fall into a priority area for clinical nursing research?

Summary of Key Ideas and Terms

The value and usefulness of the scientific approach for making real-world decisions about nursing practice are clearer if you realize that:

- Science doesn't have to be dogmatic and mechanistic.
- Science involves a process of discovery as well as a process of proof.
- Science requires interpretation of facts, and interpretations can change.
- Most of the principles and topics for nursing research exist in the practice of clinical nursing.

The *scientific approach* offers an alternative tool for making decisions and solving practical problems that can substitute for or augment trial and error and common sense, authority and tradition, inspiration and intuition, and logical reasoning.

Scientific inquiry is based on specific assumptions about the existence of a basic natural order in the world. It has the characteristics of self-correction and empiricism, and it aims to develop explanations called theories.

It is possible to classify types of nursing studies along a pure-applied continuum based on their relevance to nursing practice. Studies can also be classified according to their purpose and study design.

The **research process** is the tool of science. It involves a series of progressive steps that usually include some version of the following:

- stating a researchable problem
- defining the purpose of the research
- reviewing related literature and linking it to a theoretical context
- formulating hypotheses and defining variables
- selecting the research design
- selecting the population and sample
- conducting a pilot study
- collecting the data
- analyzing the data
- communicating conclusions

It is likely that at least understanding and using the results of nursing studies to improve practice will become an essential part of all nursing education programs.

References

American Nurses' Association. *Nursing: A Social Policy Statement.* Kansas City, Mo: ANA; 1980.

Barnard K. The effect of stimulation on the sleep behavior of the premature infant. *Common Nurs Res.* 1973,6:12–33.

Benner P. *From Novice to Expert: Excellence and Power in Clinical Nursing Practice.* Menlo Park, Calif: Addison-Wesley; 1984.

Bloch D. Strategies for setting and implementing the National Center for Nursing Research Priorities. *Applied Nurs Res.* 1990;3:2–6.

Bradley-Springer L. Nutritional support in HIV infection: A multilevel analysis. *Image.* 1991;23:155–159.

Brink PJ & Wood MJ: *Basic Steps in Planning Nursing Research.* 3d ed. Boston: Jones and Bartlett; 1988.

Coler MS & Hafner LP. An intercultural assessment of the type, intensity and number of crisis precipitating factors in three cultures: United States, Brazil and Taiwan. *Int J Nurs Stud.* 1991;28:223–235.

Cooperative Graduate Education in Nursing. *Nursing Research Television Cassettes #1.* New York: American Journal of Nursing Co.; 1975.

Diers D. *Research in Nursing Practice.* Philadelphia: Lippincott; 1979.

Diers D. Clinical scholarship. *Image.* Winter 1983;15:3.

Ferketich SL et al. The multitrait-multimethod approach to construct validity. *Res in Nurs & Health.* 1991;14:315–320.

Hall LA et al. Psychosocial predictors of maternal depressive symptoms, parenting attitudes, and child behavior in single-parent families. *Nurs Res.* 1991;40:214–220.

Kerlinger FN. *Foundations of Behavioral Research.* New York: Holt, Rinehart & Winston; 1966.

McClure ML. Promoting practice-based research: A critical need. *J Nurs Adm.* November/December 1981;11:66–70.

Medhoff-Cooper B et al. Serial neurobehavioral assessments in preterm infants. *Nurs Res.* 1991;40:94–97.

Morgan DG & Laing GP. The diagnosis of Alzheimer's disease: Spouse's perspectives. *Qual Health Res.* 1991;1:370–387.

National Center for Nursing Research. Facts about funding. Bethesda, Md: National Institutes of Health; 1990.

Polit DF & Hungler BP. *Nursing Research,* 3d ed. Philadelphia: Lippincott; 1987.

Prescott PA et al. The patient intensity for nursing index: A validity assessment. *Res in Nurs & Health.* 1991;14:213–221.

Rentschler DD. Correlates of successful breastfeeding. *Image.* 1991;23:151–154.

Sitzman J et al. Biofeedback training for reduced respiratory rate in chronic obstructive pulmonary disease: A preliminary study. *Nurs Res.* July/August 1983;32:218–223.

Snyder MC. *Calif Nurse.* September 1983;2.

Spruck M. Teaching research at the undergraduate level. *Nurs Res.* July/August 1980;29:257–259.

Stone KS et al. The effect of lung hyperinflation and endotracheal suctioning on cardiopulmonary hemodynamics. *Nurs Res.* 1991;40:76–80.

Thomas B, Price M: Research preparation in baccalaureate nursing education. *Nurs Res.* July/August 1980;29:259–261.

Wilson HS. Teaching research in nursing: Issues and strategies. *West J Nurs Res.* 1982;4:366–377.

HOW TO READ RESEARCH

HOLLY SKODOL WILSON

CHAPTER OUTLINE

In This Chapter . . .

CHAPTER OBJECTIVES

After reading this chapter, you should be able to:

- Compare and contrast four levels of reading

- Demonstrate skills of systematic skimming and analytic reading to comprehend a report of research findings

- Recognize when long or impersonal words and sentences can be translated into plain, conversational language

- Describe the arrangement of headings and subheadings in a typical research journal article

- Interpret presentations of information in each section of a journal article

2

IN THIS CHAPTER . . .

In this chapter you will be given step-by-step lessons for building the language repertoire and mental processes that will result in clear "translation" of and thinking about the research-oriented writing you read. Naturally, the arts of reading and thinking can be learned only by constant practice. This chapter encourages you to set up a training program for yourself so that reading even highly complex research literature will become second nature to you. Don't stop practicing till you reach that point.

Topics covered in this chapter include (1) techniques of reading scientific writing, (2) translating the language of science, and (3) the typical format of a research article. You don't have to be a career researcher to decipher nursing research, evaluate it, and use research findings as a basis for your clinical practice. You just have to be a master of the art of reading.

TECHNIQUES OF READING

The Art of Active Reading

In 1940 Mortimer J. Adler and Charles Van Doren published a fantastic little volume called *How to Read a Book.* It immediately became a best-seller and has since been translated into French, Swedish, German, Spanish, and Italian. The book hangs, as most good books do, on a single central idea: that *it is important for an intelligent reader to be able to read a variety of things better than he or she already does* (not necessarily faster, but with more comprehension). Adler and Van Doren introduce the reader to "the basic rules of the fine art of intelligent reading"—an essential skill if you are to apply research results from studies conducted by others to your clinical work.

A piece of scientific writing is usually complex. The amount that you comprehend often depends on the amount of active thinking that you put into the process of reading it and the skill with which you perform the separate acts involved in good reading. Active-reading skills enable you to go beyond mere reading for information to *reading for understanding.* This level of understanding is possible when you know not only what a writer has to say but also what he or she means and why. According to Adler and Van Doren, "Being informed is a prerequisite to being enlightened. The point is, however, not to stop at being informed" (p. 11). The lessons that follow are as relevant to active listening as they are to active reading and so can be put to work at conferences and symposia as well as on journal articles and books. Active reading is the opposite of passively dragging your way through seemingly endless pages of material that you don't understand. Instead, it is a process of actively questioning the material you read and of thinking about it according to an organized plan that allows you to make sense out of even the most difficult parts. Active reading lets you answer the question "What does this really say?"

The effectiveness of your reading is determined by the amount of skill you put into it. Realizing the differences between levels of reading is basic to improving your reading skill. The four levels identified by Adler and Van Doren are elementary reading, systematic skimming, analytic reading, and comparative reading (see Figure 2–1).

Elementary Reading   The first level of reading is also called initial, or rudimentary, reading. It refers to the kind of reading we do as children in passing from illiteracy to literacy. Because you are well into reading this text, we can assume that any problems you might have in reading nursing research literature are not at the elementary level.

Systematic Skimming   The second level of reading is called systematic skimming, or prereading. The aim of this level is to get the most out of a publication in a limited amount of time. When you read at this level, your goal is to examine the surface of the publication and learn everything that the surface can tell you, such as the qualifications of the author and the structure, the ingredients or parts, and the overall category of the article or book. Systematic skimming helps you decide what to read in a journal or book and in what sequence. Many of us become intimidated by research journals because we try to start at the beginning and plow through them from page 1 without even looking at the contents to see what might be relevant to our interests or work.

Analytic Reading   The third level of reading makes somewhat heavier demands on you. Here is where you begin asking questions of what you are reading so that you can truly understand it. These questions can be asked in any order, but together they form the framework for active reading.

1. *What is the book, journal, or article about as a whole?* You have to figure out what the fundamental theme or thesis of a piece is and how it is developed.

2. *What is being said in detail, and how?* Here you need to discover the author's main ideas, assertions, and arguments.

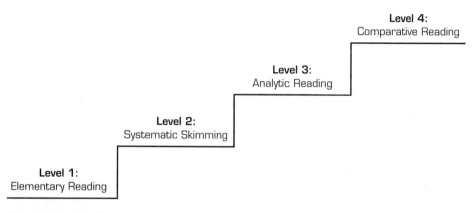

Figure 2–1   *Reading levels*

3. *Is the book, journal, or article true in whole or part?* If you have read something seriously, you must make up your own mind on this question. The strategies for conducting a formal research critique offer you an approach to doing this in the case of a report of research findings (see chapter 13).

4. *What of it?* If what you have read provides information, you ought to ask yourself about its significance. Here is where you can use your own scholarly talents to perceive clinical implications of a study even if the investigators themselves haven't done so.

Comparative Reading   The fourth and highest level of reading requires that you place what you are reading in relation to other things you have read. With comparative reading you can construct an analysis of a subject that doesn't appear in any single article or book. In short, this fourth level of reading is the most reliable way of *keeping up to date* on a topic or subject. It requires that you keep either a real or mental file of new ideas or findings in your area of clinical interest and always assess each new work that you read in light of that file of ideas. Are you reading a really new idea? a credible replication of a previously published idea? a contradiction to a prominent idea? Although this is the most difficult of the reading levels, Adler and Van Doren point out that "The benefits are so great that it is well worth the trouble of learning how to do it" (p. 20). Let us turn to a few more how tos.

Active reading, as you can see, involves engaging in a mental dialog with the authors of a book, article, or paper presentation. See Box 2–1 for some devices that can help you accomplish this fruitfully.

Guides to Systematic Skimming

Here are some basic tips to guide you when skimming a written work.

1. Quickly read the title page and preface (or abstract, if it is a journal article). Get an idea of the subject, and place the article or book in the appropriate category in your mind. Is it a theoretical treatise, an article on methodology, or an actual report of findings? If you have answered yes to the last option, is the problem under investigation of conceivable clinical relevance to the patients you are working with or might work with in the future?

2. Look carefully at the table of contents in a book or the headings in an article to get a general sense of the structure of the piece. They ought to act as a road map by alerting you in advance of where you are headed.

3. Check the book's index. Make a quick estimate of the range of topics included to see which, if any, are relevant to your interests. You can use the index in this text to get some practice.

4. Read the publisher's blurb or any boldface excerpts. Authors commonly try to summarize their main points in these spots.

5. From your knowledge of the general nature of the book's or article's contents, look more carefully at chapters or sections that seem pivotal. For

---

Box 2–1 Helpful Guides for Reading Comprehension

Underline or highlight. Get in the habit of underlining or highlighting points of major significance, particularly the central thesis of a book or article.

Use vertical lines in the margin. This is just another way of emphasizing a key paragraph or section of a page that might be too long to underline.

Put stars or asterisks in the margin to let you quickly locate the most important ideas in the piece.

Write numbers in the margin to indicate a sequence of points in the unfolding logic of an argument or to designate any other list.

Write page numbers in the margin to indicate where else in the book or article the author makes relevant or even contradictory points. Some readers use the abbreviation *cf,* which means compare, or refer to. For example, in reading a research report you might want to compare its findings to the list of original hypotheses to be sure that an investigator has not drawn unreasonable conclusions.

(cf p.25)

Write questions and reactions in the margins or at the top or bottom of a page. Here is where you can quickly summarize your own personal understanding of what you have read and how it relates to what else you have read.

I think I can use these techniques

---

example, in the case of a report of research, read the section with the heading "Findings" or "Conclusions."

6. Finally, leaf through the whole piece, dipping in here and there for a paragraph. Remember to read the last few lines, because most authors sum up what is important in their work at its conclusion.

Systematic skimming requires that you become a detective actively looking for clues about a book's or article's major theme so that you can decide whether it deserves any more of your time. You should be able to place it in your mental card catalog (or your real one) and return to it later if necessary. All of this should take anywhere from a few moments to less than an hour, even with a full-length book.

A final suggestion about systematic skimming is that you don't try to understand every page of a research report or theoretical paper the first time through, particularly if it contains unfamiliar jargon or complicated statistics. This is the most important rule. Don't be afraid to seem to be superficial at first. Read quickly through even the hardest parts. You will be much better prepared *to read it well the second time through.*

Guides to Analytic Reading

There are nine rules for analytic reading:

1. Try to discern whether a book or journal article is reporting findings that have been reached according to the canons of science or whether it is

essentially based on personal trial and error (what is often called "conventional clinical wisdom"). Examples of the former are more likely to be found in journals that have research and nursing science as their stated editorial target.

2. Try to state in a sentence or two what an article or book's main theme is. Sociologists Barney Glaser and Anselm Strauss, who have taught nurses, call this the "little logic" of a book or article. It is "little" because it can be expressed in a short space. It is "logic" because it is the hook, or central premise, that holds the piece together. In the case of a report of study findings, you often find the "little logic" in the statement of the study's purpose or the statement of the study problem.

3. Try to "x-ray" a book or article to uncover its structure and see how the major parts are organized. A study that is testing a hypothesis probably follows a fairly typical format for presentation. If you are reading an exploratory or descriptive study or one designed to develop rather than test hypotheses, or if you are reading a historical or case study report, you may encounter a wide variety of blueprints for the article or book's structure.

4. Find out what main questions or problems the article or book has set out to answer. Determine which of them are primary and which are secondary. In a research article you should be able to do this by reading the findings and conclusions and comparing them with the study purposes, objectives, or hypotheses.

5. Find the important and unfamiliar words and determine their meaning. There may be a whole new vocabulary to digest. Use the Glossary of research terms in this text to help, for example.

6. Mark the most important sentences in an article or book, and uncover the propositions they contain. A good place to practice this step is when reading the conceptual framework for a study proposal or report.

7. Locate or construct the basic arguments or premises. This rule is more likely to apply to a theoretical analysis or an expository piece than to a report of empirical findings.

8. Find out what solutions or conclusions an author has come up with. Are there other solutions?

9. Be able to say "I understand it" with reasonable certainty before you begin to criticize it. The specifics for how to critique a research study are covered in detail in chapter 13.

Guides to Comparative Reading

Comparative reading is designed to help you get a cumulative perspective on a question or topic. Use these five steps when you are comparing more than one source on a subject to establish their relationship to one another and to your own understanding of the subject.

1. Find the relevant passages that bear on your question, needs, or interests.

2. Translate the ideas of the various authors into your own terms.

3. Formulate your own set of questions, and read comparatively to determine how the respective authors do or do not address them.

4. Define any issues that emerge so that you can recognize, sort, and arrange controversies or contradictory findings in the literature.

5. Analyze the discussions you read by asking "Are they true?" and "What of it?"

A Step-by-Step Example

The best way to learn the skills of systematic skimming and analytic reading is to practice them. As an example, let us try them out on an article from *Nursing Research* written by Lim-Levy (1982).

Systematic Skimming

1. Quickly read the title and preface or abstract to get an idea of what the article is about. In Lim-Levy's article the following information appears in italics at the very beginning:

    > *A study was conducted to determine the effect of oxygen inhalation by nasal cannula on oral temperature. One hundred healthy adult subjects were randomly assigned to a control and three experimental groups that received 2, 4, and 6 liters per minute of oxygen for 30 minutes. Oral temperatures were measured before and 30 minutes after oxygen treatment. The data analysis did not show any effect of the treatment. [p. 150]*

    This is clearly a published report of an experimentally designed study. The report has implications for clinical practice—specifically, how to take the temperature of people who are getting oxygen.

2. What is the structure of the article? This article is relatively short. Its only headings are "Methods" and "Results and Discussion." We can assume that it roughly follows the typical format for presenting the results of research to test a hypothesis.

3. Check the index. Because this article does not have an index, we will look instead at the references at the end (p. 152). They give us some ideas about what else we might want to read.

4. Read any boldface excerpts. We have already read an excerpt in italics.

5. Read the pivotal and final sections. In the next-to-last paragraph, the author sums up her study findings in straightforward clinical terms:

    > *This study did not show a significant effect of oxygen inhalation on oral temperature (p. 152).*

Analytic Reading   Having inspected the research report, we can now reread it more critically at the analytic level.

Rule 1 of analytic reading is to know what kind of piece you are reading. Because of its appearance in *Nursing Research* and its format, we know that we are reading the results of an empirical clinical study. We are further told that the study was conducted by a nurse clinical specialist in medical-surgical nursing.

Rule 2 is to locate the article's "little logic." We find it on page 150 in the fourth paragraph:

> *This study sought to determine how oxygen inhalation by nasal cannula affects oral temperature. If oral monitoring is not adversely affected, there is no need for rectal or axillary procedures.*

Rule 3 is to identify the article's structure. We see by the format that it is a report of a hypothesis-testing study.

Rule 4 is to find out what the main problem or question was. We can see on page 150 that this study set out to test the following hypothesis: "Oxygen inhalation by nasal cannula of up to 6 LPM does not affect oral temperature taken with an electronic thermometer."

Rule 5 is to come to terms with the author's vocabulary. Some of the phrases that you would want to understand when reading this report would include:

- informed consent from subjects (see glossary)

- random assignment to treatment groups (see glossary)

- analysis of variance (see glossary)

- statistical significance (see glossary)

Rules 6 and 7 involve identifying the basic premises, propositions, and arguments. In this study we can extract the following line of argument.

1. Oxygen inhalation by nasal cannula is believed to affect oral temperature; in many instances, therefore, body temperature is taken by the rectal or axillary method rather than orally.

2. Many patients find that having their temperature taken rectally is uncomfortable, and nurses find that taking either rectal or axillary temperature is more time-consuming than the oral method.

3. This study of 100 healthy adult male and female volunteers ranging in age from 18 to 56 years was designed to determine whether indeed oxygen inhalation by nasal cannula of up to 6 LPM does affect oral temperature measurement when taken with an electronic thermometer.

4. The study design controlled some factors known to affect oral temperature and procedures for taking the temperature itself, in order to enhance the study's validity and reliability, respectively.

5. Findings indicated that there were no statistically significant changes between preoxygen temperatures and temperatures taken 30 minutes after the start of oxygen.

6. The clinical implication of this study is that changing from the oral method to the rectal or axillary method is unnecessary as well as inconvenient and inaccurate when charting a patient's temperature graph.

Rules 8 and 9 require you to figure out what conclusions the author has reached and make sure you understand them. Based on F and p values that were not statistically significant (see chapter 10), the author concluded that oxygen inhalation does not significantly affect oral temperature. But she recommended further research using higher oxygen concentrations, longer treatment, and febrile patients (p. 152).

If you wished to move on to the level of comparative reading, you would locate additional studies on the clinical topic of oral temperature taking.

Using the approach to reading research outlined here is one way of keeping up to date while using your reading time efficiently so that you really understand what you have read.

TRANSLATING THE LANGUAGE OF SCIENCE

The plain-talk style of writing that makes for popular magazine articles is decidedly absent in most reports of scientific research. The problem of reading research literature effectively becomes partly a matter of language translation and partly a matter of context translation.

In Pursuit of Translation

You will undoubtedly encounter multisyllable words and technical terminology in research articles you read. Here are a few preliminary strategies for understanding them when and if you encounter them:

1. Give yourself time to understand different and unfamiliar words and expressions.
2. Pause between reading heavy sentences.
3. Mentally fill in the spaces between ideas with your own reasoning about them.
4. Think of illustrations or personal rephrasings that will help you reach a personal understanding of an author's ideas.
5. Try to translate the author's sentences into your own mental, conversational talk.

Some Plain Talk about Research in Nursing

In 1976 the American Nurses' Association's Commission on Nursing Research, with the cooperation of distinguished nurse researchers, published a classic document called *Research in Nursing: Toward a Science of Health Care.* In it, using conversational, popular language and a lot of photographs, the authors explained what research in nursing is and gave some superb examples of clinical discoveries made through scientific inquiry. They describe research in nursing as

> *investigating . . . the area of knowledge where the physical and behavioral sciences meet and influence one another, in an effort to study how health problems relate to human behavior and how behavior relates to health and illness. . . . Research in nursing addresses the human and behavioral questions that arise in the treatment of diseases and the prevention of illness and maintenance of health.* [p. 1]

The document provided some selected projects conducted by nurses that represent important advances in health care knowledge and the study of people with health problems. The project descriptions are excellent examples of how technical writing styles and esoteric language can be translated into highly readable material. After reading a few of these descriptions (Examples 1–4 on pages 32–33), use the strategies in the rest of this chapter to translate some published research reports into plain talk yourself.

THE TYPICAL FORMAT OF A RESEARCH ARTICLE

Before you can evaluate the worth of a scientific article, you have to understand it. Learning what may be a new vocabulary is part of the solution. By the time you have finished this book, for example, you should have a firm grasp on the vocabulary of nursing research.

But vocabulary alone isn't all of it. We understand the meaning of even unfamiliar words when we first understand their context. What this means is that you can use terms such as *vitamin deficiency* or *wound infection* when teaching patients who may never have heard them if you put them in a context that the patients can use to interpret what they mean. Likewise, you understand unfamiliar research terminology once you grasp its context in the research process. By familiarizing yourself with the structure of a research article you are learning the context that will support your understanding of the article's meaning.

Example 1: Alleviating Pain

A series of relaxation exercises carried out once or twice a day may relieve the intensity of pain or relax patients so that they are better able to cope with pain according to results of tests by a nurse researcher. Working with three groups of patients—those having elective surgery such as gall bladder removal or hernia repairs, those having rheumatoid arthritis and cancer patients—the nurse researcher was able to validate that pain can be relieved by methods other than medication. [p. 3]

Example 2: Screening for Cystic Fibrosis

A nurse's research project has provided a breakthrough in effectively screening victims and carriers of cystic fibrosis, a process that has been impeded by lack of an efficient test system that could be readily made available to clinical laboratories. [p. 9]

Example 3: Womb Simulation for Premature Infants

Premature babies given special treatment and conditions to simulate prenatal womb life achieve a greater degree of development than similar infants provided standard conditions according to information compiled by a nurse researcher. Normal, full-term infants can usually sleep for 60 minutes at a time, while a baby who normally would be in the womb for another eight weeks lacks the nervous system development that controls sleep behavior, which in turn affects weight gain and physical development. . . . The nurse and her research team simulated womb conditions by playing a tape-recording of a heart beat for 15 minutes every hour, and rocking the mattresses of the isolettes in which the babies were placed. Those infants living in the womb-simulated situations slept more quietly and gained more weight than a group of similar babies of the same age used in comparison studies. The nursing research team is continuing efforts to determine the best time in an infant's life to begin simulation, how loud a heart beat is advantageous, the intensity of rocking that is most productive and at what point visual stimulation might be used. [pp. 10–11]

Example 4: Coping with Home Dialysis

Patients using an artificial kidney machine at home have advantages over those who continue treatment in hospitals according to a nurse researcher studying the relationships in home dialysis triads and patient outcomes. The study, which investigates how cooperation among patient, spouse, and doctor makes a difference for the patient using home dialysis, indicated that home treatment resulted in better physical health, closer adherence to medical regimen, greater amounts of work and leisure time activities, fewer hospitalized days and fewer emergencies for the patient. . . . The study of families successfully coping with dialysis is yielding information about the ways they make adaptations which maximize the quality of life for the patient and minimize the disruption of other family members. [p. 13]

Source: American Nurses' Association 1976.

Almost all research journal articles are divided into sections with headings and subheadings. The arrangement of these headings usually follows a somewhat standardized format. If you are familiar with it, you can get the most out of the time you spend reading, because you understand the context that each section intends to establish. The typical sections of a research article are arranged as follows:

1. abstract
2. introduction
   - review of the literature
   - statement of purpose
3. method
   - subjects
   - design
   - materials (data collection)
   - procedure (data analysis)
4. results (conclusions)
5. discussion
6. references

Let us examine each of these sections with a bit more care.

Abstract

An **abstract** is located at the beginning of a research article. Its purpose is to summarize the entire piece as briefly as possible. An abstract usually provides the following information about the study:

1. its purpose, objectives, or hypotheses
2. a description of the participants or sample members
3. a brief explanation of data collection and analysis procedures
4. a summary of important findings

The accompanying example is an illustration of an abstract. It offers you an overview of what you will find in the article. Because it is *located at the beginning* of an article, you can read it in a minute or two and then decide whether to systematically skim or analytically read the whole article. Because it helps you use your reading time wisely, an abstract serves a very useful purpose. It also is your first encounter with what may be some unfamiliar words. If the study is one that relates to your interest areas, you will have a chance to read about the subjects in more depth and get a fuller grasp of the meaning of terms as you go on with the article.

Sample Abstract

A national survey of a stratified random sample (n = 240) of accredited hospitals with critical care units (CCUs) was conducted in order to describe the current practice of restrictions imposed upon myocardial infarction (MI) patients. A cross-sectional correlation survey with a two-stage mailing was used.

The first-stage mailing at the institutional level was sent to the head nurses of the CCUs (n = 600). Nurses were requested to give: (a) importance and frequency ratings of selected coronary care nursing practices; (b) information about the use or discontinuance of two specific restrictions: ice water and rectal temperature measurements. Follow-ups by mail and/or telephone-yielded response rates for about 87%.

The conceptual framework, "Diffusion of Innovations," was used to assess the diffusion of the results of studies published in clinical journals. Despite findings that cast doubt on the practices of restricting ice water and rectal temperature measurement, coronary precautions are commonly practiced.

Hours spent reading and the number of journals read correlate (p less than .001) with greater levels of awareness in nurses that such restrictions are in question. Levels of awareness are not related to the importance and frequency ratings for those restrictions. Differences among nurses do not explain differences in ratings. If research is to be used, nurse researchers and managers need to actively intervene in care. Passive diffusion of research results is inadequate, unsure, and slow. [p. 196]

Source: Kirchhoff 1982.

Let's go back to the components of an abstract and figure out what we've just read. First, an abstract provides the purpose, objectives, or hypotheses of the study. In this example the purpose is "to describe the current practice of restrictions imposed on myocardial infarction (MI) patients" in CCUs throughout the United States.

Second, the sample abstract tells us that the participants in the study were a sample of 600 randomly selected nurses and head nurses from a stratified random sample of 240 CCUs in accredited hospitals throughout the country. The selection of random sampling tells us (as do the large sizes of the samples) that the investigator wanted to increase the possibilities of generalizing her findings to the total population of accredited CCUs by obtaining a representative sample, and not just to a case study of one institution or even a particular region's practices.

As far as procedures are concerned, the researcher mailed some instruments to head nurses and randomly selected staff nurses in accredited settings who were willing to participate. She asked them to provide information about the awareness and use or nonuse of coronary precautions and their typical journal-reading habits as well as some additional information. She used a statistical technique to correlate these categories of information that yielded a number called a *p* value that she compared with values in a statistical table.

Fourth, the abstract gives us a summary of important findings. Although the researcher found that nurses who spent more hours reading had greater levels of *awareness* that coronary restrictions were in question, being aware didn't seem to alter clinical practice. This finding led the author to argue for the importance of active programs to get research findings into practice.

Introduction

The introduction of a research article usually contains two parts: a review of the literature and a statement of the study's purpose. Most authors begin with a discussion of previous relevant studies that they or others have conducted. This background information is important to figure out how the study being reported relates to previous knowledge and theories in a field. It is important to ask yourself whether the study at hand is so unique and original that little or nothing of any importance has preceded it, or whether the investigator just didn't bother to look up the prior research or theoretical literature on his or her topic. The discussion of previous research and relevant theory can be as short as one or two sentences or as long as several pages. The following three paragraphs constitute the literature review in our sample study report.

Sample Literature Review

The term "coronary precautions" covers a list of restrictions imposed upon myocardial infarction patients, including restriction of: hot and cold beverages, rectal temperature measurement, stimulant beverages, and sometimes vigorous back rubs (Kirchhoff 1981).

Several clinical and laboratory studies of cardiac changes following the ingestion of ice water have been conducted (Cohen, Alpert, Francis, Vieweg, and Hagan 1977; Fitzmaurice and Simon 1974; Houser, 1976; Pratte, Padilla, and Baker 1973). The general conclusions were that a normally consumed amount of hot or ice water (200 cc) was not harmful to a recent myocardial infarction patient, although Pratte, Padilla, and Baker (1973) found that ingestion of 600 cc of ice water by normal males in the supine position was related to changes in electrical activity in the heart.

Two studies of the cardiac changes following the measurement of rectal temperature were found (Gruber 1974; McNeal 1978). Measurement of rectal temperatures did not cause bradycardia or arrhythmias. No studies were found that discounted the restriction of stimulant beverages, none were found that mentioned vigorous back rubs. Except for the findings of Fitzmaurice and Simon, and Pratte and colleagues, the results of the studies were rarely available to critical care nurses. [Kirchhoff 1982 p. 196]

Having summarized the relevant literature leading up to a current study, the author usually states the specific goals or purposes of the study. In our sample article the researcher says:

Sample Purpose

A survey of current practice was designed to assess the impact of the published studies on the practices of restricting ice water and the measurement of rectal temperature. Nurses who read these publications might have reduced the frequency of or even eliminated these practices, rendering further research meaningless. [Kirchhoff 1982 p. 196]

Translating this paragraph, the author means, "Because published studies have demonstrated that restricting ice water and rectal temperature-taking with coronary patients isn't necessary, one would expect nurses who read to have abandoned these restrictions. I decided to do a survey to find out if in fact they have." When you look for the literature review and study purpose in a research report, be prepared to find them either as separate headings or grouped together under the heading "Background" or "Introduction."

Method

This is the section of a research article where the author explains in detail exactly how he or she conducted the study. The reason for going into such elaborate detail is so that the study can be replicated. The author addresses four main questions in the method section of a research article:

1. Who participated in the study?

2. What type of research design was used?

3. What materials (data) were needed?

4. What procedures were the participants required to do?

A full description of the subjects who participated in the study and the process by which they were selected (sampling procedure) is important for the reader to know, because the conclusions of most studies are valid only for people who are similar to the subjects in the study. In our sample article the author does a good job of describing the criteria for including nurses in the sample to receive survey instruments and of the number ($n = 524$) who actually completed the data collection forms. She also explains how she selected the head and then staff nurses, using a random sampling procedure from a list provided by the head nurses of settings who met study criteria.

For any study purpose, several research designs can be used. Chapter 7 is devoted to a discussion of these designs. The design gives you an idea of the overall plan for organizing the study and enables you to make some predictions about how data might be statistically treated. Our sample article informs us that this particular study used "a cross-sectional national descriptive/correlational survey of critical-care nurses employed in acute medical-surgical hospitals." We understand that instead of a design in which two or more groups are compared on some characteristic or another (an experimental design), this study involved a survey of a national sample of critical-care nurses that correlated certain responses with other responses.

Materials are the measurement devices used to collect data from the subjects. A researcher might use a questionnaire, a thermometer, or an interview, but whatever the instrument, the article should explain whether the researcher used a new instrument constructed especially for this study or an older instrument developed by somebody else (see chapter 8). The author should describe exactly how the measurements were done and particularly report on a self-developed instrument's **validity** and **reliability.** If the instrument comes from somewhere else but is modified for use in the study being reported, the author should explain how the original was modified. In our sample article the instruments were described like this:

Sample Description of Instruments

A one-page questionnaire, printed on two sides called the Unit Form, *contained closed-ended items. The questions were designed to elicit information about the institution (hospital) and the unit (CCU). Face validity of the items was assumed on the basis of the demographic nature of the items and simplicity of the format. Pretesting of the instrument on a small national sample of hospitals (n = 24) revealed no omitted responses and no apparent inconsistencies in the data.*

The Staff Nurse Selection Sheet consisted of a one-page grid, which required the head nurse to list full-time registered nurses working the day or evening shift. . . . No changes in this instrument were needed on the basis of pretesting during the pilot study.

The Nurse Form was designed to obtain a national picture of current coronary care practices and to provide data for the analysis of the diffusion of the results of published research relating to two specific practices: the restriction of ice water and the restriction of rectal temperature measurement. The form consisted of a five-page questionnaire, divided into three parts. The first page contained explicit directions and described the clinical situation of an uncomplicated MI patient. . . . All the forms and the method were pretested in the pilot study. After the completion of the pilot study and preliminary analysis, the revised instruments were submitted to a nationally recognized cardiovascular nurse clinician for review. [Kirchhoff 1982 pp. 197–198]

The procedure section describes how the study was conducted. Remember, it is supposed to include enough detail so that a reader could replicate the study. Here's an excerpt from our sample article to give you a sense of how detailed the procedure discussion was:

Sample Procedure

A letter addressed to the director of nursing was mailed to each of the randomly selected institutions. At the sample time, a cover letter, Unit Form, Staff Nurse Selection Sheet, and a return stamped envelope were sent to the "Head Nurse, CCU" at each of the selected hospitals. A second letter and an additional copy of the Unit Form and Staff Nurse Selection Sheet along with another return envelope were sent to all head nurses who had not responded within three weeks. After another three and a half weeks, a third similar follow-up was sent to those nurses. . . . Attempts were made to contact the remaining head nurses by phone. About two months after the beginning of the first-stage mailing, with a majority of the responses from the CCU's received, the second-stage mailing was initiated. [Kirchhoff 1982 p. 198]

You can either skim through the specifics of the study's procedure quickly to move to the results, or you can use the description as a step-by-step road map to critique or replicate a study.

Results

The results of a study tend to be reported in the text, summarized in tables, or presented visually in a graph or figure. It is absolutely critical that you be able to understand and evaluate the results of any study that you read. Sometimes researchers have used a statistical test incorrectly (see chapter 10), sometimes they have drawn conclusions that go far beyond what can be justified by the sample and study design, and sometimes the tables are inconsistent with what the authors explain in the text. The results of our sample study were reported like this:

Sample Results

Avoiding the use of a rectal thermometer and restricting ice water received moderate importance and frequency ratings but large standard deviations, indicating high variability among the sample of nurses. . . . The most common origin for practice of both these restrictions is unit policy. . . . The most important nurse variable in a multiple regression is the number of years since most recent graduation, but the total explained variance despite the inclusion of 10 significant variables was only 6%. . . . Reading the American Journal of Nursing, *the number of journals read and the hours spent reading per week were significantly correlated with level of awareness that the coronary care precautions were being questioned. But the effect of awareness (reading) on persuasion (the importance ratings) and on adoption (the frequency ratings) showed no significant differences. . . .* Being aware did not affect how important the nurses thought the restrictions were or how frequently they reported practicing the restrictions. [Kirchhoff 1982 p. 200]

Discussion

The section on results presents a report of how the statistical analysis turned out. The discussion section then explains what the results mean with regard to the study's purposes and relates them to a theoretical context (see chapter 5). Many authors also use this part of a research article to explain why they think their results turned out the way they did and to suggest new types of study for future research. Sometimes the discussion section is called

"Conclusions." Our sample study conveys the nontechnical interpretation of the study findings this way:

Sample Discussion

Coronary precautions are widely practiced. The awareness of published studies has not changed practice. Although the passive diffusion [of research results] process has some effect on awareness, it has little effect on persuasion or adoption. . . . Some studies require a translation process before they are put to use. . . . Passive diffusion of research results is inadequate, unsure, and slow. A process of active intervention on the part of those nurses qualified to evaluate completed studies is needed. [Kirchhoff 1982 p. 201]

References

A research article ends with a list of books and articles to which the author referred during the study report. This list can be a useful resource if you want to tackle a comparative reading of the major ideas associated with a topic. Reading the references cited at the end of a study report can also familiarize you with the findings and logic that led the author to the study being reported. The reference list at the conclusion of our sample article includes articles and books on research utilization and communication of findings as well as on coronary care precautions.

In addition to these main narrative parts of a research article, many reports also contain visual presentations of data in the form of tables, charts, and graphs. Part of being able to get the most understanding out of a research article is being able to interpret such visuals. Methods for analyzing graphic representations of data are provided in chapter 10.

Guidelines for Critique

What is the research report about? What type of report is it?

What is the main theme ("little logic") of the report?

What is the organization of this particular report? Does it follow the typical research journal article format, or does it differ in some way?

What is the main question or problem the author set out to answer?

Are there important and unfamiliar terms that you will need to "translate" in order to understand the report?

What are the basic premises, propositions, or arguments in the report?

What conclusions has the author reached? Are there other possible conclusions?

What are the implications of the study's findings?

Summary of Key Ideas and Terms

The art of *active reading* is one set of strategies to help nurses assimilate research reports.

Reading occurs at four major levels: (1) elementary, (2) systematic skimming, (3) analytic, and (4) comparative. Each level has specific steps or rules to help nurses read for understanding.

Systematically skimming and analytically reading a sample research report can increase your ability to read and understand others like it.

You can popularize a piece of scientific writing for yourself and make it more readable by mentally translating long or impersonal sentences and words into your own plain, conversational talk.

The format for a typical research journal article usually follows these headings: (1) abstract, (2) introduction, (3) method, (4) results, (5) discussion, and (6) references.

The *abstract* summarizes the study as briefly as possible, while the *introduction* sets the stage for the study by describing previous relevant studies and stating the study's purpose.

The *method* section of the research article sets forth in detail the procedures used in the study and describes the subjects used, research design followed, and materials or measurement devices employed.

The *results* section of the report gives the findings of the study, often in the form of statistics. The *discussion* section explains what the results mean in terms of the study's purpose and relates them to a theoretical context. The report ends with a list of *references*—books and articles—to which the author referred during the study report.

References

Adler M & Van Doren C. *How to Read a Book.* New York: Simon & Schuster;1940.

American Nurses' Association, Commission on Nursing Research. *Research in Nursing: Toward a Science of Health Care.* Kansas City, Mo: ANA; 1976.

Kirchhoff KT. A diffusion survey of coronary precautions. *Nurs Res.* July/August 1982;31:196–201.

Lim-Levy F. The effect of oxygen inhalation on oral temperature. *Nurs Res.* May/June 1982;131:150–152.

DISCOVERING RESEARCHABLE PROBLEMS AND STUDY QUESTIONS

HOLLY SKODOL WILSON

SALLY AMBLER HUTCHINSON

CHAPTER OUTLINE

In This Chapter . . .

CHAPTER OBJECTIVES

After reading this chapter, you should be able to:

- Define a researchable problem and a research purpose

- Recognize sources of researchable problems

- Distinguish between researchable and nonresearchable questions

- Describe why "value" questions and "yes or no" questions are not amenable to answering with the scientific method

- Compare and contrast types of researchable problems, including factor-isolating, factor-relating, situation-describing, and situation-predicting questions

- Determine the level of a researchable question

- Describe how researchable problems are written

- Evaluate problem statements in published research reports according to the criteria of significance, researchability, and feasibility

3

IN THIS CHAPTER . . .

Research begins with a **researchable problem.** This problem may concern nursing education, nursing administration, history, ethics, or a social or natural science question related to health that interests a nurse researcher. But if it is to address the priorities cited by leaders in the profession and if it is to meet the strictest definition of nursing research, it stems most likely from nursing practice or patient care. Patient-care problems have generally been defined as difficulties or concerns experienced by patients or the nurses caring for them.

This chapter gives you insights into how researchers arrive at researchable questions and ways to differentiate between clinical problems that can be researched and those that cannot. It discusses kinds of researchable questions, how they are written, and criteria for evaluating those that serve as the basis for studies you read or hear about.

FROM RESEARCH TOPICS TO PROBLEMS AND QUESTIONS

Most nursing research begins because a nurse develops an interest in a broad topic area. Topic areas in contemporary nursing can range widely in their diversity. Sometimes the topic is the health needs of a particular population—persons who are HIV positive, low-birth-weight infants, mothers addicted to crack cocaine, the homeless mentally ill, elders with dementia, and so on. Sometimes the topic is a health care setting or context—prehospital trauma care, long-term home care, care in ICUs, care in ambulatory surgery settings, and so on. Sometimes the topic is a particular health problem—incontinence, wandering, violence, codependency, infection control, pain, medication compliance, nutrition, sleep disorders, dying, and so on.

Usually researchers must narrow these broad topic areas down to a specific researchable problem. A **researchable problem** is *a specific focus* selected from the overall topic of interest that provides the basis and direction for the study. A problem is a situation that requires a solution. A good problem statement is clear and unambiguous. It indicates to the reader the focus and direction of the research. A researchable problem may be written as a question or a declarative statement. Table 3–1 illustrates examples of general areas of interest that are narrowed down to researchable problem statements in question and in declarative forms.

The researchable problem, whether posed as a researchable question or as a declarative statement, is addressed in a study's purpose. The **purpose of a study** specifies the overall goal of the study: what will be accomplished. It lets the reader know why the study is being conducted. Clearly a study's purpose is based on the statement of a study problem, but the two are not synonymous.

Table 3–1   *Examples of Moving from Research Topic to Problem Statement*

Research Topic	Problem (Question Form)	Problem (Statement Form)
The secondary, noncognitive, behavioral symptoms of Alzheimer's disease	What are the types of secondary, behavioral symptoms of AD over the natural course of the disease?	The range and diversity of secondary symptoms of AD are unknown.
Stress and coping among families of cardiac transplant patients while waiting for the organ	What are the perceived stresses and coping strategies of cardiac transplant patients while waiting for the organ?	Perceived stress factors and coping strategies used by families of cardiac transplant patients while waiting for the organ have not been studied.

For example, a study problem might be posed as the question, "What are the effects of warm and cold applications on the resolution of IV infiltrations in healthy adults?" The study purpose would then be stated as "To determine the effects of warm versus cold applications on the speed of resolution of the extravasation of commonly used IV solutions." In a study problem posed as the declarative statement, "Biobehavioral symptoms that persist after acute withdrawal symptoms in adults recovering from alcohol dependence are unknown," the study purpose might be "To assess biobehavioral phenomena associated with late alcohol withdrawal symptoms in adults recovering from alcohol dependence."

The study problem and purpose are typically introduced at the beginning of a research report. This introductory section should let a reader know something about the researcher's thinking, should provide a background supporting the significance of the research for solving clinical practice problems or contributing to basic knowledge, and should be specific and precise enough to serve as a logical basis for the research design or plan that follows. Your ability to critique a research problem statement as a research consumer is as important as your ability to formulate one. The sections that follow in this chapter will assist you in doing both.

SOURCES OF RESEARCHABLE PROBLEMS

Valid sources of researchable problems in nursing include the researcher's experience; patterns or trends; somebody else's completed research; and the researcher's intellectual and scientific interests, which are often stimulated by reviewing existing literature.

Experience

The best source of clinical research problems is probably the investigator's own experience. Imagine yourself a practicing nurse in the following situations, and think about how questions might occur to you in the course of your clinical practice.

- You are a cardiac rehabilitation nurse and notice that many cardiac bypass patients do not comply with the suggested regimen of diet, exercises, and no smoking. You wonder what sort of nursing intervention would increase their compliance, giving them the opportunity to reap the benefits of their surgery and to live a more comfortable life.

- You are new to the medical unit of a small community hospital. You notice that hospital procedure requires the application of ice to the injection sites of patients who are receiving heparin, for 15 minutes before the injection and 15 minutes after the injection. You are told by coworkers that the ice is used to decrease bruising from the heparin. You recently worked in a hospital in the nearest large city, and ice was also applied to the heparin site there. You wonder if the ice really does what it is supposed to do.

- You work in the labor and delivery units of an urban hospital. You notice that the fathers who go through Lamaze training classes are participating in the labor and delivery process. Men who do not go through the training are excluded from the delivery room. You wonder if the two groups of fathers differ in their feelings about their partner's birth experience or their new baby.

- You read in a nursing journal that young male schizophrenics who have female counselors are more likely to keep follow-up appointments and call for help than those who have male counselors. You wonder if this is an accurate picture of the mental health clinic in which you work.

Researchable problems do not necessarily stem just from a detached, emotionless stance of objective inquiry. Strong feelings are often part and parcel of the nurse's experience in caring for clients. They can also provide energy and impetus to identify and pursue researchable questions. All of the personal reactions listed in Table 3–2 can be turned into researchable questions. By reflecting on the problems and questions that arise in your own nursing experiences, you are taking the same first steps used by nurse researchers on the road of inquiry and discovery.

Patterns or Trends

A second major source of researchable problems can be tapped when a practitioner detects a reasoned pattern from an accumulation of individual cases. It takes an inventive mind to notice the way a particular phenomenon occurs and to become involved in asking why. Such a nurse becomes an observer and interpreter of reality.

Table 3–2   *Experience as a Source of Researchable Problems*

Type of Reaction	Illustration
Wishes and desires	"I wish these children wouldn't get so upset when I come in to change the dressings on their burns."
Gripes	"There's never enough time for discharge planning with these postmastectomy patients."
Questions	"Would it be feasible to start a cardiac rehab program for post-myocardial infarction patients here?"

One curious nurse working with patients in a nursing home noted certain incidents over a three-month period (see example). This nurse's list of anecdotes and case studies extended beyond the few examples described. She eventually began to wonder whether *as a pattern* some nursing home staff members tended to use psychotropic agents continuously to ease their burden rather than episodically to ease the temporary distress of the elderly patients. Her observations of a pattern resulted in a national survey that addressed questions of misuse of psychotropic drugs in nursing homes with elderly patients. Her findings had a direct impact on changing patient care for the better.

Example: Noticing Trends in Using Psychotropic Medication Among Elderly Clients

Hazel S. came to the nursing home when her husband Sam of over 60 years was admitted because of a bout with pneumonia. Since no one else was available to look after her, she was admitted with him. Her anxiety and confusion over Sam's illness resulted in a prescription for regular Mellaril. She subsequently became stuporous and combative. She lost control of bowel and bladder function and was confined to bed. Weeks later, when her husband took her home and she was no longer oversedated, her orientation returned completely to normal.

Mary M., an 80-year-old woman with dementia, was admitted to a nursing home screaming. Thorazine was prescribed to "quiet her down." A week later we discovered that she had a fractured femur.

Jerry C., a 74-year-old man, became confused and agitated following loss of consciousness after a fall. He was given Thorazine but became more disruptive, so Haldol and Mellaril were added. He finally developed a severe parkinsonian syndrome that led to discontinuation of his drug therapy. From then on his mental status improved dramatically.

Existing Research

Researchable problems are often suggested by a review of literature that reports the work of others. Sometimes specific recommendations that a study be replicated with another group of patients or in another setting prompt research. At other times an author's suggestions for further research in the discussion section of his or her report of findings can be a source of a study question. Most often, however, study questions are stimulated when a researcher reads about contradictory results or controversial nursing issues that have limited or no empirical findings on which to base a conclusion or decision. For example, recent research on the relationship between holding and touching newborns in the delivery room and subsequent parental bonding has yielded mixed results. Similarly, questions about the advisability of a 25-pound weight gain during pregnancy, seven-day-a-week jogging, and low-sodium diets pour out of contradictory "hospital studies." Not only can a review of others' published research help investigators formulate a researchable question, it can also guide them in deciding whether replicating the work of others is useful or unnecessary.

Intellectual and Scientific Interests

The major difference between researchable questions that grow out of real-world practical problems and those that are primarily dictated by scientific interest is that the latter are less likely to involve study of a particular clinical situation for the sake of knowledge that can be used in *that situation*. Researchable problems generated from scientific interests usually concern themselves with more general and abstract explanations of phenomena. Questions that derive from this source are directed toward developing an organized accounting of the universe by discovering systematic relatedness out of what seems at times to be a bewildering collection of unconnected statements and descriptions of facts and events.

Reading theories developed in nursing and other disciplines can yield a researchable problem through a deductive process. The researcher reads theoretic schemas and conceptual frameworks published in existing literature and asks if a particular theory—such as stress and coping, adaptation, or family theory—might explain certain patterns observed under specified conditions. Theories serve as a basis for the discovery of researchable problems and the refinement of specific researchable questions. (See chapters 5 and 6 for discussions of theories and hypotheses.)

IDENTIFYING A RESEARCHABLE PROBLEM OR QUESTION

Not all questions that are personally interesting to investigators or that are clinically relevant are researchable ones. If you are going to evaluate the usefulness of research that you read, you must be able to make the distinction. *A* **researchable problem** *is one that can be investigated using the process of scientific inquiry set out in chapter 1.* Two major types of nonresearchable questions need to be differentiated from questions that can direct scientific inquiry: (1) "value" questions and (2) "yes or no" questions.

Questions of value are should questions. These seek information that reflects the values that people have or the policies that institutions have. You can recognize them because they either start with the word *should* or include it in the question. For example:

- Should all mothers be encouraged to breast-feed?
- Should all fathers participate in the experience of labor?
- Should hospital shifts be 8 hours or 12 hours in length?
- What should be the nurse's role in hospice care?

As stated, none of these questions would qualify as a truly researchable one. These are questions of value. Questions that are designed to discover what values people do hold can be researchable, but these are not the same as questions about what values people should hold. Translating this list of value questions into researchable questions requires editing out the *should*. For example:

- What percentage of newly employed staff nurses in postpartum-care settings believe that all new mothers should be encouraged to breast-feed?
- What is the extent of agreement among first-time fathers that they should participate in the experience of labor and delivery?
- What is the preferred shift length among hospital nurses?
- What definitions of the role of hospice nurse are advanced by nursing leaders in this movement?

This revised list deals with statements of fact, of *what is* or of *how things compare.* In summary, as long as a proposed researchable question is really a matter of opinion or philosophy, it can't be answered by conventional research methods without transforming it. Research can provide a basis of facts addressing the consequences or outcomes of holding one value or policy position or another, but *should* questions are better answered by logic or persuasion than by empirical investigation.

The second category of questions that does not meet the requirements of researchability consists of those that can be answered with a simple yes or no (or even maybe). Such questions may prompt collection of facts or data, but they don't really link up to a broader theoretical problem and offer explanations or predictions. What makes research *research* is its obligation to go beyond data collecting to influence theory. Examples of static yes or no questions are:

- Do most nurses in city hospitals have a baccalaureate degree?
- Are patients kept waiting for pain medication after they request it?
- Do patients rest well in ICUs?
- Do most prostate surgery patients become confused after surgery?

To qualify as researchable, these questions would have to be transformed so as to suggest a reason for collecting the information needed to answer them. For example:

- What is the relationship between educational preparation of nurses and expressed job satisfaction at city hospitals?

- What are the consequences of keeping patients waiting for pain medication after they request it?

- What conditions in ICUs contribute to diminished rest patterns for patients?

- What behavioral cues can nurses use to predict that a patient will become confused after prostate surgery?

These changes involve asking a question about the relationship of two variables associated with the topic of interest.

Questions of value, opinion, or policy and accumulations of data can be immensely valuable in clinical problem solving. But only questions that produce generalizable information for guiding practice under other conditions make a nursing problem a nursing *research* problem. Research problems reduce a complex area of interest or topic to a set of researchable questions.

Clear, significant, researchable questions become key to subsequent decisions about research design, data collection, and data analysis. An overly complex, fuzzy, or nonresearchable question bogs a study down in confusion and inconsistency. Table 3–3 summarizes some examples of researchable questions and offers an illustration of each.

TYPES OF RESEARCHABLE QUESTIONS

Categories of Practice-Oriented Questions

One system for distinguishing among the major types of researchable questions (and the types of answers they yield) has been advanced by nurse researchers and philosophers originally associated with the school of nursing at Yale University. According to the classic works of Dickoff and colleagues (1968a, 1968b), these types are

1. factor-isolating

2. factor-relating

3. situation-relating

4. situation-producing

Factor-isolating questions ask, "What is this?" They are sometimes called factor-naming questions. They isolate, describe, categorize, or name factors or situations and provide descriptive definitions. Factor-isolating questions require that the investigator characterize as fully as possible a particular phenomenon. Sample factor- or situation-isolating questions are

- What are the properties of parental bonding?

- What are the stages of the grieving process?

- What features characterize hospitals that have low turnover and high morale and function as magnets in recruiting nurses?

Factor-relating questions can be raised after factor-isolating studies have provided at least names for the important factors operating in a situation. Factor-relating questions ask, "What is happening here?" The goal is to determine how the factors that have been identified relate to one another. In some cases a factor-relating study question has not been preceded by formal factor-isolating studies. Instead, the researcher draws on his or her own experiential knowledge or on published literature to determine what the relevant factors in a given situation might be. A question such as "What is the relationship of parents' own childhood experiences to engaging in subsequent child abuse or neglect?" is a factor-relating question. Studies of drug interaction or correlates of uncomplicated postsurgical recovery are other examples.

Situation-relating questions ask, "What would happen if . . . ?" These questions usually yield hypothesis-testing or experimental study designs in which the investigator manipulates variables to see what will happen. Two examples are "Will reinforcement in the form of a token economy program decrease phobic behavior in a particular group of psychiatric patients?" and "Will biofeedback training decrease suffering among chronic-pain patients?" These questions require answers that allow the researcher to make situation-relating and explanatory statements that specify both the direction and strength of relationships (see chapter 6).

Situation-producing questions ask, "How can I make it happen?" These questions establish explicit goals for nursing actions, develop plans or prescriptions to achieve the goals, and specify the conditions under which the

Table 3–3 *Examples of Researchable Questions*

Why are things this way?	Why do some settings use primary nursing?
	Why do cancer patients without hope participate in painful experiments?
What would happen if . . . ?	What would happen if third-party payers were reimbursed specifically for nursing care?
	What would happen if all nurses were doctorally prepared?
	What would happen if sex education were taught in all schools?
Which approach would work better?	Is group or individual counseling more effective with clients who abuse alcohol?
	Does a back rub with conversation or a back rub without conversation result in greater relaxation?
Who might benefit from this?	Would laboring mothers benefit from being encouraged to choose their own position in the delivery room?
	Would hospitalized children have faster recoveries if parents were taught to participate in their care?
	Would infant mortality rates in developing countries be influenced by a prenatal teaching program?

goals will be accomplished. Most researchers agree that situation-producing questions are the most complicated ones to answer. Example questions might include

- How can I intervene to prevent postoperative vomiting?
- How can I best prepare a woman for labor and delivery?
- How can nursing services be organized to promote job satisfaction and quality of care?

Many experts believe that situation-producing researchable questions occur at the highest level of inquiry. Situation-producing, or prescribing, questions are used eventually to conduct studies that will guide activity in the environment of the practice setting. They are goal based and concerned with more than *what is*. They ask, "What must be done in order to achieve what is desired?"

Levels of Inquiry

While Dickoff and colleagues categorize questions by how they relate or isolate factors and situations, Brink and Wood (1988) view research questions as existing on three levels. One mark of a good research study is that the researchable question is written at the appropriate level given knowledge in existing literature.

Level 1 Inquiry   **Level 1 questions** are used when little knowledge is available about a topic. Level 1 questions begin with "What." These questions are used in *exploratory and descriptive research.*

Nurses often become concerned when a literature review reveals little available information on their research question. The references are often only indirectly related to their specific interest. In nursing, a dearth of information is common, because nursing is a new and evolving science and nurses have been actively engaged in research for a mere 30 to 40 years.

Writing a level 1 question is the perfect solution to the problem of minimal information. If very little information exists, the researcher can design a study to explore and describe the subject, and the findings can be the basis for subsequent higher-level studies. In this way, scientists build knowledge and develop theory. Each level of inquiry contributes to the process of maturation as a science.

To evaluate level 1 research questions, check to be sure that they have (1) one **variable,** or topic that varies, and (2) a reference to the **population** (groups to whom findings will be generalized) in which the variable or topic will be found. Table 3–4 illustrates the variables and populations for sample level 1 questions.

Level 2 Inquiry   **Level 2 questions** look for the *relationship between variables,* and they begin by asking, "What is the relationship?" A researcher might begin with the question "What is the relationship between the public's political beliefs (liberalism versus conservatism) and its image of nurses?" A literature review should support the idea that the variable *public's political beliefs* is related to the variable *public's image of nurses.* The literature will

Table 3–4 *Level 1 Researchable Questions*

Question	Variable	Population
What are the experiences of fathers who are in the delivery room with their wives?	Experiences	Fathers in the delivery room
What are nurses' attitudes toward obese patients?	Attitudes	Nurses
What do insulin-dependent diabetic patients want to know about their disease?	Desire for knowledge	Insulin-dependent diabetic patients

not specify the precise nature of the relationship between the variables, but it will give the researcher enough information to make a conceptual leap in assuming that the relationship might logically exist. For example, the literature may report that people who have conservative political views tend to prefer that women remain in traditional roles. Those with liberal political views are better able to see women in a variety of roles. A researcher can assume, then, that conservative people may view nurses (97% women) in the traditional role of dependent handmaiden to the physician. In contrast, those with liberal views may more readily see the nurse as being autonomous, creative, and professional. Table 3–5 summarizes other examples of level 2 research questions.

Level 2 questions make reference to two variables. (Remember, level 1 questions have only one variable and identify the population in which the variable is of interest.) A **variable** is any factor that varies (see chapter 6). In the variables listed in Table 3–5—patient education, patient compliance, in-service education, and turnover rate—every factor can vary. There may be a patient education program or the absence of such a program—thus, the variability. Patients may or may not comply, or they may comply in part. There may be continuing specific in-service education, no education, or just general education. The turnover rate can be stated as a percentage of nurses leaving over a certain period of time.

Table 3–5 *Level 2 Researchable Questions*

Question	Variables	Population
What is the relationship of patient education to patient compliance in a cardiac rehabilitation program?	(a) Patient education (b) Patient compliance	Cardiac rehab patients
What is the relationship of continuing in-service education in their specialty to turnover rate of cardiac care unit nurses?	(a) In-service education (b) Turnover rate	CCU nurses

If a researcher asked, "What is the relationship of the discussion method of in-service education to the nurse turnover rate?" he or she would soon recognize that the factor of "discussion method of in-service education" does not vary as stated. Consequently, the researcher would need to change the "variable" to the more general category of "method of in-service education," which would allow him or her to examine the discussion method versus the lecture method versus videotape, demonstrating the variability of methods.

Level 3 Inquiry   Level 3 inquiry assumes a relationship, either causal or influential, between two variables and asks "Why?" or "How?" For example, "Why does a behavior modification program decrease the acting out of adolescent patients on a psychiatric unit?" This question is based on learning theory (classical conditioning) used to predict how rewards (for not "acting out," for "good" behavior) act as a stimulus to elicit the desired response of more "good" behavior.

Level 3 questions require (1) two variables, one that is predicted to be causal and one that is the effect, or outcome, variable; (2) a population; and (3) a predicted direction (see Table 3–6). If there is a theory to predict the nature of the relationship between the variables, then researchers should use a level 3 question.

Table 3–7 summarizes and integrates this section using examples of questions.

HOW RESEARCHABLE PROBLEMS ARE WRITTEN

A Four-Step Approach

A research problem can be inspired by any of the sources discussed earlier in this chapter. Let's take the nurse's *wish* that burned children she took care of

Table 3–6   *Level 3 Researchable Questions*

	Variables			
Question	*Causal*	*Effect*	*Population*	*Direction*
Why do self-care behaviors increase the feelings of well-being in patients with chronic illness?	Self-care behaviors	Feelings of well-being	Patients with chronic illness	Increase
Why does attending Alcoholics Anonymous meetings decrease the drinking behavior of alcoholics?	Attending AA meetings	Drinking behavior	Alcoholics	Decrease

Table 3–7   *Matching Types of Researchable Questions to Level of Inquiry*

Type of Research	Level of Inquiry	Example
Factor-isolating	1	What factors influence diabetic patients so that they will learn self-care?
Factor-relating	2	What is the relationship between hope and remission in cancer patients?
Situation-relating	3	Will an egg-crate mattress decrease the number and severity of decubiti on quadriplegic patients?
Situation-producing	4	How can humor be used to mediate the suffering of patients in chronic pain?

wouldn't get so upset when she came in to change their dressings.* To transform her wish into a researchable problem, all she would need to do is to turn that wish around and ask, "Why can't I get my wish?" In other words, step 1 is to *clearly state the discrepancy* between nursing practice as it is and what would be desirable. Step 2 is to *identify the constraints that contribute to the discrepancy.* This involves thoughtful periods of brainstorming, consultation with others, and review of the literature, which might yield the following list of constraints:

1. fear

2. prior experience of pain

3. lack of familiarity with the nurse

4. lack of trust in the nurse

5. fatigue

6. separation from parents

7. lack of information about what to expect

8. being caught off guard

9. low pain threshold

10. emotionally expressive personal style

Constructing a list like this one is, in effect, specifying the possible variables that might be studied. Once the list of constraints has been completed, a researchable problem can be formulated in step 3 by *focusing on the most likely explanations.* Step 4 involves *rephrasing the problem in conceptual terms* to determine the impact of different approaches on burned children's levels of "being upset." So the hope that began as "I wish they wouldn't get so upset when I come in to change their dressings" becomes a researchable problem stated as the following question:

---

*Adapted with permission from Cogen Television Cassettes, University of Nevada, Reno, 1975.

> *Will burned children be less upset by a dressing change if they have already*
> *met the nurse and been prebriefed about the procedure than if they have not?*

The steps involved in refining a general topic or area of clinical interest into a researchable problem, then, are the following:

1. Clearly state the discrepancy between actual and desired practice.

2. Identify all plausible constraints or explanations.

3. Narrow the focus by selecting a few specific high-priority variables.

4. Rephrase the problem in conceptual terms.

A Two-Stage Approach

Lindeman and Schantz (1982) offer an alternative system for moving from interest in several broad topics to a narrowed, formal problem statement or question that will guide the conduct of the study: Stage 1 is formulating the question, and stage 2 is refining it.

Stage 1: Formulating the Question   Most authors agree that researchable questions have two components: a stem and a topic. The basic *stem* words used in formulating research questions are

- *Who?*
- *What?*
- *When?*
- *Where?*
- *Why?*

When the stem word that is attached to a substantive topic changes, the entire direction of the study changes. *Who* questions require that the researcher describe and categorize such information about populations as ethnicity, sex, age, social class, race, health status, and so on. *What* questions are either specific descriptive questions or more complex *what if* questions that demand a description of relationships. *When* and *where* questions again require specific descriptive answers, including a time frame and a location. *Why* questions seek an explanation, as do *how* questions. I began my own doctoral dissertation many years ago by asking, "How is social order possible under conditions of espoused freedom in an antipsychiatric community?" My master's thesis several years earlier asked a *what* question: "What is the meaning of current dance forms to adolescent girls?"

The *topic* is the other part of a research question. In nursing it may be nursing interventions, attitudes, behaviors, feelings, beliefs, people, families, communities, health care problems, and so on. The important point about your topic is that the researcher must be able to specify how he or she intends to measure it through working, or **operational, definitions.** Some of the phenomena of interest to nursing are easier to measure than others. The further away a topic is from some observable indicator for it, the harder it is to operationally define.

Stage 2: Refining the Question   The second stage of writing a good research question is refining it. In the refinement stage, the researcher must build a bridge between current research-based knowledge related to the topic and the steps or study the researcher intends to undertake. Organizing existing literature and integrating it helps the researcher decide whether to formulate the researchable question as an experiment or as a nonexperimental study. This process also helps the researcher make decisions about instruments and about methods for controlling extraneous variables.

EVALUATING RESEARCHABLE PROBLEMS

To evaluate the potential usefulness of any particular study's question or problem statement, consider using the following criteria:

- significance
- researchability
- feasibility

Significance

Kaplan (1964) recalls an anecdote involving a drunkard searching under a street lamp for his house key, which he has dropped some distance away. Asked why he isn't looking for it where he dropped it, he replies, "It's lighter here." Much research, according to Kaplan, is conducted in much the same way as the drunkard's search. Important problems are not always those that are most interesting to the researcher or easiest to study.

The problem studied should advance knowledge of phenomena that are objects of inquiry in the field. Even though a question may reflect an individual researcher's thoughts and imagination, it must be articulated in a conceptual system that is understandable to others in the scientific community. Significant researchable problems yield contributions to the science or the discipline of nursing in a meaningful way. Insignificant study questions are trivial, obvious, or expedient.

Researchability

Researchability demands that a study problem imply the possibility of empirical testing. This means not only that a question about the possibility of a relationship between variables is asked but also that the variables under scrutiny must somehow be measurable. As we saw earlier in this chapter, certain questions of value or policy may be important to philosophers and administrators but cannot be studied using empirical testing procedures.

A researchable problem is stated clearly and unambiguously as either a question or a statement. For example, an investigator can ask, "What are the effects of group meetings on locus of control among inpatient psychiatric clients?" Other ideas can be best stated in a declarative sentence: "Little is known about the nursing interventions that help patients achieve behaviors necessary for control of their hypertension" or "The effect of episodic apnea on sleeping patterns in chronic respiratory patients have not been determined." Questions have the advantage of putting study problems in a simple and direct way. For that reason, I recommend asking a question. A problem put in statement form is also easier to confuse with the statement of a study's purpose, and the two are not the same.

A researchable problem or question follows logically and consistently from a review of what is already known about a topic. It is the next logical question to pursue given what has been learned in the past (Lindeman & Schantz 1982).

Feasibility

Polit and Hungler (1987) remind us that a good study problem should be feasible in terms of

- *Time.* The problem should be sufficiently restricted that enough time will be available to study it.

- *Availability of subjects.* There must be enough participants with the desired characteristics who will be willing to cooperate.

- *Cooperation of others.* The problem must be one that host settings and approval boards are likely to endorse.

- *Facilities and equipment.* Research problems must be framed in such a way as to be possible given the space, office equipment, transportation, consultation, and computer facilities available.

- *Money.* Study questions not only must be proposed in the context of sufficient budget but also must be sufficiently worthwhile to justify the anticipated cost of studying them.

- *Experience of the researcher.* The problem should be chosen from a field about which the investigator has some prior knowledge or experience. Furthermore, the investigator should either possess the requisite skills to collect and analyze data or have access to those who do.

- *Ethical considerations.* A research problem may not be feasible if it poses unfair or unethical demands upon potential subjects.

ANNOTATED RESEARCH EXAMPLE

Citation

general topic / area of interest

Miller MP: Factors promoting wellness in the aged person: An ethnographic study. *Adv Nurs Sci* 1991;14(4):38–51.

— study at level 1

Study Problem/Purpose

Little information is available on factors that might contribute to the wellness state in elders. The aim of this study was to obtain a broad, detailed view of the aged person's perception and interpretation of his or her state of wellness, as well as the perceived factors responsible for the present state of wellness.

[handwritten margin left: This implies a what question.]

[handwritten margin right: — declarative statement of researchable problem]

[handwritten margin right: Factor-isolating is the purpose]

Methods

An ethnographic study design involved four to six interviews with a volunteer group of healthy members of the Grey Panthers, who were between the ages of 70 and 81. Transcribed interviews were analyzed using content analysis methods to identify factors that subjects believed to be responsible for their present level of wellness.

[handwritten margin left: study design was based on problem and purpose.]

Findings

Major factors that emerged from the subjects in this study were categorized as altruism (a concern for others), resiliency (the ability to bounce back), drive or ambition, hardiness (a firm courage), global concern, and, finally, meta-aging (a form of self-actualization that fuels motivation for continued personal growth).

[handwritten margin left: findings have implications for nursing activities to foster wellness in elders.]

[handwritten margin right: — findings report factors identified.]

Guidelines for Critique

Is the statement of the problem clearly presented early in the report?

Have the investigators placed the study problem within the context of existing knowledge and prior work on the topic?

Are the concepts or variables that are included in the study problem measurable?

Is the researchable question written at the appropriate level?

Is the problem significant to the development of knowledge about the discipline or the practice of nursing?

Can a feasible study design be developed to address the question?

To sum up, knowledge of the characteristics of a good researchable question will help you, as a research consumer, select study findings that have scientific merit to put into practice.

Summary of Key Ideas and Terms

Important sources of research problems include (1) the researcher's own experience, (2) patterns or trends, (3) somebody else's completed research, and

(4) the researcher's intellectual and scientific interests, often stimulated by a review of the literature.

A researchable problem can be differentiated from a "value" question or a "yes or no" question by its ability to be solved using the process of scientific inquiry.

Most researchable questions in nursing fall into the categories of factor-isolating questions, factor-relating questions, situation-relating questions, or situation-producing questions. Researchable questions may also be written at three different levels of inquiry.

Writing a researchable problem involves four steps:

- Step 1: Stating a discrepancy between what exists and what is ideal or desired.
- Step 2: Identifying the constraints that contribute to a discrepancy between what goes on and what outcome is desired.
- Step 3: Focusing on the most likely explanation.
- Step 4: Rephrasing the problem in conceptual terms.

Narrowing the focus of a researchable problem can be seen as comprising two stages: (1) Formulating the question, including the stem and the topic, and (2) refining the question.

- The criteria for evaluating a researchable problem are significance, researchability, and feasibility.

References

Brink PJ & Wood MJ. *Basic Steps in Planning Nursing Research, from Question to Proposal.* 3d ed. Boston: Jones & Bartlett;1988.

Dickoff J et al. Theory in a practice discipline. Part I: Practice oriented theory. *Nurs Res.* September/October 1968(a);17:415−435.

Dickoff J et al. Theory in a practice discipline. Part II: Practice oriented research. *Nurs Res.* November/December 1968(b);17:545−554.

Kaplan A: *The Conduct of Inquiry.* San Francisco: Chandler;1964.

Lindeman CA & Schantz D. The research question. *J Nurs Adm.* January 1982;6−10.

Polit DF & Hungler BP. *Nursing Research.* 3d. ed. Philadelphia: Lippincott;1987.

THE LITERATURE REVIEW

HOLLY SKODOL WILSON

SALLY AMBLER HUTCHINSON

CHAPTER OUTLINE

In This Chapter . . .

CHAPTER OBJECTIVES

After reading this chapter, you should be able to:

- Specify the rationale for a literature review

- Critically examine a literature review

- Specify the steps in a literature review

- Specify the scope of a literature review

- Demonstrate familiarity with nursing's primary research journals

4

IN THIS CHAPTER . . .

Both nursing research that is designed to solve practical clinical problems and studies that are conducted to test or yield knowledge for knowledge's sake must be placed in the context of any scientific work that has gone before. Even Sir Isaac Newton paid tribute to his predecessors by commenting that he had been able to see some things that others had not because he had stood on the shoulders of giants. A review of relevant literature is included in a research article to accomplish several purposes:

1. It presents the theoretical framework or organizing schema of which the study is a part.

2. It offers not a mere bibliography but an analytic and critical appraisal of the important and recent substantive and methodological developments in the researcher's area of interest and indicates how the study will refine, revise, extend, or transcend what is now known.

3. It informs and lends support to the researcher's assumptions, operational definitions, and even methodological procedures by demonstrating that the study has profited from the scholarly and scientific work that has preceded it.

This chapter explains why the literature review is needed. It also describes how a researcher conducts a literature review and outlines the variety of sources that a researcher may consult in the course of the review.

WHY REVIEW?

You may wonder why a review of literature is important when doing a research study. Why can't researchers formulate their own questions, conduct their study, and report their findings? Remember that the purpose of science is to build theory and that research is the tool of science (chapter 1). Although many studies do not directly contribute to theory—for reasons that will become clear in the next chapter—they need to have contextual links. That is, a study in isolation cannot be clearly evaluated for significance and meaning, whereas a study that links up with previous research or theory provides a sense of context and a sense of history. We can analyze and understand the extent of existing knowledge and can determine where we should go in the future. The relevant books and articles that researchers read are the references that form the foundation and rationale for their own research.

READING THE LITERATURE REVIEW

The literature review can sometimes be the first major barrier to the reader's ability to grapple with a scientific research study. Without a patient and attentive reading, you might develop the feeling that the literature review is simply a parade of citations to demonstrate that the researcher had done the "requisite" amount of reading before tackling the real problem.

The well-executed literature review will not, of course, deserve such an evaluation. It will clearly announce its reason for being by describing a context—theoretical, methodological, or thematic—into which the study should be placed.

Go back and reread the sample literature review in chapter 2 (p. 36). Here are the citations Kirchhoff (1982) referred to:

Cohen IM et al. Safety of hot and cold liquids in patients with acute myocardial infarction. *Chest.* April 1977; 71:450–452.

Fitzmaurice JB & Simon MB. A comparison of the effects of iced and tap water on selected cardiac parameters in patients following acute myocardial infarction. *Circulation.* October 1974;50(Sup 3):254.

Gruber PA. Changes in cardiac rate associated with the use of the rectal thermometer in the patient with acute myocardial infarction. *Heart Lung.* March/April 1974;3:288–292.

Houser D. Ice water for MI patients? Why not? *Am J Nurs.* March 1976;76:432–434.

Kirchhoff KT. An examination of the physiologic basis for coronary precautions. *Heart Lung.* September/October 1981;10:874–879.

McNeal GJ. Rectal temperatures in the patient with an acute myocardial infarction. *Image.* February 1978;10:18–23.

You will notice that Kirchhoff grouped these studies thematically—that is, by the research problem that the studies addressed. The studies focus on either the effects of ice water or the effects of rectal temperature-taking on patients with acute myocardial infarction. Kirchhoff's point is that there do not seem to be any ill effects. This provides appropriate and necessary background for the focus of Kirchhoff's study, which has already been discussed in chapter 2.

Another literature review, organized somewhat differently, comes from an article that reflected the place of nursing research a decade ago.

Introduction and Review of Literature

The research of a number of nurse educators has suggested that the teaching of research methods for nurses must begin at the undergraduate level to be properly assimilated into the student nurses' repertoire of skills and attitudes (American Nurses' Association 1975, Bree 1981, Burkhalter 1976, Carnagie 1974, King 1972, National League for Nursing 1978, Schlotfeldt 1975, & Verhonick 1973). Nurse educators generally agree that research methods should be part of the undergraduate nursing curriculum. Nevertheless, it is well recognized that nursing students have difficulty seeing the relevance of research in their future work (Kissinger & Youngkin 1975, Noble 1980, Reed 1976, Schare 1977, & Spruck 1980).

Student attitudes toward statistics and research methods in general have been studied by a number of educators in nursing and other related health professions. The attitudes toward statistics among graduate students in a school of public health were analyzed by measuring attitude change before and after a basic statistics course using a questionnaire with Likert scale items. There was no significant improvement in student attitudes toward statistics before and after the course (Kleinbaum & Kleinbaum 1976). A similar tool was used on nursing graduate students in a statistics course revealing no change in attitudes after the course. Another study also using a similar attitude questionnaire to measure attitudes toward research among graduate nursing students found significant differences between pre- and post-test scores. No similar studies were found on undergraduate nursing students.

There were no other studies found in the literature which examined undergraduate nursing students' perceptions of how they actually used the content from their research course in other courses during their program. Also, there were no studies found which addressed how much students actually retained from their research courses if examined on the research content at a later point in their program of study. Furthermore, there has been no apparent assessment of whether students perceive any need for further content on research in their future plans for education and career development. Consequently, this study examined some of these related issues along with an assessment of student attitudes toward research.

Source: Swenson & Kleinbaum 1984. Reprinted by permission.

The citations in this literature review constitute the authors' entire reference list:

References

American Nurses' Association. Resolution on priorities in nursing research. In *Summary Proceedings, ANA House of Delegates, 49th Convention, June 9–14, 1975, San Francisco, California.* Kansas City, MO: ANA; 1975.

Bree N. Undergraduate research. *Nurs Outlook.* January 1981;39–41.

Burkhalter P. The honors program approach to undergraduate research in nursing *J Nurs Ed.* January 1976;15:21–25.

Carnagie ME. The research attitude begins at the undergraduate level (editorial). *Nurs Res.* March/April 1974;23(2):99.

King K. Research in a basic baccalaureate program. *Can Nurs.* May 1972;21–23.

Kissinger JF & Youngkin EO. One approach to teaching clinical inquiry. *J Nurs Ed.* April 1975;14:5–9.

Kleinbaum DG & Kleinbaum AP. A teaching approach for systematic design and evaluation of visual oriented modules. In JR O'Fallin & J Service (eds.). *Modular instruction in statistics: Report of the American Statistical Association study of modular instruction.* Washington, DC: American Statistical Association; 1976:115–121.

National League for Nursing, Council on Baccalaureate and Higher Degree Programs. *Characteristics of baccalaureate education in nursing.* New York: NLN;1978.

Noble MA. Teaching clinical research: Idealism vs. realism. *J Nurs Ed.* 1980; 19(2):34–37.

Reed J. Teaching research by the tell, show and do process. *J Nurs Ed.* January 1976; 15(1):18–20.

Schare BL. An undergraduate research experience. *Nurs Outlook.* March 1977;25(3): 177–180.

Schlotfeldt R. Research in nursing and research training for nurses: Retrospect and prospect. *Nurs Res.* May/June 1975;24(3):177–183.

Spruck M. Teaching research at the undergraduate level. *Nurs Res.* 1980;29(4): 257–259.

Verhonick PJ. Research awareness at the undergraduate level. *Nurs Res.* May/June 1973;20(3):261–265.

This literature review discusses studies in which the focus of attention is students' attitudes toward nursing research. As the authors explain in their last paragraph, they did not find any studies that addressed the particular questions that they themselves had. The reader could reasonably infer that the authors hoped to help fill a gap in the literature with this study. An important question for the reader to ask at this point is, "Is this a gap that needs to be filled?" As seen in chapter 3, a researchable problem needs to be significant. Given the importance of nursing research to the nursing profession, the attitudes of tomorrow's nurses should certainly be of interest to today's nursing educators, the audience for this particular journal.

A problem and possible flaw of this literature review is that the second paragraph seems to refer to two studies that are not named. As these two studies seem to be more similar to the authors' own study than the ones named in the first paragraph, they might well be of interest to the reader, who unfortunately has no way of finding them.

Another possible flaw of this review is the omission of a relevant article:

> Thomas B & Price M. Research preparation in baccalaureate nursing education. *Nurs Res.* July/August 1980;29:259–261.

This omission may or may not be significant. In the ideal world the critical reader should notice such omissions and decide whether they make a difference. It would be important to note, for instance, whether the author has left out studies that would contradict the results of the author's own work. Unless the reader is as familiar with the topic as the author, however, or is willing to do an exhaustive literature search when reading an article, such a critical perspective is too much to expect. If you were preparing a more formal critique with an eye toward evaluating the study's applicability to clinical practice, you might well decide to survey the literature related to a particular study.

> *Authors: Mishel, Merle & Murdaugh, Carolyn*
>
> *Title: Family Adjustment to Heart Transplantation: Redesigning the Dream*
>
> *Source: Nursing Research, 1987, 36: 332–338*
>
> *Research Question or Hypothesis:*
> *What are the processes used by the family members to manage the unpredictability elicited by the need for and receipt of heart transplantation?*
>
> *Method: Field study (grounded theory): Twenty family members were sampled. They attended support groups conducted by the investigators. The groups focused on any topic of concern to the family members and met for 12 weeks for 1½ hours. The aim was to generate substantive theory.*
>
> *Findings: The integrative theme, Redesigning the Dream, described how family members gradually modify their beliefs about organ transplantation and develop attitudes and beliefs to meet the challenge of living with continual unpredictability. Three concepts central to the theory are immersion, passage, and negotiation; these parallel the stages of waiting for a donor, hospitalization, and recovery.*

Figure 4–1   *Sample research note card.*

Source: Mishel & Murdaugh 1987. Reprinted with permission. Copyright 1987 by American Journal of Nursing Company.

CONDUCTING THE LITERATURE REVIEW

Once a researcher has formulated a researchable question, the next step is to go to the research literature to find out more precisely what is known about the chosen topic. A common way to begin the literature review is with a computer search. Some of the most commonly used computerized searches include **MEDLINE/MEDLARS, HEIRS, PAIS, ERIC,** and **DATRIX.** These search biomedical and nursing, health education, psychology, education literature, and dissertation abstracts. The researcher selects a few key words from his or her question and discusses with a reference librarian the appropriate terms to put into the computer. The review should include all variables (key terms) relevant to the study. For example, a researcher interested in the question "Why do self-care behaviors increase the feelings of well-being in patients with chronic illness?" would look up Orem's theory of self-care (1980), articles on self-care behaviors in patients with chronic illness, and articles on patients' feelings of well-being. Reference librarians are incredibly helpful in selecting key words that elicit relevant printouts of references. (The researcher should be aware that there is usually a fee for this computer service.)

The next step is to check the appropriate indices—medical, nursing, sociology abstracts, and the like—depending on the nature of the question (see Box 4–2). Because there are only a few nursing research journals, the researcher can quickly hand search the last few years and determine what types of research question have been asked in his or her problem area. An exhaustive search should cover at least the last five years to give a true indication of the state of knowledge on a particular topic. The aim of the search is to place the researchable question in the context of existing knowledge.

The real work of the literature review is taking notes. Figure 4–1 shows a sample note card. Although note taking may seem like a lot of work at the time, it is necessary and will save the researcher from the fate of one nurse who read approximately 100 articles but took no notes because she felt none of the articles was particularly relevant to her study of fathers' perceptions of their pregnant wives. At the end of weeks of work, she had nothing recorded. After reexamining the research purpose and rethinking her study, she recognized that her readings were indirectly related to the topic and thus supported the need for her research. Consequently, she had to start all over again.

A literature review requires not just the ingestion of large amounts of information but a criticism of each piece. Research articles are critiqued for their credibility and soundness. If a study has a sample size of five yet makes generalizations to a larger population, a reader should be skeptical of it. In composing the literature review, the researcher mentions the serious flaws that may affect his or her rationale for doing the particular study. For example, if a study used five subjects in an effort to understand the problems these subjects had feeding their cerebral palsied children, a researcher might want to replicate the study using a larger sample. Or if a study used an inappropriate method of data analysis or did not sample the appropriate population, a replication study would be acceptable.

As with most steps of the research process, no rigid rules exist for all studies. At each stage the researcher makes many decisions. As he or she critically analyzes the books and articles, he or she makes decisions about what information is vital and relevant to include in the literature review.

THE SCOPE OF A LITERATURE REVIEW

A literature review should include six major types of literature:

1. Relevant nursing research. (Sources of nursing research findings are described later in this chapter.)

2. Theoretical literature (see chapter 5).

3. General and specialty nursing literature. The general nursing literature—*American Journal of Nursing, Heart and Lung, Maternal Child Nursing,* and the like—and other non-research-oriented specialty journals may

provide insights into a researchable topic. In a study on the experiences of young women with cancer, the researcher found no scientific articles relating to experiences but did find several anecdotal articles in the general nursing literature describing a nurse's experience as a patient with breast cancer.

4. Methodological literature. If a researcher notices that all the studies on his or her subject use a certain method of analysis, the researcher may want to read something on the method to gather new ideas or sources for criticisms of the method.

5. Research literature from other disciplines. Most nursing research can benefit from research done in other related disciplines—sociology, psychology, anthropology, political science, physiology, or economics, depending on the nature of the question. Nursing can be viewed as an applied science, so literature in social and natural science may be relevant. Society's pressing problems today are both political and economic, so literature from these disciplines may offer a broad yet relevant perspective on certain nursing research questions.

6. Popular literature. This category includes books like *First You Cry, Anatomy of an Illness, In the Company of Others,* and *Heartsounds.* These are written by patients or family members and in journalistic fashion describe a hospitalization or illness through the eyes of involved participants or subjects. Often newspaper (professional and popular) and magazine articles deal with health issues. The American Medical Association newsletter and the Associated Press reported on a California case in which two physicians were tried for murder for discontinuing life support systems on a patient. Articles such as these would be relevant for a study focused on ICU nurses' experiences in caring for nonviable patients. These studies add context and history and emphasize the rich descriptive nature of the problems. They also help in identifying particularly relevant variables, such as the legal aspects, ethical aspects, and physicians' perceptions versus nurses' perceptions of discontinuing life support, for example.

Only those articles and books that are used for the actual written review are listed in the references for the final research article.

SOURCES OF RESEARCH LITERATURE

Literature that may be relevant to nursing practice often cuts across traditional disciplinary boundaries. Box 4–1 summarizes indexing and abstract resources that are useful for locating literature in fields related to nursing. The key sources for nursing literature itself are summarized in Box 4–2. A good place to begin a literature search is the *Cumulative Index to Nursing and Allied Health Literature,* which can be found in any school of nursing or hospital library.

Locating reports of research that may be relevant to clinical practice will

---

Box 4–1 Indexing and Abstract Resources for Fields Related to Nursing

Abstracts for Social Workers
Bibliography of Reproduction (Cambridge, England)
Bibliography of Suicide and Suicide Prevention
Child Development Abstracts and Bibliographies
Dissertation Abstracts (microfilm from Ann Arbor, Michigan)
Excerpta Medica
Hospital Abstracts
Hospital Literature Index
Index Medicus
International Index
National Library of Medicine Catalogue (monthly holdings of the National Library of Medicine, Bethesda, Maryland)
Psychological Abstracts
Research Grants Index (U.S. Government Printing Office, Washington, DC)
Sociological Abstracts

---

become a lot easier once one is familiar with nursing's primary research journals. As of publication of this text, at least six are well known: *Nursing Research, Advances in Nursing Science,* the *Journal of Research in Nursing and Health,* the *Western Journal of Nursing Research, Applied Nursing Research,* and the *International Journal of Nursing Studies.* Research studies are sometimes published in the general-practice and specialty nursing journals, and social science and medical literature also often contains information that can be useful to nursing. The *Cumulative Index to Nursing and Allied Health Literature,* as well as the *International Nursing Index,* the *Cumulative Medical Index,* and computerized biographical literature searches such as MEDLINE, are resources that can help keep you up to date with these references. Other computerized literature searches and data bases appear in Box 4–3.

Nursing Research (*Nurs Res*) is nursing's oldest and most widely circulated professional journal in the U.S. whose "preferred subject content" is research. It is published six times a year by the American Journal of Nursing Company in New York City. There are about ten full-length articles per issue.

Despite the fact that *Nursing Research* is nursing's oldest and most widely read source of research findings, its circulation pales when compared with that of nursing's most popular general-practice journals, such as *Nursing, The American Journal of Nursing,* and *RN.* We can expect these statistics to change, though, as the value of nursing research to improving clinical practice is increasingly recognized. As of 1992, *RN* magazine is adding a research column as a new feature to its publication which is read by many nurses. Investigators will be expected to make the practice implications of their research more explicit, service settings will benefit by developing systems for using research findings in practice, textbook authors will include research findings, and all nurses will need the skills required to read, understand, and interpret research-oriented literature.

Box 4–2 Abstracts, Indices, and Reviews of Nursing Literature

Annual Review of Nursing Research—Initiated in 1983 to critically review important work so that students, faculty, and other scholars can recognize the advances made, the existing gaps, and the areas that need further work. Volume 1 is *Human Development Through the Life Span;* volume 2, *The Family;* and volume 3, *The Community.*

Cumulative Index to Nursing Literature—Published quarterly with annual compilations since 1956 that draw from 54 journals in nursing and related fields.

Facts About Nursing—Published by the American Nurses' Association in Kansas City, Missouri. It includes information on numbers and distribution of nurses, their employment status, types of education programs, student characteristics, graduates, and the major nursing organizations.

Indexes to Nursing Periodicals—Published annually and in cumulative form.

International Nursing Index to Periodical Literature—Published by the American Journal of Nursing Company.

Nursing Research Abstracts—Between 1959 and 1978, a regular feature of *Nursing Research.*

Nursing Studies Index—Published by J. B. Lippincott, Philadelphia. It contains an annotated guide to reported studies and methodology papers from more than 200 sources.

Advances in Nursing Science (*Adv Nurs Sci*) is published quarterly by Aspen Systems in Maryland. The primary purpose of this journal is "to stimulate the development of nursing science." *Advances in Nursing Science* focuses on empirical research, theory construction, concept analysis, practical application of research and theory, and investigation of values and ethics that influence the practice and research activities of nursing science. Since the first issue was published in October 1978, it has targeted all its issues to specific topics. Each issue has approximately seven full-length articles. Notices of upcoming research or scientific conferences are included near the end.

The *Journal of Research in Nursing and Health* (*Res in Nurs & Health*) is published quarterly by John Wiley & Sons of New York City. The titles of articles in this journal are indexed in the *Cumulative Index to Nursing and Allied Health Literature, Social and Behavioral Science Index, Index Medicus, International Nursing Index, Public Health Reviews, Social Science Citation Index,* and *Sociological Abstracts.* The first issue of *Res in Nurs & Health* was published in April 1978.

This journal's intent is to publish nursing theory, nursing research, and scholarly and analytic works that lead to improvement and refinement of both theory and research. *Res in Nurs & Health* also publishes significant inquiries into nursing administration and education, as well as inquiries into the nature of health. The journal's goal has always been to publish what is "new, true, and important." Each issue includes approximately five feature-length articles.

The *Western Journal of Nursing Research* (*West J Nurs Res*) was begun in 1979 by Phillips-Allen Publishers of Anaheim, California, and its first editor, Pamela Brink. The *West J Nurs Res* was initiated to serve the growing need of nurses in the western United States to share information about what they are doing. It has a three-pronged editorial philosophy:

1. The communication and dissemination of nursing research can be practical.
2. Nursing research is only good if it is used.
3. Talking about research makes it more useful.

To these ends, *West J Nurs Res* serves three different functions:

1. It publishes completed research papers.
2. It disseminates information about research conferences, grants available, and developing research projects.
3. It provides "how to" comments on the research process and its functions.

The journal is correspondingly divided into three distinct sections:

1. Three or four feature articles, each followed by at least two commentaries and an author's response.
2. The Information Exchange, including a meeting calendar, grant deadlines, brief news reports, brief conference reports, research briefs, requests for assistance, and book reviews.
3. Technical notes, problems in doing research, ethical issues, research utilization, and strategies for teaching research, each written by an expert in the area.

Box 4–3 Primary Computerized Literature Searches

1. DATRIX (Direct Access to Reference Information)—Contains more than 150,000 dissertation abstracts on university microfilms

2. ERIC (Educational Resources Information Center)

3. HEIRS (Health Education Information Retrieval System)

4. MEDLINE/MEDLARS—Indexes more than 2,900 biomedical and nursing journals

5. National Clearing House for Mental Health Information of the National Institute of Mental Health

6. NEXUS—American Association for Higher Education's telephone information referral service

7. PAIS, PATELL, PADAT (Psychological Abstracts Information Services)—Available through tape leasing, direct access terminal, and printout

8. SSIE (Smithsonian Science Information Exchange)

9. U.S. Commerce Department's National Technical Information Service

West J Nurs Res also publishes the proceedings of the annual conferences of the Western Society for Research in Nursing in its summer issue.

Applied Nursing Research (*ANR*) was first published in May 1988 by W. B. Saunders Company of Philadelphia. It expressly emphasizes applications to practice of research studies across all clinical specialties and strives for a lively, readable style. Features include "Ask the Experts," "Research Briefs," "Clinical Methods," "Book Reviews," news and announcements related to research conferences and funding opportunities, and an editorial.

The *International Journal of Nursing Studies* (*Int J Nurs Stud*) is published quarterly in Oxford, England by Pergamon Press. Its primary purpose is to enhance the practice of nursing through the promotion of international debate. It is supported by an editorial board comprising members from 11 different countries. In addition to refereed articles on subjects including nursing administration and education, each issue contains a book review section.

THE REVIEW ARTICLE

Sometimes the literature review constitutes the entire study. Such articles are called review articles. *Annual Review of Nursing Research* is devoted to this kind of article. Review articles can be extremely valuable to both researchers and nurses interested in applying research findings to a particular practice area. They are often written by experts in the specialty and offer both a broad survey of what has been done and a critical perspective on it.

Review articles can be broad in scope, such as the classic article "When the Practical Becomes Theoretical" (O'Toole 1981), which surveys significant research in psychiatric nursing. They can also have a more specific focus, such as appears in the "State of the Science" feature in the journal *Image*. Recent examples of review articles include Brown's 1990 appraisal of the quality of diabetes research published in the *Journal of Research in Nursing and Health,* Kuhlman and colleagues' 1991 critical review of literature on Alzheimer's disease published in *Nursing Research,* and Lindenberg's 1991 review of the literature on cocaine abuse in pregnancy, also published in *Nursing Research.*

ANNOTATED RESEARCH EXAMPLE

Alzheimer's Disease and Family Caregiving: — *Review article* [handwritten]
Critical Synthesis of the Literature and Research Agenda

Citation

Kuhlman GJ, Wilson HS, Hutchinson SA, & Wallhagen M. *Nurs Res.* November/ December 1991;4(6):331–337.

focus of search [handwritten] — This paper is a synthesis of knowledge about Alzheimer's disease (AD) and *parameters of search* [handwritten] AD family caregiving published over the last decade (approximately 1979–

critique this area, methodological difficulties, unclear findings, and gaps, particularly with regard to inclusion of ethnic minority populations, persist. The current research priority on evaluating intervention programs represents a worthy direction, yet such a focus may be premature until basic knowledge builds on, *conclusions drawn* extends, and transcends the foundation established in the past decade.

Guidelines for Critique

Is the article's literature review simply a "laundry list," or does it offer critical appraisal of relevant research?

Does the literature review indicate how the present study will refine, revise, extend, or transcend existing knowledge?

Has the author consulted literature from other disciplines besides nursing?

Has the author cited theoretical literature as well as research studies?

Are the primary sources from reputable, sound journals or publishers?

Are all the cited sources relevant to the study, or are many simply marginally related?

Does the literature review appear to have been exhaustive, or was it perhaps cursory?

Are cited sources up-to-date?

Is the literature review well organized, with an obvious summary?

Summary of Key Ideas and Terms

The review of literature included in a research report serves several purposes:

- It presents the theoretical framework of which the study is a part.
- It offers a critical analysis of developments relating to the study's topic.
- It lends credence to the study by showing that there is a tradition of research preceding it.

Reviewing the literature is important because it provides a link between the current research study and previous research or theory, thereby giving the study a context and meaning.

Conducting the literature review involves (1) doing a computer search, (2) checking appropriate indexes, (3) taking notes on the relevant articles located through the search, and (4) doing a critical analysis of each article.

A literature review should include six major types of literature:

- relevant nursing research

- theoretical literature

- general and specialty nursing literature

- methodological literature

- research literature from other disciplines

- popular literature

Most nursing research is reported in a number of key journals: *Nursing Research, Advances in Nursing Science,* the *Journal of Research in Nursing and Health,* the *Western Journal of Nursing Research, Applied Nursing Research,* and the *International Journal of Nursing Studies.*

References

Brown SA. Quality of reporting in diabetes education research: 1954–1986. *Res in Nurs & Health.* 1990;13:52–62.

Kirchhoff KT. A diffusion survey of coronary precautions. *Nurs Res.* July/August 1982;31:196–201.

Kuhlman GJ, Wilson HS, Hutchinson SA, & Wallhagen M. Alzheimer's disease and family caregiving: Critical synthesis of the literature and research agenda. *Nurs Res.* November/December 1991;4(6):331–337.

Lindenberg CS. A review of the literature on cocaine abuse in pregnancy. *Nurs Res.* March/April 1991;4(2):69–75.

Mishel M & Murdaugh C. Family adjustment to heart transplantation: Redesigning the dream. *Nurs Res.* 1987;36:332–338.

Orem D. *Nursing Concepts of Practice.* New York: McGraw-Hill;1980.

O'Toole AW. When the practical becomes theoretical. *J Psychosoc Nurs.* December 1981;19(12):11–19.

Swenson I & Kleinbaum A. Attitudes toward research among undergraduate nursing students. *J Nurs Ed.* November 1984;23(9):380.

THE THEORETICAL BACKGROUND

SECOND EDITION
REVISION BY
HOLLY SKODOL WILSON

CHAPTER OUTLINE

In This Chapter . . .

Based on or including material from *Introducing Research in Nursing* First Edition by Linda E. Moody and Sally Ambler Hutchinson

CHAPTER OBJECTIVES

After reading this chapter, you should be able to:

- Explain the terms *theory, concept, proposition,* and *construct*

- Discuss the use of theoretical and conceptual frameworks in nursing research

- Describe purposes of theory in a discipline

- Discuss major issues in nursing theory

- Analyze and evaluate nursing theories by applying three basic questions

- List and interpret the ten criteria for theory evaluation

- Understand the intellectual contributions of historically important nurse theorists

5

IN THIS CHAPTER . . .

One goal of research is to extend the scope of our knowledge. To do this successfully, a research study must be placed within a theoretical context or be designed to develop one. When a study is placed within a theoretical context, the theory guides the research process from the researchable question, through the design, to a discussion of the results. Words such as *theory, concept, construct, theoretical framework,* and *nursing theory* frequently evoke anxiety, confusion, and dismay. This chapter aims to make these terms understandable and relevant to the nursing student and practicing nurse who is interested in research. The chapter discusses the use of theories from other disciplines and also emerging nursing theories in the research process. You may wonder how a nursing theory differs from any other theory. How do you know a good theory from a poor one? Where do theories come from? And what *is* a theory, anyway? These questions constitute the focus of this chapter, and examples drawn from nursing research serve as illustrations.

VOCABULARY OF THEORY

As you read about theories and their relationship to nursing research, you will immediately become aware of the frequent use of some new language. An understanding of this vocabulary is essential for you to be able to appreciate and apply the ideas in your reading and in your practice and research.

Theory

What is a theory? The word **theory** comes from the Greek *theoria,* which means vision. Most people expect theories to be fact, but they really are systematic views on the truth or reality of some phenomena. Theories are viewpoints or ways of perceiving. Kerlinger (1973) gives us a more formal definition of *theory:* "A theory is a set of interrelated constructs (concepts), definitions, and propositions that present a systematic view of phenomena by specifying relations among variables, with the purpose of explaining and predicting the phenomena" (p. 9). Examples of theories you have probably heard about and perhaps have even used in your practice are psychoanalytic theory, the theory of relativity, the theory of evolution, the theory of gravity, learning theory, systems theory, the theory of homeostasis, and stress and coping theory.

Concept

Concepts are the building blocks of theories. Concepts may be concrete (patient blood loss, height and weight, temperature elevation) or abstract (wellness, grief, stress, quality of life) and must be clearly defined so researchers understand their real meaning and can attempt to measure them. A concept's

operational definition links that concept to the real world so it can be observed, controlled, and measured through the research process. Concepts allow you to organize and categorize observations. **Propositions** describe the relationship of two or more concepts.

Construct

When you read about concepts and theories, you may also read about *constructs*. **Constructs** are concepts that are derived from existing theory. Familiar examples of constructs are society, socioeconomic status, and self-concept. Some authors distinguish constructs from concepts by stating that they are "invented or constructed" by researchers and are more abstract and less observable. Generally, the terms are used interchangeably.

Putting Them All Together

Before nursing can claim to have its own unique theories, it first must have concepts, propositions, and constructs. Theories, concepts, propositions, and constructs, aim to describe pieces of reality. Most scientists believe that there is a reality "out there" and that it is worthwhile to obtain knowledge about it. Theories and their component parts refer to, explain, describe, and predict reality in more or less concrete or abstract ways. Kaplan (1964) describes an empirical-theoretical continuum that allows us to view the relationship between what is observed empirically and what is described theoretically (see Figure 5–1).

Concepts may vary from the empirical, or observable (such as blood loss) to the theoretical, or abstract (such as grief); constructs tend to be more symbolic (such as social loss) and are generally derived from specific theories (such as ego, id, superego, individuation, or reinforcement). Recognition of this continuum from the empirical to the theoretical should help when you read theories and attempt to understand how they are linked up with observable reality.

THEORETICAL OR CONCEPTUAL FRAMEWORKS AND NURSING RESEARCH

Nursing theories both guide nursing research by yielding hypotheses to be supported or refuted and are generated from nursing research. Approaches to theory building that begin with an existing theory and test hypotheses deduced from that theory—such as the Roy Adaptation Model (Roy & Andrews 1991)—are often called **deductive**. Approaches to theory building that generate hypotheses and explanatory schema from observations, interviews, and other data are often called **inductive**.

The **theoretical framework** for a particular study is an essay that places the study in the context of existing related theory based on the literature that has been reviewed. The framework of background knowledge is called a

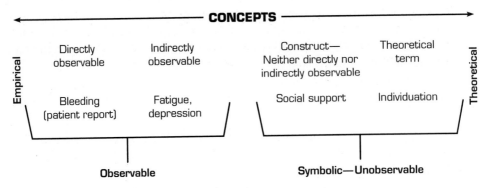

Figure 5–1   *An empirical-theoretical continuum.*
Source: Adapted from Kaplan 1964 pp. 57–60. Reprinted with permission.

conceptual framework when it does not contain a specific theory that explains the expected relationship between variables in a study but does synthesize possibly relevant literature and sensitizing ideas. In many cases these two terms are used interchangeably.

THE PURPOSES OF THEORIES

The Need for Nursing Theories

Why does nursing need theories? Leininger (1991) identifies eight uses for nursing theories.

1. Nursing theories, coupled with research findings, provide a perspective, a common framework, and a sound basis to guide nurse clinicians' thinking, decisions, and actions.

2. Nursing theories provide a holistic or comprehensive perspective of human beings under varying life situations or environmental conditions and prevent nurses from viewing humans simply as organs, or body systems, or in other partial, fragmented ways.

3. Nursing theories with substantiated and cumulative research findings on nursing phenomena are essential for supporting the judgments and actions of nurses and for improving nursing care practices.

4. Nursing theories are a powerful means for stimulating the intellectual, clinical, and humanistic dimensions of nursing practice so that nursing does not become a boring or highly ritualized technical practice that leads to burnout among nurses.

5. With the use of nursing theories, not only will the quality of nursing care improve, but also there will be a decrease in costs and an increase in consumer satisfaction.

6. With the use of nursing theories and concomitant research findings generated from the theories, important differences and solutions to current problems in nursing practice will become more readily apparent—alleviating many problems, such as nurse shortages and other concerns.

7. The use of nursing theories provides a common referent language that facilitates communication, provides common goals and plans for nursing care.

8. Nursing theories can be among the strongest and most lasting means for identifying and supporting differentiated role practices and role responsibilities in nursing administration.

For these reasons, one can predict some highly promising and still largely unknown or unrecognized clinical nursing practices in nursing. Most assuredly, nursing theories can provide a strong position for differentiated or even undifferentiated nursing practice (pp. 28–29).

Issues in Nursing Theory

We have established that the discipline of nursing needs theories, but of what type? Questions raised in recent literature include:

1. Is nursing research basic or applied?

2. Is nursing theory borrowed or unique?

3. What paths to knowledge and development exist?

Although many diverse opinions and beliefs on these issues coexist, there appears to be unity around several points.

Basic or Applied Research? Debating whether nursing knowledge is basic or applied raises the question of whether nursing research should aim to discover new knowledge (thus expanding the knowledge base for the sake of acquiring more knowledge) or to develop knowledge that can be used expressly to guide nursing practice. An example of research in nursing that contributes to our knowledge may be a physiological study about how respiratory exchange works with cardiopulmonary disease patients. Early on, this research may not have a clear application for practice, but ultimately its utility would be recognized once scientists understood the process. Such understanding surely would suggest appropriate nursing intervention measures.

This example illustrates a point that many nurse scientists make: It is foolish and wasteful to spend time discussing the philosophical questions about whether nursing research is basic or applied. Rather, nursing needs all kinds of research, basic *and* applied, and inevitably most basic research in nursing results in practical suggestions that will affect patient care.

Borrowed or Unique Theory? A second question asks if nursing theory is borrowed or unique. There is agreement among nurse scientists that nursing theory is *both* borrowed and unique. That is, nurses use knowledge from many disciplines (psychology, sociology, physics, physiology, education);

however, this knowledge only becomes integrated into nursing theory if nurses adapt it and alter it to fit the unique needs and perspectives of nursing. Nursing theories are those that are systematically derived from studies of nursing practice and that reveal a unique nursing perspective.

What Paths to Knowledge?   A major goal for nursing research is to decide what questions are relevant to and significant for nursing. A related goal is the application of investigative methodologies that are appropriate to these significant questions and congruent with nursing's philosophy. The debate here often puts the methods borrowed from the natural sciences (which attempt to objectively measure phenomena), termed **positivist** or **empiricist,** in competition with the methods borrowed from social sciences and humanities, termed **naturalistic** or **interpretive.** Many authorities argue that nursing research needs both and urge what is termed methodologic **triangulation,** or the usefulness of multiple "slices of data" on the same phenomena or variables.

EVALUATION AND ANALYSIS OF THEORIES

You can use three main questions to make informed decisions about the value of proposed nursing theories: (1) Is it a theory? (2) Is it a nursing theory? (3) Is it any good?

Is It a Theory?

For a theory to be considered a theory, the following components must be present:

1. concepts that describe the empirical world
2. definitions of concepts
3. propositions or constructs
4. links among the concepts and constructs that explain and predict phenomena

Developing a theory is complex, laborious, and time-consuming work requiring superior conceptual abilities. Only the mature sciences can boast that they have confirmed theories to guide them in research. In nursing, this work has just begun.

Is It a Theory Unique to Nursing?

Contemporary debate focuses on the feasibility and desirability of developing theories unique to nursing. On one side are those scientists who believe that one's interests should dictate the pursuit of knowledge. Therefore, regardless of one's discipline, any scientist is free to explore and study any phenomenon, ultimately making a contribution to knowledge in general that may be useful to nursing or to the other sciences. Another group, also opposed to working toward developing nursing theories, believes that theories do not and will not have special relevance for nursing. Rather, theories from other disciplines (physiology, psychology, anthropology, and economics) can be modified and applied to nursing problems.

In the opposite camp are those who advocate working toward unique nursing theories. They are fearful that scientists outside of nursing will not have the depth of interest and effort required to generate nursing knowledge. And unique nursing knowledge is mandatory to guide our practice. Borrowing from other disciplines will not contribute comprehensive in-depth knowledge necessary for scientifically based practice. Later in this chapter we will look at some theories that do meet the criterion of being unique to nursing.

How Good Is It?

Stevens (1979) presents one set of standards for theory evaluation. She advocates both internal criticism (how theory components fit with each other) and external criticism (how theory relates to the real world). The following four criteria are used to judge internal construction of a theory:

1. *Clarity.* Is the theory presented in such a way that the definitions of concepts and propositions and their relationships are easily understood?

2. *Consistency.* Is the theory consistent in the meaning of terms, interpretations, principles, and methods of reasoning?

3. *Logical development.* Does the reasoning process lead logically to conclusions?

4. *Level of theory development.* Is it a conceptual analysis, a descriptive theory, a situation-relating theory, or a more advanced situation-producing theory?

The next six criteria are used in judging the *external* aspects of a theory—that is, how it relates to the world of people, health, environment, and nursing (the four key variables in most nursing theories):

1. *Adequacy.* Does the theory satisfactorily deal with the nurse scientist's perspective of nursing? There must be adequacy of principles, interpretations, and methods. Do you accept the basic principles that are the foundation of the theory? Does the theorist's perception or interpretation of nursing make sense and accurately mirror the real world? Does the method of the theory permit research, and if so, what types of research are appropriate (deductive, philosophical)?

2. *Utility.* Is the theory useful in education, research, or practice?

3. *Significance.* Does the theory address issues basic and relevant to nursing and aim toward increasing nursing knowledge?

4. *Discrimination.* Does the theory clearly define its boundaries so that its relatedness to nursing is obvious? The theory must discriminate between what nursing is and what it isn't.

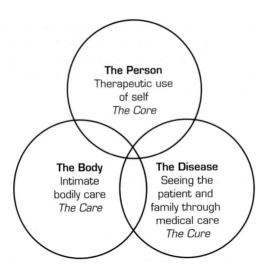

Figure 5–2   *Hall's three aspects of nursing.*
Source: Nursing Theories Conference Group 1980 p. 44. Reprinted by permission of Prentice-Hall.

5.   *Scope.* Is the focus of the theory narrow or broad?

6.   *Parsimony.* Does the theory explain as much as possible with the fewest possible variables? This is sometimes called the power of a theory. A powerful theory is one that makes few assumptions and that clearly separates the critical variables from the diffuse background. Some scientists believe that in aiming for parsimony, one may miss the essence. Rather, one should strive for complexity because it examines the relationship between many variables. In fact, the nature of the subject matter should dictate to what degree a theory is complex or parsimonious. (Stevens 1979)

These criteria offer a useful structure for you to evaluate any theoretical model for nursing.

NURSING THEORIES—SOME EXAMPLES

This section offers you a brief overview of several of the best-known nursing theories. Perhaps one or more of these theories will catch your interest, and you can read in more depth by going directly to the writings of the particular theorist or an authoritative source on nursing theory such as Meleis (1991) or Stevens (1984).

Lydia Hall

Hall's theory presents the three "aspects of nursing": the person (or the core of nursing), the disease (or the cure of nursing), and the body (the care of nursing) (see Figure 5–2). Her philosophy developed from her work at the Loeb Center of Montefieore Hospital in the Bronx, where patients had recovered from their acute illnesses and were recuperating in this long-term, patient-centered treatment center. Depending on the patient's problems, each of the three aspects of nursing might be emphasized or deemphasized, demonstrating the changing nature of their relationships.

Hildegard Peplau

Peplau, a psychiatric nurse, presented her theoretical model in *Interpersonal Relations in Nursing* (1952). According to Peplau, nursing is a "significant therapeutic interpersonal process. . . . Nursing is an educative instrument, a maturing force, that aims to promote forward movement of personality in the direction of creative, constructive, productive, personal, and community living" (p. 16).

Peplau's theory focused on the four phases of the nurse-patient relationship (see Figure 5–3).

1. *Orientation.* The nurse and patient meet in response to the patient's "felt need."

2. *Identification.* The patient responds to the nurse if he or she offers needed help.

3. *Exploitation.* The patient uses the nurse as a resource person.

4. *Resolution.* When the patient's needs are met, he or she relinquishes ties to the nurse.

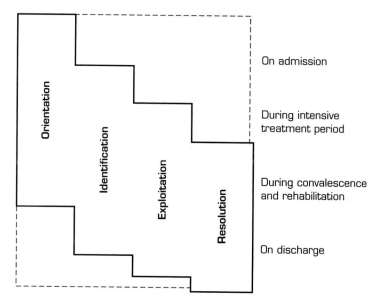

Figure 5–3 *Peplau's conception of overlapping phases in nurse-patient relationships.*
Source: Peplau 1952 p. 21. Reprinted with permission.

Dorothea Orem

Orem's theory of self-care appeared in the nursing literature in 1959. Her theory centers on the individual: "Self-care is the practice of activities that individuals personally initiate and perform on their own behalf to maintain life, health, and well-being. . . . It is an adult's personal, continuous contribution to his own health and well-being" (1971 p. 13).

Orem proposes six categories of universal self-care requisites:

1. air, water, and food

2. excrement

3. activity and rest

4. solitude and social interaction

5. hazards to life and well-being

6. being normal

She has identified four concepts that best express the properties and actions of persons in need of nursing:

1. self-care

2. therapeutic self-care demand

3. self-care agency

4. self-care deficit

Additionally, she has defined the nursing agency and nursing system as concepts that express the properties and actions of nurses.

Self-care refers to the activities that individuals initiate and perform on their own behalf to sustain life, health, and well-being. Self-care is viewed as a form of deliberate action that is learned within a sociocultural context.

Therapeutic self-care demand is defined as the measure of care required at certain moments to meet existent requisites. Orem identifies three categories of self-care requisites: universal, developmental, and health-deviation. These three categories of requisites represent the types of purposeful self-care that persons may require at various phases of the life cycle and in various states of health.

The human capabilities for self-care are conceptualized as *self-care agency. Agency* is used here in the sense of power or capacity. Thus, self-care agency refers to the complex set of acquired abilities that are specific to the performance of the actions of self-care (Orem 1985).

The fourth concept in this category is *self-care deficit,* which refers to a specific relationship between the concepts of self-care agency and therapeutic self-care demand in which self-care agency is not adequate to meet the therapeutic self-care demand (Orem 1985). According to the theory, the presence of an existing or potential self-care deficit identifies those persons in need of nursing.

Thus, Orem's self-care deficit theory explains when and why nursing is required and provides criterion measures for identifying those who need nursing. The theory of self-care explains why these forms of care are necessary for life, development, health, and well-being. Finally, Orem's theory of nursing systems explains how persons can be helped through nursing. Clearly, the work of this theorist differentiates nursing from other forms of human service and provides a basis for structuring nursing knowledge and nursing practice.

Martha Rogers

Rogers published her book *An Introduction to the Theoretical Basis of Nursing* in 1970, drawing on knowledge from anthropology, sociology, religion, philosophy, mythology, and general systems theory. Her theory has changed somewhat and has become clarified over the years. At the present time, she views the "unitary" person as the basis of nursing's uniqueness. The science of nursing is "the study of the nature and direction of unitary human development and the derivation of descriptive, explanatory, and predictive principles that are basic to nursing practice." The practice of nursing is "the use of the body of knowledge in service to people." The purpose of nursing is "to help individuals and groups achieve maximum well-being within the potential of each" (Rogers 1982).

Rogers views science as humanistic, not mechanistic. People and the environment are two energy fields that are always open, have pattern and organization, and change continuously and creatively.

Myra Levine

Levine (1967, 1971) proposes four conservation principles that aim to alter patients' adaptation processes in positive ways. The nurse first identifies the patient's specific pattern of adaptation and then uses the following principles to plan nursing intervention:

1. *The principle of the conservation of patient energy.* Nursing intervention is based on conserving the individual patient's physiological and psychological resources.

2. *The principle of the conservation of structural integrity.* Nursing intervention is based on conserving the individual patient's body form and function.

3. *The principle of conservation of personal integrity.* Nursing intervention is based on conserving the individual patient's self-identity and self-respect.

4. *The principle of conservation of social integrity.* Nursing intervention is based on conserving the individual patient's ethnic, religious, and subcultural affiliations.

Levine views her principles as offering new directions for holistic approaches to patient care.

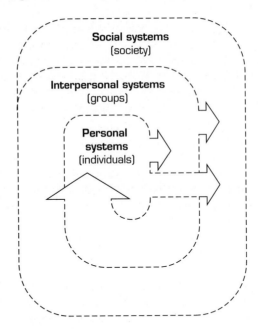

Figure 5–4   *King's conceptual framework for nursing.*
Source: King 1981. Reprinted with permission.

Sister Callista Roy

Roy's adaptation theory (1976) views us as biopsychosocial beings who have to continually engage in a life process of adaptation to a variety of stimuli, which she calls *focal, contextual,* and *residual* (p. 12). The focal stimulus has to do with a degree of change (for example, a temperature variation); contextual stimuli include other stimuli present (for example, humidity); and residual stimuli involve beliefs and attitudes that affect a given situation (p. 13). Roy identifies four adaptive modes that help people cope with the changing environment: basic physiological needs, self-concept, role function, and interdependence. These four adaptive modes are essentially methods of coping that appear between a need and a behavior. For example, if the environmental temperature changes, a person may be hot or cold, and these feelings elicit an adaptive mode. The person feels the need and acts to address the need. Roy views basic needs as underlying the adaptive modes. The nursing process is used to promote the patient's adaptation in each mode. In her books, Roy gives examples of nursing interventions for specific adaptation problems and identifies indicators of effective adaptation (Roy 1990, Roy & Andrews 1991).

Imogene King

King (1978) proposes a general systems theory about the human level of functioning. People, environment, nursing, and health are her four basic concepts.

She postulates three dynamic interacting systems (see Figure 5–4). Each individual is a *personal system.* Individuals interact among one another to form *interpersonal systems,* such as dyads, triads, and groups. The interpersonal systems then form *social systems,* which are comprehensive levels of functions of human beings. A person's personal system is dependent largely on his or her perception of self. These perceptions directly influence behavior. The nurse-patient nursing process is implemented in the interpersonal system. The social systems—family, religious, educational, and health care systems (King 1981)—provide a context in which nurses work. To help patients achieve goals, nurses must interact effectively with social systems. King views her theory as "organizing complexity and variety in nursing . . . [and] in looking for relationships within this complexity and variety" (p. 15).

Betty Neuman

Neuman (1982) proposes a health care systems model that views the person as a complete system with parts and subparts that interrelate. Neuman sees human beings as subject to stressors, which she identifies as intrapersonal, interpersonal, and extrapersonal and as having flexible lines of resistance that help defend against these stressors (see Figure 5–5). Nursing assessment focuses on gaining information about the relationship among physiologic, psychologic, sociocultural, and developmental variables; nursing intervention can be primary, secondary, or tertiary. The nursing process, including nursing diagnosis, nursing goals, and nursing outcomes, is expected to facilitate the use of the model.

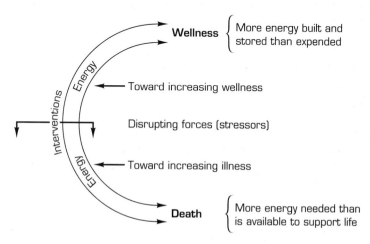

Figure 5–5 *Neuman's wellness-illness continuum based on a systems model.*
Source: Neuman 1982 p. 11. Reprinted with permission.

Rosemarie Rizzo Parse

Parse's theory of human becoming posits that humans are open, unitary beings in mutual process with the world, cocreating patterns of becoming. The human-world-health process is the phenomenon of concern to nursing. Parse's theory focuses on the meaning of lived experiences.

Three major principles identify *human becoming* (Parse 1981):

1. structuring meaning multidimensionally through imaging, valuing, and language

2. cocreating rhythmical patterns of relating through revealing/concealing, enabling/limiting, and connecting/separating

3. cotranscending possibilities through empowerment that originates in transformation

QUESTIONING NURSING MODELS

In a quest for useful theories for nursing research, Cronenwett and Brickman (1983) discussed four models of helping and coping in childbirth. After describing each theory and its assumptions and the pros and cons, they concluded the article by raising some relevant questions for nursing research. Some or all of these questions could be adapted and asked about many other theories for nursing.

1. Are some theories generally better than others?

2. Are different theories best for different clients?

3. Are client-provider teams using the same (congruent) theories most effectively?

4. Is it better to apply one theory to a client consistently or to change as the client's needs, situations, and skills change?

5. Are some theories better for providers?

6. Do organizational structures determine the choice of a theory?

7. Does professional role socialization determine the choice of a theory?

8. Has there been a historic evolution of the dominant nursing theories?

The search for theories and models for many areas of nursing is a most useful endeavor. Cronenwett and Brickman's beginning look at models generates many varied ideas and approaches for further study. The American Academy of Nursing devoted its 1990 annual conference to the topic of differentiating nursing practice into the twenty-first century using nursing theories.

This chapter has emphasized the interdependence of nursing theory, research, and practice. Developing a body of knowledge about nursing and for nursing practice is critical if we are to move from a discipline based on tradition and authority to a discipline based on science. Placing nursing studies within the context of our evolving theoretical base is essential to that goal.

ANNOTATED RESEARCH EXAMPLE

Citation

— study was designed to generate — not test — theory.

Swanson KM. Empirical development of a middle range theory of caring. *Nurs Res.* May/June 1991;40(3):161–166.

Study Problem/Purpose

The purpose of this study was to describe the inductive development and refinement of a middle range theory of caring. Prior literature reveals that a universal definition or conceptualization of caring does not exist.

— Relevant literature was reviewed.

Methods

Twenty-two women who had recently miscarried were interviewed on two occasions, 33 interviews with 19 care providers in a newborn ICU were combined with participant observation, and eight additional interviews were conducted with mothers who had been recipients of a long-term public health nursing intervention. The transcripts of these textual data were subjected to phenomenologic steps for interpretation, including bracketing, intuiting, analyzing, and describing.

Findings

The study resulted in five subdivisions or categories of caring: (1) knowing, (2) being with, (3) doing for, (4) enabling, and (5) maintaining belief. Caring as defined through these perinatal studies is related to prior literature on caring such as Watson's carative factors and Benner's helping role supports. Future research beyond perinatal situations is urged.

Research generates conceptual notions) which in turn can guide further research

Discussion links findings with existing knowledge.

Guidelines for Critique

Is the theoretical background of the research study clearly stated in the report's review of the literature?

Are theoretical concepts, propositions, and constructs defined and related to the research at hand, or are concepts generated?

Is the research based on a theory or a conceptual framework appropriate to the research?

Does the research draw solely on nursing theory, or does it draw on theory from other disciplines?

Does the research report successfully demonstrate the relationship between theory and research findings?

Summary of Key Ideas and Terms

A **theory,** according to Kerlinger (1973), is "a set of interrelated constructs (concepts), definitions, and propositions that present a systematic view of phenomena by specifying relations among variables, with the purpose of explaining and predicting the phenomena" (p. 9).

Concepts are the building blocks of theories and may be concrete (such as a patient's blood loss) or abstract (such as wellness). **Propositions** describe the relationship of two or more concepts.

A **construct** is a type of concept that is constructed from theory and is usually abstract.

The empirical-theoretical continuum demonstrates the relationship between what is observed empirically and what is described theoretically.

Theoretical and conceptual frameworks from nursing and from other disciplines can be used to guide nursing practice and nursing research and can be generated from nursing research.

Dominant issues in nursing theory include answers to the questions (1) Is nursing research basic or applied? (2) Is nursing theory borrowed or unique? and (3) What paths to knowledge and development are preferred?

A proposed nursing theory can be analyzed in terms of three broad questions: (1) Is it a theory? (2) Is it a theory unique to nursing? (3) How good is it?

A theory may be evaluated on four criteria that refer to its internal construction: (1) clarity, (2) consistency, (3) logical development, and (4) level of theory development.

A theory may be evaluated on six criteria that refer to its external aspects: (1) adequacy, (2) utility, (3) significance, (4) discrimination, (5) scope, and (6) parsimony.

Nursing theories have been proposed by a number of thinkers, including Lydia Hall, Hildegard Peplau, Dorothea Orem, Martha Rogers, Myra Levine, Sister Callista Roy, Imogene King, Betty Neuman, and Rosemarie Rizzo Parse.

References

Cronenwett L & Brickman P. Models of helping and coping in childbirth. *Nurs Res.* 1983;82:84–88.

Kaplan A. *The Conduct of Inquiry.* San Francisco: Chandler;1964.

Kerlinger N. *Foundations of Behavioral Research.* New York: Holt, Rinehart & Winston;1973.

King I. The "why" of theory development. In *Theory Developments: What? Why? How?* New York: National League for Nursing;1978.

King I. *Toward a Theory for Nursing.* New York: Wiley;1981.

Leininger, M. Nursing Theories to Guide Differentiated Nursing Practices. *Differentiating Nursing Practice into the Twenty-First Century.* Edited by Irma E. Goertzen. Kansas City, Mo: American Academy of Nursing;1991:27–29.

Levine M. The four conservation principles of nursing. *Nurs Forum.* 1967;6:45–59.

Levine M. Holistic nursing. *Nursing Clinics of North America.* 1971;6:253–264.

Meleis A. *Theoretical Nursing: Development and Progress.* 2d ed. Philadelphia: Lippincott;1991.

Neuman B. *The Neuman Systems Model.* Norwalk, Conn.: Appleton-Century-Crofts;1982.

Nursing Theories Conference Group. *Nursing Theories: The Base for Professional Nursing Practice.* Englewood Cliffs, NJ: Prentice-Hall;1980.

Orem D. *Nursing: Concepts of Practice.* New York: McGraw-Hill;1971.

Orem D. *Nursing: Concepts of Practice.* 2d ed. New York: McGraw-Hill;1985.

Parse RR. *Man-living-health: A Theory of Nursing.* New York: Wiley;1981.

Peplau H. *Interpersonal Relations in Nursing.* New York: Putnam;1952.

Rogers M. *An Introduction to the Theoretical Basis of Nursing.* Philadelphia: F. A. Davis;1970.

Rogers M. *Nurse Educators' Conference.* New York: National League for Nursing; December 1982.

Roy Sister C. *Introduction to Nursing: An Adaptation Model.* Englewood Cliffs, NJ: Prentice-Hall;1976.

Roy Sister C. Dialogue on a theoretical issue: Strengthening the Roy Adaptation Model through conceptual clarification response. *Nurs Sci Quarterly.* 1990;3(2):64–66.

Roy C & Andrews H. *The Roy Adaptation Model: The Definitive Statement.* Norwalk, Conn.: Appleton & Lange;1991.

Stevens B. *Nursing Theory: Analysis, Application, Evaluation.* 2d ed. Boston: Little, Brown;1984.

VARIABLES AND HYPOTHESES

HOLLY SKODOL WILSON

SALLY AMBLER HUTCHINSON

CHAPTER OUTLINE

In This Chapter . . .

CHAPTER OBJECTIVES

After reading this chapter, you should be able to:

- Distinguish between independent and dependent variables

- Explain the importance of operationalizing variables

- Discuss the need for controlling for confounding variables

- State two criteria for hypotheses

- List the components of a hypothesis

- Distinguish between simple and complex hypotheses, directional and nondirectional hypothesis, and research and statistical hypotheses

6

IN THIS CHAPTER . . .

It is impossible to begin collecting data for a study until the researcher has clearly defined the specific concepts to be studied unless the study is designed to discover concepts and theory. These concepts are called **variables.** A variable is, as the name suggests, any factor that varies. For example, age, weight, height, temperature, pCO_2 values, stress, political beliefs, and attitudes are all variables, because all vary to some degree. Gender varies from male to female and is an example of a **dichotomous variable**—that is, a variable with only two categories. Age, weight, height, and pCO_2 values have a range of variability and are examples of **continuous variables.**

Variables are often labeled as *dependent* or *independent*. The **dependent variable** (DV), also called the output or criterion variable, is the study variable that is under investigation and is usually symbolized as Y. It's the one that the researcher determines *as a result* of conducting the study. In some cases it is the *effect* or *outcome* of an experimental procedure. The variability in the dependent variable presumably *depends* on the cause or conditions that may be manipulated by the researcher in the study. In most studies, the dependent variables are the ones that the researcher is intending to understand, explain, or predict. They constitute what the researcher measures about the subjects *after* they have experienced or been exposed to the independent variable.

Independent variables (IVs), usually symbolized as X, on the other hand, are the causes or conditions that the investigator manipulates or identifies to determine the effects or outcomes. Their values are established independently ahead of time by the investigator. They constitute the *input* of an experiment and precede the measurement of the dependent variable.

It is not usually too hard to spot the difference between the independent variables and the dependent variable(s) in a research study. Sometimes they are alluded to in the study title: "A Diffusion Survey of Coronary Precautions" means that the study is about the impact of the diffusion of research knowledge about coronary precautions on the practice arena. The statement of study purpose sometimes reveals that an investigator has set out to establish the effects of something (IV) on something else (DV)—for example, the effects of preoperative teaching on postoperative recovery or of therapeutic touch on perception of pain. The same statement is sometimes made in reverse order: "This study was conducted to see whether a client's self-esteem (DV) was affected by changes in levels of physical exercise (IV)." In both cases, though, the investigator is doing the same thing: manipulating or selecting an IV or several of them to determine whether it (they) affects or changes measurements in the DV(s).

This chapter briefly reviews the role of the statement of purpose for a study and then goes on to examine not only the nature of variables but also the role of hypotheses, which are statements about predicted relationships between variables in research.

> **Box 6–1 Study Levels and Their Statements of Purpose**
>
> Level 1   In a study that asks the question "What are the eating habits of bulimics?" the purpose can be expressed in the statement "The purpose of this research is to explore and describe the eating habits of bulimics."
>
> Level 2   In a study that asks the question "What is the relationship between smoking and prematurity in primiparous mothers?" the purpose is written as "The purpose of the study is to answer the question 'Is there a significant relationship between smoking and prematurity in primiparous mothers?'"
>
> Level 3   In a study that asks the question "Why does the teaching of self-care strategies increase the feeling of well-being in chronically ill patients?" the purpose is written as "The purpose of this study is to test this hypothesis: Chronically ill patients who are taught self-care techniques will have higher scores on feelings of well-being than those who do not receive the teaching."

STATEMENT OF PURPOSE

Planning research begins with formulating a problem statement or a researchable question (chapter 3), moves through a review of the related literature (chapter 4), and culminates with a concise statement of purpose.

The statement of purpose answers the question "Why do the study?" Researchers hold different views about stating a purpose for the research. Some believe that a question or hypothesis is sufficient and that including a statement of purpose is redundant. Others believe that both a statement of purpose and a researchable question or hypothesis are necessary. Brink and Wood (1988) suggest that the purpose be written as a statement for a level 1 study, as a question for a level 2 study, and as a hypothesis (or hypotheses) for a level 3 study. Box 6–1 illustrates this approach.

VARIABLES

Nurse researchers are interested in studying variables, particularly how they vary in relation to one another. When studying relationships between variables, the researcher is asking "Is X related to Y? For example, how does alcohol abuse vary with different types of treatment methods? How does surgical patients' anxiety vary with different types of anesthesia? Table 6–1 provides some examples of variables and their types of variations.

As noted earlier in this chapter, an independent variable can stand alone, whereas a dependent variable depends on another variable. In some studies, independent variables are thought to influence dependent variables in a cause-and-effect fashion; for example, exposure to the sun over time may cause

---

Table 6–1   *Variables and Their Types of Variations*

Variable	*Type of Variation*
Reconditioning	Patients receive reconditioning or don't receive reconditioning.
Bladder dysfunction	The bladder is dysfunctional or it is not.
Preoperative education	Patients receive preoperative education or they don't.
Postoperative experiences	Unusual sensory experiences are present or they are not.
Feelings about the post-operative experience	Patients can feel comfortable or in control of the unusual sensory experience or not.
Type of surgery	Surgery can be mastectomy, hysterectomy, or biopsy.
Amount of depression	Depression can range from none to severe.
Health belief scores	Scores may range from high to low.
The practice of breast self-examination	Women may or may not practice BSE.
Sleep-wake patterns	Sleep-wake patterns may vary in terms of times and duration.
Head injury	Patients may be preinjury or postinjury.

---

skin cancer. Independent variables are those that the researcher manipulates. Thus, a researcher could study people with much sun exposure and people with little sun exposure, manipulating the independent variable. Or the researcher could introduce a cardiac rehabilitation education program (independent variable) and study patients' understanding (dependent variable) of their illness.

A researcher conducting a level 3 inquiry will have an independent and a dependent variable. Since level 1 studies are exploratory, the relevant variables are not all known at the outset. All variables are assumed to be independent until there is enough of a knowledge base to predict the nature of the variables. In level 2 studies, in which the researcher asks whether there is a significant relationship between variables—for example, "Is there a significant relationship between women's age and sleep patterns?"—there is the underlying assumption or hunch that women's age (independent variable) does affect sleep patterns (dependent variable). But until the research is completed, one cannot justifiably predict a strong pattern of association.

It is important to note that variables are not inherently independent or dependent. A variable that is considered the independent variable in one study can be the dependent variable in another based on the role it plays. Studies may have more than one independent or dependent variable. For example, in a study of experienced burden, use of humor, and mental health among family caregivers of Alzheimer's disease victims, the use of humor can be an independent, an intervening, or a dependent variable.

Defining Variables

Once a research statement, question, or hypothesis is written clearly, with the appropriate delineation of variables, the researcher needs to write **operational definitions** for the variables. Operationally defining variables requires clearly specifying them and stating how they will be measured.

If the variable is age, how will the researcher collect data on the subjects' age? Ask them? Have them write it on a questionnaire? Here, for example, is an operational definition of age: "The age of the subject will be asked during the interview session and will be recorded in number of years and months." An operational definition of sleep pattern is: "Sleeping electroencephalograms will be recorded over one eight-hour period, and the pattern will be assessed according to the Bannon Sleep Pattern Instrument." In both examples, you can see clearly what variable is being studied and how it will be measured. The operational definition permits you to go from the abstract idea of variables to a concrete definition of how to measure the specific variables. (See Box 6–2 for examples of operationalized variables from three publications of nursing research.)

Variables can be concrete (gender, age, height) or more abstract (stress, depression, political beliefs, spiritual beliefs). Abstract variables can be measured using many different instruments (see chapter 8). Stress and depression can be measured psychologically or physiologically; depression can be studied by projective techniques, self-report, observation, or laboratory test. Political and spiritual beliefs can be assessed by in-depth interviews or questionnaires.

Understanding how the researcher has operationalized the variables in a study is crucial to your evaluation of that study's results. This is especially true with abstract variables. If you think about some of the terms we use to describe our experiences in nursing—empathy, caring, support, adaptation, communication—you can see that many "variables" that nurse researchers might wish to study are intangible qualities, rather than concrete quantities such as blood pressure, temperature, and healing time. The latter are also important objects of attention for nursing research and are often studied.

With abstract variables you must take the time to evaluate the researcher's operational definition and selection of measurement tool. Take empathy as an example. Everyone would seem to know what it is, but how can one "measure" empathy? How could one quantify whether one nurse has "more" empathy than another? Scrutinizing the operational definitions of abstract variables will help you decide whether the measurements taken in the study do in fact measure the concepts the researcher claims to be measuring.

Uncontrolled, or Confounding, Variables

When planning a research study, an investigator not only must define relevant variables but also must take into consideration other variables that might have effects on the DV other than or in addition to the IVs. If these other variables are not taken into account, they can confuse the interpretation of a study's results, because they confound the effects of the IV. Not surprisingly, they are

Box 6–2 Examples of Operational Definitions in Nursing Studies

Purpose/Question/Hypotheses

The purpose of the study was to examine the behavioral effects of releasing restraints on the hospitalized elderly, and the feasibility of caring for patients considered at risk if left unrestrained. One researchable question was: Do the amount of nursing time and the number of nursing contacts increase when the patient is unrestrained?

Operational Definitions

1.   Nursing time: Measurement in seconds whenever a staff member was on camera (subjects were being videotaped).

2.   Nursing contacts: Number of times a nurse attended the patient to provide care to the subject during an eight-hour shift.
    Source: Morse & McHutchion 1991.

Purpose/Question/Hypotheses

Subjects receiving antiemetic therapy via a patient-controlled pump will report the same amount of nausea, will experience the same amount of vomiting, and will experience less sedation than subjects receiving antiemetic therapy via mini-bags administered by the nurse when measured 1 hour, 12 hours, and 24 hours following moderate emetic potential chemotherapy.

Operational Definitions

1.   Nausea was measured using a self-report one-item visual analogue scale. The scale consisted of a 100-mm horizontal line anchored at one end by "not at all nauseated" and at the other by "extremely nauseated." Each subject's score was determined by measuring the distance from the end of the line marked "not at all nauseated" to the slash mark placed by the subject on the line.

2.   Vomiting was measured by self-report and by nurse observation using a tool that consisted of a 5-point Likert scale with points labeled from 0 to 4. Zero was defined as no emesis, while 1 indicated less than 5 retches with or without emesis, 2 indicated 5–9 retches with or without emesis, 3 indicated 10–15 retches with or without emesis, and 4 indicated intractable vomiting.

3.   Sedation was measured by nurse observation using a tool that consisted of a 5-point Likert scale with the points labeled from 0 to 4. Zero was defined as wide awake, 1 was drowsy, 2 was dozing or sleeping less than 50% of the time, 3 was sleeping more than 50% of the time, and 4 was awake only when deliberately aroused.
    Source: Edwards et al 1991.

Purpose/Question/Hypotheses

The purpose of the study was to examine the perceived well-being of persons who are smokers, are nonsmokers, or are quitting smoking. Subjects' well-being

Box 6–2 (*continued*)

was examined controlling for the effects of daily hassles and selected demographic differences.

Operational Definitions

1. Well-being was measured by the subjects' general perception of health (single, self-reported item), the affective state (Bradburn Morale Scale), physical symptoms (Physical Symptom Survey), and psychological symptoms (Symptoms Checklist 10).

2. Daily hassles were measured with a modified version of the Hassles Scale. The 4-point Likert-type scale ranging from "none" to "a great deal" was modified to include a "not applicable" option for ratings of the 49 items that describe things that may annoy, bother, upset, or anger a person. The sum of the subjects' ratings was used, with both "none" and "not applicable" scored as 0.

3. Demographic characteristics were measured by a Subject Characteristics Questionnaire developed by the investigator.

    Source: Macnee 1991.

therefore called **confounding variables;** if they are not controlled in the study design or procedure, they may be called **uncontrolled variables. Extraneous variables** is yet another term that may be used to refer to these factors.

In the sample study reported in chapter 2, Kirchhoff (1982) concluded that the effect of nurses' level of awareness about coronary precautions on persuasion and on adoption, as determined by a statistical test called analysis of variance (see chapter 10), was not significant or meaningful. That is, reading or being aware of research that challenged the value of the coronary-care precautions did not affect how important the nurses thought the precautions were or how frequently they practiced them. The investigator decided to take a look at any possible confounding variables that might account for her study findings. In doing so, her statistical analysis allowed her to add the following information about potential confounding variables:

1. Larger medical centers in urban locations, with educational programs for nurses, had significant but weak relationships to lower ratings on the frequency and importance of the two questioned coronary-care precautions.

2. Federal and nonprofit institutions had lower importance and frequency ratings for the rectal temperature-measurement.

3. Nurses employed in units that used special procedures for measuring cardiac output (thermodilution technique) had lower ratings for restriction of ice water.

Including both head nurses and staff nurses and reporting these additional findings about practices on the unit that were not among the independent variable measurements on the list were part of this researcher's attempt to "control" for potentially confounding variables.

How researchers control for various extraneous variables is examined in greater detail in the next chapter, where we explore how studies are designed.

HYPOTHESES

A hypothesis is a statement of a predicted relationship between two or more variables. In the level 3 example in Box 6–1, the variables are teaching versus nonteaching and feelings of well-being. The hypothesis suggests that there is a relationship between teaching self-care techniques and patients' feelings of well-being. The hypothesis predicts that those receiving the teaching will have higher scores on a measure of feelings of well-being. Hypotheses are generally deduced by researchers from theories. By testing hypotheses, the researcher can judge the value of a theory.

Criteria for a Hypothesis

Polit and Hungler (1987) suggest that the following criteria are required if a statement is to be considered a hypothesis:

First, it must be testable. In order for a hypothesis to be testable, there must be a predicted relationship between variables. For example: "Nursing schools with flexible curricula will retain and graduate more students." Here, there is only one dependent variable (retention and graduation of students), making the hypothesis untestable because there is nothing to compare. If the hypothesis were rewritten as "Nursing schools with flexible curricula will retain and graduate more students than nursing schools without flexible curricula," the hypothesis is testable. You can measure the retention and graduation rates of schools with both curricula—flexible and inflexible (the other variable)—and compare them.

A hypothesis can be tested only if the variables can be observed or measured. An **operational definition** specifies what the researcher does to make the variable observable or measurable. For example, you may wonder what a "flexible curriculum" is. A flexible curriculum can be operationally defined as a curriculum that allows the students to (1) take a test to demonstrate knowledge of lower-level courses, (2) challenge upper-level courses, and (3) meet at a variety of times and places for classes. An inflexible curriculum refers to programs without these three criteria. Because of this clear definition, the variables *flexible curriculum* and *inflexible curriculum* can be measured. Many studies are criticized primarily on the approach the researcher has used to operationalize concepts that are being studied. It is the researcher's job to try to make his or her operational definitions plausible in the eyes of critical readers.

Second, a hypothesis must be justifiable. This means that the researcher has derived the hypothesis from existing theory. For example, if you read that

Table 6–2 *Example Hypotheses and Their Parts*

Hypothesis	Experimental Group	Expected Result	Comparison Group
Prevalence of substance abuse is higher among registered nurses than among nonnurses (Trinkoff et al 1991).	nurses	will have greater incidence of substance abuse	nonnurses
Dysmenorrheic women will report higher levels of all gastrointestinal symptoms at menses than nondysmenorrheic women (Heitkemper et al 1991).	dysmenorrheic women	greater incidence of GI symptoms	nondysmenorrheic women
Children age six or younger who develop acute lymphocytic leukemia will have a greater degree of aberrant palmar creases than their relatives (Edelstein et al 1991).	children age six or younger who develop ALL	greater degree of aberrant palmar creases	healthy relatives

behavior modification is more effective in encouraging weight loss in obese people than lectures on nutrition and dieting, you can write a hypothesis to that effect. For example: "Obese people who participate in behavior modification training lose more weight than obese people who attend lectures on nutrition and dieting." This hypothesis is clearly derived from a behavioristic theoretical framework. However, suppose you have an idea that meditation might help people lose weight, and you write a hypothesis that proposes to look at the relationship between meditation and weight loss in two groups (one with meditation classes and one without). This hypothesis does not strictly meet the criteria of being justifiable, because it was not deduced from a theoretical framework. Rather, the idea was merely a whimsical thought or personal hunch.

Components of a Hypothesis

Hypotheses must be written clearly and concisely. Each word should add meaning to the hypothesis and have a purpose. Brink and Wood (1988) identify the three components that are essential to a well-written hypothesis: (1) the experimental group, (2) the expected result, and (3) the comparison group. Table 6–2 shows the different parts of hypotheses in studies published in *Nursing Research*.

Types of Hypotheses

Hypotheses can be

- simple
- complex
- directional
- nondirectional

- research

- statistical

A **simple hypothesis** predicts the relationship between one independent variable (IV) and one dependent variable (DV), whereas a **complex hypothesis** predicts the relationship between two (or more) independent variables and two (or more) dependent variables. Note the examples in Table 6–3.

As the words imply, a simple hypothesis is easier to test, measure, and analyze than a complex hypothesis. Because nursing research deals with human beings, who are complex, however, a lot of nursing research uses complex hypotheses. The most important considerations for the researcher to think about are (1) What type of hypothesis is best for the study? and (2) Is the study feasible? That is, if a complex hypothesis would be appropriate for the study but data cannot be collected to test it, a simple hypothesis is more appropriate.

A **directional hypothesis** specifies the direction of the relationship between variables, whereas a **nondirectional hypothesis** only predicts that there is a relationship. Note the difference:

- *Directional hypothesis:* Pregnant women who have higher levels of information about breast-feeding have more successful breast-feeding experiences.

- *Nondirectional hypothesis:* There is a relationship between information level about breast-feeding in pregnant women and their success with the breast-feeding experience.

In the example of the directional hypothesis, the word *more* is the key feature that indicates a direction. Other words and phrases that indicate the direction of a hypothesis include *less, greater, negative* or *positive relationship, higher,* or *lower.* In the example of the nondirectional hypothesis, the neutral phrase *There is a relationship* reveals that the researcher does not want to posit the direction of the relationship and simply wishes to describe whatever relationship is discovered through the research study. *There is a difference* also indicates nondirection.

A **research hypothesis** states the anticipated relationship between variables; all the examples to this point have been research hypotheses. A **null,** or **statistical, hypothesis** is a hypothesis written in the form that predicts *no relationship* between the independent and dependent variables: "There is no relationship between modes of intervention and weight loss in obese people" is an example of a null hypothesis. Principles used in statistical inference require that all research hypotheses be tested in the null form. The probability used to do statistical tests works under the assumption that there are no differences between variables, thus the use of the null (see chapter 10). For clarity in research studies, however, hypotheses should be stated in the research form, which clearly indicates the thinking of the investigator. Note the difference between a null hypothesis and a research hypothesis in the following example.

Table 6–3 *Example Hypotheses and Their Independent and Dependent Variables*

Simple Hypothesis	*Independent Variable*	*Dependent Variable*
The prevalence of cigarette smoking in Hispanic women of childbearing age will be higher than the national average for women (Pletsch 1991).	cultural group	prevalence of cigarette smoking

Complex Hypotheses	*Independent Variables*	*Dependent Variables*
Mothers of children hospitalized with acute physical conditions who know what events to expect and have some control over those events will experience less anxiety and expend less effort coping with the stressful event than mothers who do not know what to expect or do not have control (Schepp 1991).	predictability of events, control	anxiety, coping
Maternal confidence, maternal health, mother-in-law disapproval, baby behavior, solid foods, and formula will accurately predict adequate/inadequate supply of breast milk as reported by the mother (Hill & Aldag 1991).	maternal confidence, maternal health, mother-in-law disapproval, baby behavior, solid foods, formula	reported supply of breast milk
A suction catheter inserted into the endotracheal tube versus a suction catheter inserted with the application of negative pressure on PaO_2 causes changes in heart rate prior to and following vagal blockade (Gunderson et al 1991).	catheter insertion alone, catheter insertion with the application of negative pressure on PaO_2	heart rate prior to and following vagal blockade
Maternal confidence is positively related to maternal behaviors and skills and to infant temperament (Zahr 1991).	maternal confidence	maternal behaviors and skills, infant temperament
Perceived work environment, demographic variables, and work-related variables will predict burnout among nurses (Robinson et al 1991).	perceived work environment, demographic variables, work-related variables	burnout

- *Research hypothesis:* Chronically ill patients who are taught self-care have more feelings of well-being than those who are not taught self-care.

- *Null or statistical hypothesis:* There is no difference in the amount of well-being felt by chronically ill patients who are taught self-care and those who are not taught self-care.

Thus far we have discussed various kinds of relationships that hypotheses posit between variables. Some posit a specific relationship (directional) while others posit a more general one (nondirectional). If you review each of the hypotheses used as examples in this section, however, you will not find one that explicitly states the relationship to be *causal*. The concept of causation will be taken up in more detail in the next chapter, when we discuss experimental designs, but it is important to point out here that to show a causal relationship requires a great deal of rigor in the methodology of a research study. It may be very tempting for the novice reader of research to interpret an association between two variables—especially a *strong* association—as being causal, but the temptation should be resisted unless the study explicitly includes a causal effect as part of the hypothesis and unless the study is shown to have successfully demonstrated the relationship.

In any case, a hypothesis is almost never "proven" definitively. The findings of a successful research study may support a hypothesis; successful replications of the study would lend further support. Over time a strong case can accumulate in favor of the validity of the hypothesis. However, the attitude of skepticism that is intrinsic to all scientific inquiry does not usually permit the conclusion that a hypothesis has been proven beyond question.

ANNOTATED RESEARCH EXAMPLE

Citation

Wright SM. Validity of the human energy field assessment form. *West J Nurs Res.* 1991;13:635–647.

Study Problem/Purpose

Assessment is an integral part of the Therapeutic Touch process, and clinicians gather much information through that process. The *purpose of this study* was to establish construct validity of the human energy field assessment form, which was developed to record basic findings of the energy field assessment. The following hypotheses were generated:

1. There will be an association between the *location of energy field disturbance as assessed by the investigator* and the *location of pain as assessed by the patient*.

2. There will be an association between the overall strength of the energy field disturbance and fatigue and/or vigor and/or depression.

3. There will be an association between the intensity of the energy field disturbance and the intensity of the pain.

Operational Definitions

Human energy field assessment is a subjective recording of sensations felt by a trained observer approximately two to four inches from the skin's surface.

Location of energy field disturbance is reported by the observer as assessed by the body diagram that delineated 21 separate body areas on the energy field assessment form. Pain location is the patient's reported location of pain, as assessed by the body diagram on the Brief Pain Inventory. Overall strength of the energy field is the observer's reported strength of the overall field, as assessed by a 100-mm visual analogue scale on the energy field assessment form.

Fatigue is a mood marked by weariness, inertia, listlessness, and/or low energy level, as assessed by Factor F on the Profile of Mood States.

Vigor is a mood marked by feelings of high energy and vitality, as assessed by Factor V on the Profile of Mood States.

Depression is a mood marked by feelings of personal worthlessness, hopelessness, sadness, guilt, discouragement, unhappiness, and/or loneliness, as assessed by Factor D on the Profile of Mood States.

Intensity of the energy field disturbance is the observer's reported intensity of the field disturbance, as assessed by a 100-mm visual analogue scale on the energy field assessment form.

Pain intensity is the patient's present, worst, least, and average pain, as assessed by the 100-mm visual analogue scales on the Brief Pain Inventory.

Method

A convenience sample of 52 outpatients with chronic nonmalignant pain was used in the study. The patients had experienced pain for two months or longer, had consented to participate in the study, and had a diagnosis of musculoskeletal pain, fibrositis/fibromyalgia, or osteoarthritis only. *Data related to pain, its effects, and mood* were collected through a self-administered study questionnaire that contained the Brief Pain Inventory and the Profile of Mood States. *The findings of the energy field assessment* were systematically collected and recorded on the energy field assessment form.

All data were collected from two sites: a suburban chiropractic practice and an urban rheumatology practice.

Findings

The sample was 65% female and 88% Caucasian. About half of the sample were married, and more than half had children. The average length of time in pain was 83.4 months (range: 2 to 480 months). The sample consisted primarily of people with back and neck pain. Hypothesis 1 was partially confirmed where body areas showed 75% to 100% agreement between the location of the disturbance and the location of the pain. Hypothesis 2 was partially confirmed. Scatter plots of all pairs indicated no nonlinear relationships. The relationships for fatigue and vigor were confirmed, but the relationship to depression was not. Hypothesis 3 was not confirmed. There was no significant relationship between the intensity of the field disturbance and any of the four measures of pain intensity.

Implications

The relationship of the overall strength of the energy field was confirmed with respect to fatigue and vigor; both occurred in the theoretically expecte directions: more fatigue, less strength. Future study may include more than one measure of these constructs, because fatigue is a significant clinical problem in chronic pain. A primary consideration in future studies should be to increase the sample size. A group of people with chronic pain and documented clinical depression could be studied to make a determination on the relationship between the overall strength of the energy field and depression. Future development of the energy field assessment form will see the deletion of the field intensity construct as well as some changes in format. Approximately 10,000 nurses in the United States have learned Therapeutic Touch, but the percentage who use it in their daily practice is unknown. Indeed, no systematic record of the Therapeutic Touch assessment was maintained prior to this study. The addition of a valid and reliable form on which these findings can be recorded may help to add valuable information to the Therapeutic Touch data base.

Guidelines for Critique

Does the study include a statement of purpose? If so, at what level of inquiry is it written?

Are all variables given clear operational definitions?

Are variables concrete or abstract? Has special care been taken to operationalize abstract variables?

What confounding variables have been taken into account?

Are hypotheses testable, justifiable, and related to the study purpose?

Are hypotheses written clearly and concisely? Do they contain the three essential components of a good hypothesis?

Are the hypotheses simple or complex? Directional or nondirectional? Researchable or statistical?

Summary of Key Ideas and Terms

The statement of the research purpose derives from the level of inquiry. The purpose of a level 1 question is written as "The purpose of this research is to explore and describe . . ." The purpose of a level 2 question is written as "The purpose of this study is to answer the question . . ." The purpose of a level 3 study is written as "The purpose of this study is to test the hypothesis . . ."

Independent variables (IVs) are the causes, conditions, and inputs that are established or manipulated before measuring the dependent variable(s).

Dependent variables (DVs) are measures of outcome and consequences that depend on exposure to the independent variable.

After identification of the variables, operational definitions are written that specify how the variables will be measured.

Confounding, extraneous, or uncontrolled variables are all those variables that might also affect the dependent variable and confuse your interpretation of the effects of a study's independent variable(s).

Hypotheses are statements of relationship that the investigator expects to find between a study's independent and dependent variables.

For a hypothesis to be testable, the variables must be able to be observed and measured. The dependent variable must be observed under at least two different conditions; variables, to be measured, require operational definitions.

A hypothesis requires three components (Brink & Wood 1988): an experimental group, the expected result, and a comparison group.

Hypotheses can be simple or complex, directional or nondirectional, and stated as research or statistical hypotheses.

References

Brink J & Wood MJ. *Basic Steps in Planning Research.* 3d ed. Boston: Jones and Bartlett;1988.

Edelstein J et al. Dermatoglyphics and acute lymphocytic leukemia in children. *J Ped Oncology Nurs.* 1991;8:30–38.

Edwards JN et al. Comparison of patient-controlled and nurse-controlled antiemetic therapy in patients receiving chemotherapy. *Res in Nurs & Health.* 1991; 14:149–157.

Gunderson LP et al. Endotracheal suctioning-induced heart rate alterations. *Nurs Res.* 1991;40:139–143.

Heitkemper M et al. GI symptoms, function, and psychophysiological arousal in dysmenorrheic women. *Nurs Res.* 1991;40:20–26.

Hill PD & Aldag J. Potential indicators of insufficient milk supply syndrome. *Res in Nurs & Health.* 1991;14:11–19.

Kirchhoff KT. A diffusion survey of coronary precautions. *Nurs Res.* July/August 1982;31:196–201.

Morse JM & McHutchion E. Releasing restraints: Providing safe care for the elderly. *Res in Nurs & Health.* 1991;14:187–196.

Pletsch PK. Prevalence of cigarette smoking in Hispanic women of childbearing age. *Nurs Res.* 1991;40:103–106.

Polit DF & Hungler BP. *Nursing Research.* 3d ed. Philadelphia: Lippincott;1987.

Robinson SE et al. Nurse burnout: Work related and demographic factors as culprits. *Res in Nurs & Health.* 1991;14:223–228.

Schepp KG. Factors influencing the coping effort of mothers of hospitalized children. *Nurs Res.* 1991;40:42–46.

Trinkoff AM et al. The prevalence of substance abuse among registered nurses. *Nurs Res.* 1991;40:172–175.

Zahr LK. The relationship between maternal confidence and mother-infant behaviors in premature infants. *Res in Nurs & Health.* 1991;14:279–286.

RESEARCH DESIGNS

HOLLY SKODOL WILSON

CHAPTER OUTLINE

In This Chapter . . .

- Matching Research Design and Research Purpose
- Historical Study Designs
    - External Criticism
    - Internal Criticism
    - Steps in a Historical Research Design
    - Advantages and Disadvantages of Historical Research
- Case Study Designs
    - Steps in a Case Study Design
    - Advantages and Disadvantages of the Case Study
- Naturalistic/Interpretive Study Designs
- Survey Research Designs
    - Steps in Survey Research
    - Advantages and Disadvantages of Surveys
- Experimental Study Designs
    - Strengths of Experimental Designs
    - Internal and External Validity in an Experiment
    - Types of Experimental Design
    - Steps in Experimental Designs
    - Advantages and Disadvantages of Experimental Designs
- Quasi-Experimental Designs
    - The Nonequivalent Pretest-Posttest Control Group Design
    - The Time Series Design
    - Advantages and Disadvantages of Quasi-Experimental Desig
- Ex Post Facto Study Designs
- Methodological Studies
- How Designs Fit Study Problems

CHAPTER OBJECTIVES

After reading this chapter, you should be able to:

- Evaluate the match between a study's design and its overall purpose

- Specify the major steps in each type of study design

- Compare the advantages and disadvantages of each major type of study design

- Recognize correctly the type of study design used in reports of nursing research

- Explain the hallmarks of true experimental study designs

- Discuss the concepts of reliability and validity in relation to experimental study designs

- Formulate design remedies to counter potential threats to the internal and external validity of experimental designs

- Describe the major types of experimental design

- Compare and contrast quasi-experimental designs with experimental designs

- Account for the major disadvantages of ex post facto study designs

- Discuss the purpose of methodological research

7

IN THIS CHAPTER . . .

Suppose you are responsible for providing nursing care to a 50-year-old woman during her postoperative recovery from gallbladder surgery. What do you do first? What do you avoid? How much of anything is going to be enough to prevent postoperative complications? What strategies will work? To help you answer these questions and accomplish the clinical goals set for this patient, you need to devise a *workable plan*. The plan is customarily called a nursing care plan. It offers you and the other clinicians working with this patient a blueprint, or organized design, for achieving certain specified objectives, such as the prevention of wound infection, pneumonia, thrombosis, and other complications that can follow such surgical procedures. The plan would take on quite different configurations if it were intended to accomplish an alternate purpose, such as decreasing a patient's anxiety or teaching someone about a diabetic diet.

Designs accomplish much the same thing for scientific research. Research designs suggest what observations or measurements to make, how to make them, and what to make *of* them. In effect, **research designs** *imply a set of instructions that tell an investigator how data should be collected and analyzed in order to answer a specified research problem*. There are almost as many designs as there are possible approaches for attempting to establish that something is or is not true. But as is the case with nursing care plans, certain designs are better suited to certain levels of inquiry, research purposes, and types of problem than are others. Thus, you as a reader must be prepared to evaluate critically not only the type of design that was used but also the wisdom of selecting it.

What follows in this chapter is an overview of the range and diversity of study designs. We will compare and contrast nonexperimental, true experimental, and quasi-experimental designs and examine examples of nursing studies that have used various approaches. We will also take a look at the advantages and disadvantages of each type of design within the framework of the key concepts of *validity* and *reliability*.

MATCHING RESEARCH DESIGN AND RESEARCH PURPOSE

Every study has its own specific substantive purpose. You might find, for instance, that a study is designed to determine whether structured preoperative teaching will significantly increase a postsurgical patient's ability to cough and deep breathe. Or a study might be designed to identify the mental health care needs of the deinstitutionalized elderly or to describe the influence of religion on nursing in Western civilization. Most investigators think of research purposes as falling into several main groups, or categories (see chapter 1). Diers (1979) uses the following categories of research studies in nursing:

1. *Factor-naming, or factor-searching, studies.* These studies describe, name, or characterize a phenomenon, situation, or event in order to gain familiarity with it or achieve new insights.

2. *Factor-relating, or relation-searching, studies.* These studies are done to develop links among variables and describe the relationships that are found. These studies go on at the second level of inquiry after a phenomenon has been explored, named, and described.

3. *Association-testing studies.* Also called explanatory or correlational studies, these studies seek to determine what factors occur or vary together without either changing the natural situation (manipulating it) or attempting to reach conclusions about whether one causes another.

4. *Causal hypothesis-testing studies.* These studies test a causal relationship between variables and are also called true experiments.

In the first two types of studies the major emphasis is on discovery, and the research design must be flexible enough to permit the investigator to use any strategy that might be helpful in obtaining rich and broad-ranging data on a phenomenon. In studies that are aimed at the third and fourth purposes, the prime issues are of control and accuracy. Thus, the design must minimize bias, control variance, and enhance the reliability and validity of the evidence obtained.

When reading a report or proposal for a study, you may not always find its purposes as clear-cut as this discussion might lead you to expect. In actual practice, a study may have some overlap of purpose. But the distinctions made by sorting studies into four types by purpose are helpful as we turn our attention to understanding the various types of study design.

HISTORICAL STUDY DESIGNS

Most scholars agree that history is an activity engaged in for the purpose of learning the truth about the past. History is also a discipline of study that has established methods for collecting and evaluating evidence about the past. In fact, the clearest characteristic of the historical research method is that its data already exist. The purpose of **historical research** is to explain the present or to anticipate the future based on a systematic collection and critical evaluation of data pertaining to past occurrences. Historical study designs call for a prescribed approach to examining and interpreting data contained in historical sources such as diaries, letters, documents, and journals. Hockett (1955) emphasized the importance of efforts to establish the validity and reliability of historical research when he wrote:

> The aim of historical research is to ascertain facts, as they must be made
> the basis of all conclusions. . . . Statements are the raw materials with which
> the historian works and the first lesson he must learn is that they must not be

mistaken for facts. They may be facts but that cannot be taken for granted. . . . In view of the possibilities for error, it becomes the duty of the historian to doubt every statement until it has been critically tested [p.14].

Christy (1975) echoed this warning by reminding us that "the danger lies in the fact that we tend to believe anything in print, especially if it is found in an old document." Use of a historical design, therefore, requires that the researcher employ two separate processes to establish the validity and reliability of the data before using them to reach a conclusion: external criticism and internal criticism. These processes are hallmarks of sound historical research.

External Criticism

External criticism refers to examination of the historical data sources (maps, letters, books, documents, inscriptions, artifacts, and the like) for their validity, genuineness, or authenticity. Documents cannot be taken to reflect the truth unless they are really what they appear to be rather than forgeries or frauds. Techniques that historical researchers use to establish the authenticity of their data sources include consideration of the age of the paper, the kind of ink used, the appearance of watermarks, the match with other samples of handwriting, the congruity with other evidence of the author's or originator's ideas, or the use of a variety of laboratory procedures that determine characteristics (age, composition, and so on) of materials. In the case of book or article manuscripts, the historian must determine who the true author was. Questions that help establish authorship include:

- Is the manuscript an original or a copy?

- Is it dated?

- Could it have been written by anyone else?

- Might it be a forgery?

Other problems with which a historian must deal in the process of evaluating data for their validity include the possibility that a previous historian misidentified a document, the chance of errors due to translations or even transcriptions from other languages, and the likelihood that documents have been altered or changed. Canons of historical research require that the historian get to original, primary sources in order to minimize the chance of distortion and error.

Internal Criticism

Once the validity of data sources is established, the historical researcher turns his or her attention to determining the accuracy of the statements contained within the documents or historical material. The process involved in making such a determination is called **internal criticism.** It requires the following steps:

- The researcher must be certain that he or she understands the information contained in the documents. As with all other designs discussed in this chapter, being aware of one's own biases and expectations is a basic requirement to avoid interpreting statements so that they provide false support for one's own hypotheses or pet notions.

- The investigator must be knowledgeable about the meaning of terms and statements in their historical and cultural context. Consultation with translators and linguists can sometimes help in this area. Words take on different meanings in different cultures, eras, and social settings. *Goodynurse,* for example, at the time of the Salem witch trials referred *not* to a nurse but to a married, middle-class woman in the Puritan community.

- The researcher must subject the statements to a phase of negative criticism in which efforts are made to corroborate the truth reflected in them. Most authorities believe that the further an author moves from reporting an eyewitness account, the less reliable are the statements. Establishing the reliability of a rendition of what occurred usually requires two independent primary sources that corroborate each other. Comparing accounts of the same events and finding agreement increases confidence in the data. Evidence is considered "probable" when the researcher has information from one primary source that passes the tests of authenticity and finds no substantial evidence to the contrary. If neither of these routes to confidence in the truth of the data is available, the historian is dealing from the substantially weaker position of "possibility." Historical research requires the ability to find evidence, group it, evaluate it, interpret it, and communicate it in relation to important questions, themes, or hypotheses.

Steps in a Historical Research Design

The historical researcher begins a study with a clearly stated researchable problem that has resulted from narrowing down a broader, more general area of interest. Christy (1969), a nurse historian, studied "the impact of the leadership of the Nursing Department at Teachers' College, Columbia University, on changes and major events in American nursing during the first half of the twentieth century." Data in historical research such as Christy's study consist of evidence about events, people, situations, and so on that were created in the past. Instead of manipulating variables or designing data-collection tools, the historian must rely on documents from the past. Such documents are considered either **primary sources** (firsthand information) or **secondary sources** (second- or thirdhand accounts). Examples of primary sources include letters, eyewitness accounts, diaries, photographs, and legal or public documents. These are materials that existed at the time of the event. Secondary sources might be newspaper articles, reference books, and hearsay. These are the end products of studying primary data. Once the problems of data availability, data gaps, and evaluation of data validity and reliability are surmounted, the final step in a historical research design is synthesis, analysis, and articulation of the findings. This last step involves the historian in building into a related whole the facts that have been verified. Determining the meaning of facts, discovering relationships among them, and presenting them in a way that is interesting to the reader are among the challenges. Obviously, documentation in the form of footnotes and references is critical to verifying sources used by a historian to reach his or her conclusions. The steps implicit in the process of historical research described above are:

1. Formulate a researchable problem that is best approached with a historical research design.

2. Specify the data needed to address the researchable question.

3. Determine that sufficient data are available.

4. Collect known data, new data, and previously unknown data sources (primary and secondary).

5. Evaluate data sources through external and internal criticism.

6. Initiate the descriptive synthesis of findings in a written report while continuing to collect data.

7. Draw interpretive conclusions with respect to the original research question.

Advantages and Disadvantages of Historical Research

The value of historical research to nursing has only recently been recognized. The orientation to the past of historical research has as its major advantage the potential for illuminating a current question through the intensive study of carefully selected material that already exists.

Disadvantages of the historical research design include the following:

- The investigator must rely on finding data that already exist and cannot develop new data.

- The investigator cannot alter the form in which data appear but must attempt to understand them in the form in which they are found.

- The investigator must analyze and interpret the meaning of data without the advantage of being able to ask clarifying questions.

- The data may be incomplete and have gaps in crucial areas.

- The investigator must be able to translate concepts, terms, and ideas in light of their historical period and context.

- The investigator must overcome obstacles of time, resources, freedom of movement, and language to search for and evaluate data resources.

- The investigator cannot predict an accurate timetable for completion of a historical study. Not only must data be located and evaluated, but insights that tie together these masses of data must ultimately be reached.

A historical study is noted in the example following. Such studies can serve to interpret the past and supply perspective to contemporary problems and issues by suggesting parallels, differences, and trends. For example, the emergence of specific nursing leaders, the establishment of nursing education in hospitals or institutions of higher learning, and the proliferation of nursing functions are all studied against a background of social needs, economic constraints, and the political climates of given periods.

CASE STUDY DESIGNS

A **case study** provides an in-depth analysis of a subject for investigation, such as an individual patient, a family, a hospital ward, a health care agency, a professional organization, or a group such as Recovery Incorporated or Alcoholics Anonymous. A case study is customarily done under natural conditions. It examines only a single subject or a small number of subjects with respect to a number of variables pertaining to history, current characteristics, and interactions. The case study design is useful in accomplishing the following purposes:

- gaining insight into little-known problems
- providing background data for the planning of broader studies
- developing explanations of social-psychological and social-structural processes
- offering rich descriptive anecdotes or examples to illustrate generalized statistical findings

---

Example: Historical Design in Nursing Research

In a study entitled "Factors influencing high rate of 'born-before-arrival' babies in Nigeria," Reuben Fajemilehin (1991) wanted to identify factors that might explain the rate of nonhospital births and identify postdelivery problems that motivated the seeking of medical care. Medical records from the maternity center at one of two main hospitals in the city were analyzed. Of 12,373 deliveries, recorded from 1982 to 1985, an analysis was done of the 377 cases born-before-arrival at the unit. The two most common reasons for not delivering in the hospital were inability to pay and inadequate transportation. The two most common reasons for seeking medical care immediately after delivery were bleeding with the retainment of the whole placenta and bleeding with a noncontracting uterus. The author suggested the implications for the study in terms of primary health care needs of the population.

Steps in a Case Study Design

Case studies, by definition, are both more flexible and more vulnerable to bias than many other designs, in that the investigator must make judgments about sources, amounts, and credibility of data without many rules or guidelines. In general, however, the steps involved in a sound case study design are as follows:

1. Determine the purpose of conducting a case study.

2. Identify the unit of analysis (individual, family, group, aggregate, organization, community).

3. Determine how data sources will be selected.

4. Specify the data-collection plan and methods.

5. Collect, analyze, and interpret data.

6. Write a report of findings.

7. Suggest directions for further research on the basis of these findings.

Example: Case Study Design in Nursing Research

Mildred Roberson (1992) desired to study the concept of compliance from the viewpoint of a group of African-American adults in South Carolina. She interviewed those who lived with a chronic physical illness. The subjects were asked to express their understanding of the meaning of chronic illness and the treatment and their self-care activities. The information gained is imbedded in the life realities of a people in a particular place. The author suggests that reports of self-care by these black subjects are similar to reports obtained through previous studies of white populations and that health care providers need to consider the clients' views of compliance and efforts to live well with their chronic disease.

Advantages and Disadvantages of the Case Study

Researchers who are working in a relatively unstudied area of investigation where there are few prior studies on which to base design decisions have often acknowledged the value of intensely studying selected case examples in order to stimulate insight and suggest hypotheses or even directions for future research. Much that is known in anthropology and medicine has depended for its start on the case study method. Psychoanalytic theory is based for the most part on Sigmund Freud's carefully documented case studies of psychiatric patients. Case studies can often provide information that is rich and otherwise difficult to come by. They are also well suited for studying a process over time.

Descriptive single-subject research has indeed made valuable contributions to knowledge in psychopharmacology, psychotherapy, and medicine. Behavior modification studies are cited by Holm (1983) in the areas of weight control and childhood eating disorders as bringing research and practice closer together. Other descriptive case studies report how particular patients respond to specific situations or nursing approaches. See the accompanying example.

The major disadvantages of the case study design are still its problems with generalizability. It is difficult to argue with certainty that what is learned from a single case is representative of patterns or trends in the entire population. Furthermore, the methods for compiling case study data are not as rigorously prescribed as those for data collection under other study designs, resulting in what to critics may appear to be outright ambiguity. Considered from the other side of the coin, however, this very ambiguity may provide the flexibility necessary to bring inventive approaches to gathering a rich array of data and arriving at insightful interpretations of them.

The other disadvantages of a case study design are those associated with its flexibility and lack of rigor and control. To elaborate:

- Investigators have no guidelines to help them decide whether they have collected enough data.

- Because most of the data collected in case studies are based on interviews and observations obtained by the investigator and the circumstance is often one of a relatively long-term and close association between the investigator and the subject or subjects, the possibility of researcher bias influencing the findings and conclusions is always present.

- The cost-effectiveness of case studies is open to criticism, because some authorities believe that the costs in terms of money and time are high relative to the value of the information obtained.

- A case study design is not adequate for testing causal hypotheses and is definitely unsuited for trying to establish scientific cause and effect.

NATURALISTIC / INTERPRETIVE STUDY DESIGNS

When nursing research emphasizes discovery, naturalistic and interpretive study designs are often selected. Such research includes ethnographic field studies rooted in anthropology, ethology studies rooted in observational science, content analysis, grounded theory, and phenomenology. Because these forms of "qualitative" methodology are growing in their applicability to nursing, chapter 11 has been devoted to them.

SURVEY RESEARCH DESIGNS

Survey research designs involve studying populations or universes based on the data gathered from a sample drawn from them. The data are often gathered using a questionnaire completed by the study subjects. Survey research generally serves the purpose of describing characteristics, opinions, attitudes, or behaviors as they currently exist in a population, although other purposes are possible. The word **survey** means that information is being collected from a variety of subjects who resemble the total population on the characteristic(s) of interest to the researcher. For example, a nurse working in the field of psychogerontology might conduct a national survey of factors that affect access to health care resources among elderly women with Alzheimer's disease. When a survey studies a sample of the total possible population, it is technically called a **sample survey.** If the entire population is studied—for example, all doctorally prepared nurses in the United States—the survey may be called a **census.**

Steps in Survey Research

Surveys may take a variety of forms, from face-to-face interviews to mailed questionnaires, and they may be designed to serve a variety of purposes, from determining a group's attitudes to evaluating the effectiveness of a program. In general, all survey designs require that these steps be addressed:

1. State the researchable question.
2. Ascertain that the researchable question can be addressed with a survey design.
3. Decide on the type of survey to be used.
4. Translate the objectives of the survey into categories of question or item.
5. Identify the population of respondents or settings.
6. Use sampling procedures to identify a representative sample.
7. Design data-collection procedures.
8. Plan for analysis of data.
9. Pilot test the data-collection and analysis approaches.
10. Modify as indicated.
11. Collect and analyze data.
12. Write descriptive, comparative, or evaluative findings and draw conclusions.

Advantages and Disadvantages of Surveys

The strength of the survey design lies in its ability to combine flexibility of content and purpose with elements of precision and control. It can be used to gather information from a large number of subjects with comparatively minimal expenditure of time and money. Its methodology can be explicitly stated, making it easier to evaluate and to replicate in comparison with alternative designs that are high in flexibility. It can take advantage of existing standardized scales and questionnaires and can be structured so that data analysis can be accomplished using a computer.

Results .

Limitations of survey designs include

1. the possibility of a low return rate due to the impersonal approach that often characterizes survey research

2. the possibility that preconceived questions are irrelevant or confusing to the respondents and therefore yield meaningless data

3. the necessity of developing a system for storing and keeping track of a vast amount of data

4. the tendency of data obtained to be relatively superficial

5. the fact that survey data do not allow an investigator to answer cause-and-effect questions about related variables

---

Example: Survey Design in Nursing Research

Seymour and Buscherhof (1991) surveyed 1,000 nurses, randomly drawn from the membership of the American Nurses Association, to identify the factors for differences in the achievement patterns of professional nurses. Subjects were asked to complete a 22-page questionnaire and were invited to write about factors that had influenced the course of their careers. The authors concluded, from both the frequency and the strength of the writers' accounts, that the counterproductive conditions under which nurses work and the poor remuneration they receive are those in most urgent need of comprehensive nationwide remedy. They further state that if these perceived problems are not addressed, the number who choose to leave nursing is likely to grow.

EXPERIMENTAL STUDY DESIGNS

The term *experiment* is sometimes used interchangeably in everyday conversation with *study* or *research project*. In the language of science, however, an experiment, or **experimentally designed study,** has a very specific meaning. It refers to a kind of study in which the researcher *manipulates*—and thus controls—one or more independent variables and observes the dependent variable or variables for the consequences, change, outcome, or effect. Furthermore, in a true experiment, the investigator has the *power to assign subjects to either an experimental or a control group* and ideally has the *power to use random sampling procedures to select them* in the first place. Summarizing, then, true experiments are characterized by the following features:

1. manipulation of at least one independent variable by the investigator

2. random selection of sample members

3. random assignment of sample members to experimental and control groups

In the opinion of many philosophers of science, the true experiment is the ideal study design, because it measures relationships among variables with the most precision, rigor, and control. The control accomplished with an experimental design is best understood in terms of the idea of *control over variance*. The experimental study design can

1. maximize systematically introduced experimental variance

2. control extraneous variance

3. minimize error variance

Let's look at each of these notions in a bit more detail, because they represent the assets of a true experimental design.

Strengths of Experimental Designs

Maximizing Experimental Variance   A typical experiment begins with a hypothesis about the existence of a relationship between an independent variable and a dependent variable. The hypothesis, for example, may be that holding a newborn at time of delivery (independent variable) will be related to postpartum bonding behaviors in first-time fathers during the first three days after a baby's birth (dependent variable) (Toney 1983). The investigator then randomly selects a sample of first-time fathers who meet specific inclusion criteria—for example, married, aged 20 to 32, father of a baby without deformities, delivery uncomplicated, and the like. At delivery, the fathers who meet the sample criteria are randomly assigned to two groups by the investigator. The fathers in the experimental group are offered their newborn infant to hold for 10 minutes during the first hour after delivery. The fathers in the control group don't hold their babies until 8 to 12 hours after delivery. The null hypothesis tested in the study is that there will be no significant difference in the frequencies of father-infant bonding behaviors between fathers who have early contact and those who do not.

An experimental study design is selected because it can most accurately determine how much variance in the dependent variable (father-infant bonding behavior) can presumably be due to manipulation of the independent variable (holding or not holding an infant at birth). In an experimental design, the variance in the dependent variable due to the independent variable is separated from the total variance in the dependent variable, which can be due to a lot of things, including chance. An experiment maximizes the experimental variance by operating according to a precept of *planning and conducting the research so that the experimental and control conditions are as different as possible*. In the case of our example study, holding the newborn for ten full minutes was contrasted to not holding the infant at all. Every effort was made to avoid introducing the ambiguity of holding for a few seconds or even touching for a moment.

Controlling Extraneous Variables   Controlling extraneous variables means nullifying, or eliminating, that variance in the dependent variable which might be due to something other than the influence of the independent variable. This goal is accomplished in an experimental design in five ways:

1. A researcher can eliminate extraneous variables altogether as variables in the study. For example, if the researcher studying bonding had suspected that years of college education might have an effect on the dependent variable of father-infant bonding, he or she might have selected sample members for both her experimental and control groups who had zero years of college. In short, to eliminate the variance that might be due to some extraneous factor, the investigator can select sample members who are homogeneous for that particular factor or variable.

2. The investigator can control the influence of extraneous variance through random selection of sample members and random assignment of subjects to the experimental and control groups. Proper randomization allows the investigator to assume that the experimental and control-group members are statistically equal on all possible extraneous variables.

3. The researcher can build an extraneous variable into the design of the experiment as yet another independent variable and collect data about its effect on the dependent variable (and its interaction with other independent variables).

4. The experimenter can match subjects in the control and experimental groups on the variable in question. Because matching can also have some disadvantages (including the possible loss of subjects from the study group), randomization and analysis of covariance (points 2 and 3) are sometimes considered better controls.

5. Finally, certain statistical methods can isolate and quantify the amount of extraneous variance (see chapter 10).

Minimizing Error Variance   Error variance can be associated with individual differences among subjects and what are commonly called measurement errors, such as those due to test fatigue, lapse of memory, fleeting feelings, and other unpredictable phenomena. The primary precept that experimental designs reflect to reduce error variance is that *to increase the reliability of measures is to reduce error variance.* This means that the less scores or values are allowed to fluctuate randomly on subsequent administrations of an instrument and the more repeatable and consistent they are, the more *reliable* and free of error variance they are.

The more reliable and accurate the measures are, the easier it is to identify systematic variance in the dependent variable; thus, systematically controlled testing circumstances and procedures are also a requisite in an experimental design. In our sample study, the researcher's trained observers observed both the experimental and control-group fathers for the same amount of time (ten minutes) while the fathers changed the infants' shirts and diapers. They assessed the father-infant bonding using an instrument for interaction assessment that had been tested in a number of prior studies.

Internal and External Validity in an Experiment

The ability of an experimental design to control variance contributes to what is called its **internal validity.** Internal validity refers to whether or not the manipulation of the independent variable really makes a significant difference on the dependent variable. The study we have used as an illustration found no statistically significant differences in bonding behaviors between fathers who had contact for ten minutes with their newborn infants in the first hour after delivery and those who did not. The author explained this finding by reflecting on the possibility that certain demographic and situational factors that were not controlled in her design may have detracted from the study's internal validity.

External validity refers to the representativeness or generalizability of a study's results. In our study, the author acknowledged that, without cross-cultural replication, her study findings were limited to predominantly middle-class Caucasian fathers who were married and had some college education. She acknowledged that cross-cultural sampling would be indicated to increase her study's external validity, because different subcultures have different beliefs and methods of expressing affection and attachment. The basic experimental study is designed with control and experimental groups and pre- and posttests (often called a 2×2 design), and its variables are structured as they are to increase the experiment's internal and external validity.

Campbell and Stanley (1963), in their classic resource on experimental and quasi-experimental designs, list seven classes of extraneous variables that can represent threats to an experiment's internal validity. Table 7–1 presents these. Not only are the seven threats to internal validity the ones that occur in the conduct of an experimental design, but most authorities agree with Waltz and Bausell (1981) that they occur as the most common extraneous variables.

Many of the strategies in true experimental designs are intended to control or prevent their influence or the influence of yet another set of factors that act as threats to *external* validity. Most researchers deal with the threats to internal validity first because altering features of experimental designs makes them easier to control than are many of the threats to external validity. The primary threats to external validity derive from (1) population validity problems, (2) ecological validity problems, and (3) pretest sensitization.

Population Validity   The concept of **population validity** is that the researcher can reasonably generalize from his or her actual sample to all possible sample members and likewise to the total population of interest to the investigator. If, for example, a nurse researcher were to conduct an experimental study to determine the effects of touch as a means of communication with profoundly retarded children, he or she would want to be sure that

- the responses obtained from sample members would be representative of potential responses from the target population

- results for subsets in the sample (for example, different sexes or age groups) would occur similarly in the population

Two strategies designed to minimize problems with population validity are to (1) define the accessible population as broadly as possible and then randomly sample as many subjects as is feasible, and (2) use sampling procedures to increase the likelihood that the sample has the same constituencies (or characteristics) as the target population. If a researcher designs an experiment without employing these two sampling strategies and instead simply grabs subjects in a single setting as they become available, the sample will likely be

---

Table 7–1   *Extraneous Variables That Can Threaten Internal Validity*

Classes of Extraneous Variables	*Remedy and Rationale*
History, defined as the influence of events that occur during the course of the experiment that might affect the dependent variable	Randomly assign subjects to experimental and control groups, because both groups could be assumed to have had exposure to the events that occur.
Maturation, referring to processes that go on within the respondents themselves as a function of the passage of time	Complete the experiment in as short a time as possible to minimize developmental changes. Randomly assign to control groups for the same reason as for #1.
Testing, defined as the effect of having taken the test previously on retest scores	Don't test the same subjects. Build in a second control group that is tested the same number of times as the experimental group so as to be able to account for amount of change due to subjects becoming test-wise.
Instrumentation, referring to lack of reliability or consistency in the way scores are assigned to a dependent variable	Keep scorers "blind" to which subjects are experimental-group and which are control-group members. Use standardized procedures and protocols for rating or scoring, to avoid biases. Give scorers as much practice as possible before they work with actual research data.
Statistical regression, meaning the tendency for subjects who score at extremes of a distribution to have less extreme scores when they are retested	This is only a factor when subjects are chosen for a study *because* of their extreme scores. It can be taken care of through random assignment to control and experimental groups.
Selection, referring to a tendency for certain types of subject to be alike if they are not randomly assigned to experimental and control groups	Avoid volunteers, and randomly assign to treatment groups to try to make groups as much alike as possible.
Differential loss of subjects from treatment groups during the course of an experiment	Little can be done about this factor except to document it as a potential limitation of the study when it occurs and try to prevent it by making every ethical effort to enable willing subjects to continue participating in the study.

Source: Campbell and Stanley 1963. Adapted with permission from Houghton Mifflin Company and American Educational Research Association.

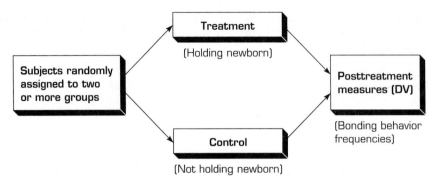

Figure 7–1   *An after-only study design.*

systematically biased or different from the population to whom he or she hopes to generalize the findings, and the study's external validity will be compromised.

Ecological Validity   A study is ecologically valid if the experimental environment in which it is conducted is explicit, clear, and consistent enough to be replicated by another investigator. Replication is said to be the final arbiter of all external validity questions (Waltz & Bausell 1981). In the study of touch with profoundly retarded children, the investigator would need to spell out in detail the nature of the touching (IV) and the indicators of responsiveness (DV), so that another researcher could replicate the study with different subjects or under different circumstances. Furthermore, the researcher would need to counteract effects that might be due just to the subjects' knowing about participating in a study. This phenomenon is referred to as the **Hawthorne effect** because it was first observed in the Hawthorne plant of the Western Electric Company, where it was discovered that productivity or job satisfaction could change temporarily whenever management made a change of any kind. The Hawthorne effect can occur in all kinds of study situations when data reflect the effects of the study itself. To control it, researchers can keep caregivers blind as to the exact indicators being recorded (without, of course, violating ethical research conduct).

Pretest Sensitization   The final threat to external validity occurs when subjects are pretested (for example, on an attitude scale) and become sensitized to the experimental intervention to follow. For example, nurse practitioners being studied for their attitudes toward caring for homosexuals before and after a series of workshops designed to clear up misconceptions and decrease prejudice might be tipped off about the researcher's interests or even the desired responses by the test taken before the workshops.

   The design strategy used to counter this tendency is to include a second control group that does not receive the workshops but receives only the posttest. Comparing this second control group's posttest scores with the posttest scores of the first control group—who were both pre- and posttested (but who did not attend the workshops)—should allow the researcher to estimate how much change in the dependent variable (attitudes) could be attributed to the pretesting itself.

Types of Experimental Design

All true experimental designs contain four strategies in one configuration or another. These typical experimental design strategies are

1. manipulation of the independent variable (IV)
2. an experimental group that is exposed to the IV and at least one control group that is not exposed to the IV
3. random selection of sample members and random assignment of them to control or experimental groups
4. measurement of the effects of an IV (or IVs) on the dependent variable

The logic of experimental designs is to structure the situation so that you have a sound basis for determining how much of the effect on a dependent variable is related to the independent variable and how much is due to chance.

The **after-only,** or **posttest-only, design** is the simplest experimental design. In it, the investigator assigns subjects to an experimental group or a control group but collects data only at the end of the treatment or exposure to the independent variable. The soundness of the design relies on the two groups being comparable. The design's weakness is that one must assume this comparability at the beginning of the study without testing for it. From what we've seen earlier in this chapter, random sampling and random assignment to the two groups help the investigator to have confidence in this assumption.

An example of an after-only experimental design appeared in Toney's 1983 study of the effects of holding the newborn on paternal bonding. She randomly assigned 37 married, first-time fathers attending uncomplicated deliveries of normal infants to experimental and control groups (those who held and did not hold their infants at delivery). From 12 to 36 hours after the babies were born, bonding behavior frequencies were recorded during ten minutes of father-infant interaction. Her findings revealed that early contact (IV) did not appear to enhance bonding behaviors (DV) in this study. Her study necessitated, by virtue of the nature of her question, an after-only design (see Figure 7–1).

In a **before–after design,** subjects are measured before the experimental treatment on the same variables as after the treatment.

A variation on the after-only design involves assigning subjects to experimental and control groups *after they have been ranked* with respect to some variable that is important to the dependent variable. For example, in a study of preoperative teaching methods and their respective effect on patient recovery rates, subjects might be matched according to the extensiveness of their surgical procedure before being assigned, one to the experimental group and one to the control group, by the flip of a coin. This is called a **randomized block posttest design** (see Figure 7–3).

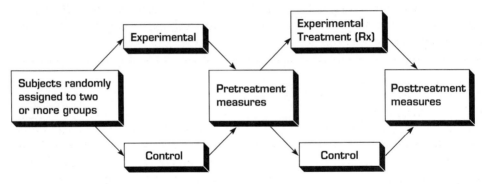

Figure 7–2   *A before-after study design.*

Example: Experimental Design in Nursing Research

*Gortner and Jenkins (1990) tested the question of whether combined inpatient
and outpatient teaching and monitoring programs might enhance efficacy
expectations for recovery at 12 weeks after cardiac surgery.*

*First-time and repeat cardiac surgery patients from two surgical centers
were included in the study. Following surgery, consenting subjects were randomly assigned to an experimental or a control group. The accrued sample
consisted of 125 male and 31 female patients. At induction, no statistically
significant differences were noted between control and experimental patients.
Before surgery, interviews and self-reports of activity were used for both experimental and control patients to obtain efficacy assessments for four behaviors:
walking, climbing, lifting, and general activity.*

*Nurses provided both experimental and control subjects with routine in-
formation on recovery while they were in the hospital. Additionally, experimental subjects viewed a slide/tape program on family coping and conflict
resolution followed by a brief counseling session. Both groups were appraised
for efficacy expectations just prior to discharge.*

*Nurses followed the experimental group by telephone on a weekly basis
for four weeks to monitor recovery, to reinforce risk-factor reduction, to coach
toward activity, and to provide reassurance to spouses as well as to patients.
Between the fourth and eighth weeks of home convalescence, calls were made
at two-week intervals.*

*At 4, 8, 12, and 24 weeks, nurses telephoned both groups to obtain effi-
cacy assessments and self-reports of activity.*

*Nurses found dramatic rises in perceived efficacy for walking, climbing,
lifting, and general activity in the early surgical recovery phases in the experimental group. Further, the differential perceptions for walking efficacy between experimental and control patients suggest that the experimental interventions may have had a sustained effect on perceived capability for activity
through the 12th week of recovery after surgery. That being coached in re-*

hypothesis tested

random subject design with control group

intervention or treatment

posttreatment data collection

findings

covery activities was a significant predictor of later activity, as were efficacy expectations, reinforces verbal persuasion and modeling as important sources of efficacy enhancement.

When matching is done based on a nominal variable that can't be rank-ordered—for example, sex or race—but that is still assumed to have an effect on the dependent variable or to interact with the independent variable, a **factorial design** is used. Factorial designs can be constructed using three or four variables, which results in increased numbers of cells and the need for larger samples. The basic 2×2 factorial posttest design appears in Figure 7–4.

The types of experimental design we have examined generally reflect a comparison of the experimental treatment or intervention with *no* treatment or intervention. Sometimes, control groups receive an alternative treatment or intervention (for example, "standard practice"), because receiving no treatment or a placebo would not be ethical. In this case, what is typically called the control group may be called the **comparative group.** As long as two groups are randomly assigned to experiences that differ from each other in an important way, the conditions for an experimental design have been met. This is true even when a second independent variable, such as race or sex, is not randomly assigned to subjects, as occurs in a factorial design. Study designs with posttest only and no control group have neither pretesting nor the potential for comparison and are considered weak, or **preexperimental, designs.** The design with pretest, posttest, and no control group is considered the second weakest. It has a few advantages over preexperimental designs in that changes in the DV can be identified, but without a control or comparative group, it's impossible to determine which of all the possible extraneous or error variances might have caused the change.

Steps in Experimental Designs

Although experimental designs vary, all involve these steps:

1. State the researchable problem.
2. Determine that an experimental design is well matched to the problem.

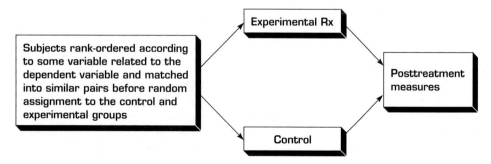

Figure 7–3   *A randomized block posttest design.*

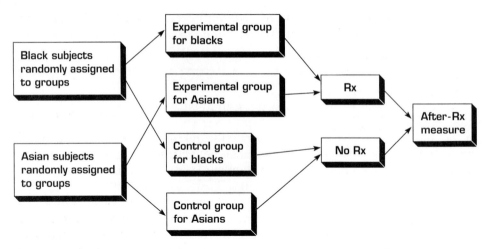

Figure 7–4 *A 2 × 2 factorial design.*

3. Operationalize the independent and dependent variables.

4. Formulate the hypothesis to be tested.

5. Identify measures for the dependent variable.

6. Specify the full range of potential intervening variables and decide which should be controlled, which can be permitted to vary, and which can be ignored.

7. Design the experiment to test the hypothesis, including selecting the sample.

8. Collect data on "before" measures.

9. Implement experimental and control conditions.

10. Collect data on "after" measures.

11. Analyze data.

12. Present findings in relationship to the hypothesis being tested.

13. Prepare a discussion of conclusions, limitations, and implications for further study.

Advantages and Disadvantages of Experimental Designs

The rigor, precision, and control properties of experimental designs enable them to be the most powerful way for scientists to establish cause-and-effect relationships or to test causal hypotheses. Causal relationships are important to science because they allow us to predict and explain. For example, an experimental design could tell us if using a dry-abraded skin preparation causes poor-quality EKG signals. Or it could tell us if using sterile saline solution and K-Y jelly causes an increase in the number of pathogens at the meatal introitus of male patients with an indwelling urinary catheter. *Causation* in the scientific sense requires three criteria:

1. A cause must precede an effect in time.

2. Evidence must indicate that the causal variable (IV) and the dependent variable (DV) are associated.

3. Evidence must rule out other factors as possible determining conditions for the dependent variable.

The scientific notion of causality acknowledges that in most cases a multiplicity of determining conditions together make up the necessary and sufficient conditions for an event. A **necessary condition** is one that *must* occur if an effect is to occur. For example, trying drugs is necessary for drug addiction to occur (except, of course, for newborns). A **sufficient condition** is one that is always followed by the effect. For example, destruction of the optic nerve is a sufficient condition for blindness. Some phenomena are both necessary and sufficient, but these are rare (Sellitz et al 1976). The experimental design's strategies of (1) manipulation, (2) comparison, and (3) randomization help the investigator to rule out alternative causal explanations for changes in dependent variables.

Disadvantages of experimental designs also exist:

- Some variables are not feasible or ethical to manipulate. For example, assigning pregnant women to take a new drug found to be dangerous to fetal development in animal studies would not be ethically possible.

- Randomization and otherwise equal treatment of control and experimental groups can occur in a laboratory, but these conditions do not resemble what goes on under real-world conditions, and experimental findings can therefore be based on rather artificial circumstances.

- Experimental designs attempt to reduce variables to measurable terms. Many of the phenomena that are important to science in nursing are complex, multidimensional, and holistic and defy the reductionism that has worked reasonably well in the physical or natural sciences.

Despite these limitations, however, the evolution of nursing's research and theory base will probably yield increasing numbers of studies that employ experimental designs in the years to come.

QUASI-EXPERIMENTAL DESIGNS

When it is not feasible for a researcher to implement all of the characteristics of an experimental design—for example, random assignment to control and experimental groups—alternative designs, usually called **quasi-experimental designs,** are selected. We will now take up some of the most familiar quasi-experimental options.

The Nonequivalent Pretest-Posttest Control Group Design

The most basic quasi-experimental design uses nonequivalent pretest and posttest and a control group. This type of quasi-experimental design is useful when a researcher cannot randomly assign subjects to different treatments but must rely instead on comparative groups. Collection of the pretreatment data allows the investigator to determine how similar the groups are on the variable of interest even though it cannot be assumed that the experimental and comparison groups are equal. This type of quasi-experimental design is described in the following example.

Example: Quasi-Experimental Design

In order to study the effects of maternal employment status on family functioning and on the preterm infant's development at three months chronological age, Youngblut et al (1991) recruited a convenience sample of 110 families from a larger, longitudinal study of premature infants. Study subjects were self-selected based on whether or not the mother chose to (or had to) work. Controls were those mothers who did not work. Data were collected in a 2.5-hour home visit and through hospital chart reviews. The findings suggest that maternal employment does not adversely affect the preterm infant's development at three months of age.

The Time Series Design

The **time series design** is used when the investigator can study only one group but uses "before" measures to establish a baseline against which to compare the posttreatment measure of the dependent variable. Even though some authors include the time series design as a quasi-experimental design, Campbell and Stanley (1963) consider it to be preexperimental, because it fails to control so many confounding or extraneous variables. Expanding the design so that it includes a more extended time series and multiple data collection points both before and after introduction of the independent variable is an adaptation that they say qualifies as a quasi-experimental design with considerable integrity, because it strengthens the researcher's ability to attribute change in the dependent variable to the experimental treatment or manipulation.

Advantages and Disadvantages of Quasi-Experimental Designs

From the point of view of controls for internal validity, quasi-experimental designs are thought to be superior to preexperimental designs. Their disadvantages, however, include the facts that they

- cannot test causal hypotheses
- do little to ensure external generalizability
- are more susceptible to the effects of both testing and experimental settings because of the frequent testing schedules

EX POST FACTO STUDY DESIGNS

An **ex post facto study** is one that attempts to study something after the fact. Instead of introducing or manipulating an independent variable, the investigator selects subjects who have undergone some life experience. He or she then attempts to describe or explain the experience and, often, its possible relationships to some variable. Such correlations might be the presumed causes, but this cannot be confirmed, only tentatively suggested. Without the control that is possible in an experiment, the investigator must take things as they have already occurred and try to untangle them. Many nursing studies use ex post facto study designs.

The major disadvantage of ex post facto studies is that the investigator cannot establish cause-and-effect relationships, only correlational ones. This disadvantage is due to three weaknesses in the ex post facto design: (1) The researcher cannot actively manipulate the independent variable, (2) the researcher cannot randomly assign subjects to experimental treatments, and (3) the possibility for misinterpretation of study results is high. Suggesting the plausibility of cause-and-effect links when strong correlations are found can be very tempting when an investigator discusses conclusions in an ex post facto study. It takes a sharp and critical reader to recognize that a researcher has gone beyond the data when writing up a study's interpretations.

METHODOLOGICAL STUDIES

Generally speaking, **methodological studies** are those that are designed to develop, validate, or evaluate research tools or techniques. Of particular interest to nurse researchers engaged in methodological studies has been the effort devoted to constructing approaches to measuring the quality of nursing care. Some have focused on structural variables (that is, on the organization of the patient-care system); others have emphasized the actual process of giving care; and yet others have examined outcome as reflected in patient welfare. Some of the instruments developed for this purpose are the Slater Nursing Competencies Rating Scale (Wandelt & Steward 1975), which measures the competencies displayed by a nurse; the Quality Patient Care Scale (QUALPAC) (Wandelt & Ager 1974) for measuring the quality of nursing care received by a patient while care is being given; and the Nursing Audit (Phaneuf 1972) for measuring the quality of nursing care received by a patient after a cycle of care has been completed and the patient has been discharged.

HOW DESIGNS FIT STUDY PROBLEMS

Earlier chapters in this text considered questions such as "What do nurses study?" and "Why are such topics important?" The emphasis in this chapter has been on "How are nursing research questions studied?" If you as a research consumer expect to have confidence in the credibility of research findings, you must be convinced that the plan or blueprint for conducting the study itself is one that effectively fits the question being asked. The design must not only suit the study purposes and answer the question but also control for unwanted variance.

As you may surmise, research designs can be simple or quite complex. By now, you should have a good sense of the range, diversity, advantages, and disadvantages of the ones that are used most frequently in nursing research.

ANNOTATED RESEARCH EXAMPLE

Citation

Gardner K. A summary of findings of a five-year comparison study of primary and team nursing. *Nurs Res.* 1991;40(2):113–117.

Study Problem/Purpose

"team nursing" as a control group

In the past two decades, primary nursing has emerged as a major nursing delivery system for acute-care hospitals. The purpose of the current study was to add to the previous evaluations of primary nursing by comparing primary and team nursing on quality of nursing care, nurse retention and stress, and costs over a four-year period.

"primary nursing as treatment independent variable

Methods

type of design: quasi-experimental

A quasi experiment was conducted of three primary and two team units in a 526-bed urban teaching hospital. Patients chosen to be observed for the quality of patient care were on the unit for more than two days, understood English, and fit into one of three cardiac Diagnostically Related Groups (DRGs). Quality of care was assessed by support and stress scales. For example, trained nurse raters used Ager's quality patient care scale, among other scales, to measure quality of care.

quality of care, nursing stress, and cost as dependent variables

Gray-Toft's nursing stress scale was used to measure the degree of change over time of the primary nursing staff stress level.

Nursing cost was defined as the personnel cost actually expended to provide nursing care on each unit. This cost included salaries and fringe benefits for the direct care providers and support persons.

The study was carried out in three phases: a preintervention phase (phase I) and two postintervention phases (phase II at 12 months and phase III at 30 months after implementation).

Findings

Using the quality patient care scale, the findings show that there were statistically significant higher scores for quality of care for primary nursing over team nursing in phases II and III. Between phases II and III there was no difference in amount of direct care activity. However, in phase III, the percentage of direct care activities increased by 4% for both days and evenings, statistically significant when compared with the other primary nursing units. There were no differences for the nurses' stress scores between primary and team nursing. Retention of registered nurses was studied over three years. The staff members on the primary units were retained significantly longer than the staff members on the team units. This study supports the founders of primary nursing who advocated primary nursing as a delivery system to promote professional practice and to facilitate the nurse-patient relationship.

Guidelines for Critique

What type of design has been used in the study?

Is the design carefully described in the methods section?

Has the researcher examined the strengths and weaknesses of this particular design approach?

Is the design well suited to the researchable problem? To the purpose of the study?

If the design is a case study, what procedures has the researcher used to try to impose order on the data collection?

If the design is historical, have rules for external and internal criticism been met?

If the design is a survey, were survey questions relevant to the research problem? Was the return rate sufficient to draw meaningful conclusions?

If the design is experimental, what methods were used to control for extraneous variables? What attempts were made to keep research conditions the same for all subjects? Does the design demonstrate internal validity? External validity?

If the design is quasi-experimental, why was this approach chosen? What steps were taken to try to mitigate the disadvantages of this type of design?

If the design is ex post facto, has the researcher gone beyond the data in drawing conclusions from the study?

Summary of Key Ideas and Terms

Study designs are the overall plans, or blueprints, for collecting and analyzing data in order to answer researchable questions as validly and reliably as possible and to control for unwanted variance.

An intelligent reader of research findings should be able to recognize the design used in a study report and evaluate its suitability for addressing a study's purpose.

Designs for *factor-naming* and *factor-relating studies* emphasize flexibility and discovery; designs for *association-testing* (explanatory) and *causal hypothesis-testing studies* rely on control and accuracy.

Historical study designs explain the past and its implications for the present and future by systematically collecting, evaluating, and interpreting evidence—such as letters, maps, books, artifacts, diaries, and public documents—that already exists.

Case study designs provide in-depth analyses of a single subject of investigation such as an individual patient, a family, a hospital ward, a professional organization, or the like in order to gain insight, provide background information for broader studies, develop explanations of human processes, and provide rich, descriptive anecdotes.

Interpretive study designs examine and explain human experience and practices under natural conditions.

Surveys are also called *nonexperimental designs* by some authorities, because they lack the control associated with true experiments. In general, they involve collecting information from a variety of sample subjects and generalizing the findings to the population of interest to the investigator.

In a true *experimental design* one finds the following hallmarks: (1) control over at least one independent variable and manipulation of at least one independent variable, (2) random selection of sample members, and (3) random assignment of sample members to experimental and control groups.

The strengths of an experimental design are that it can (1) maximize systematically introduced experimental variance, (2) control extraneous variance, and (3) minimize error variance.

The ability of an experimental design to control variance contributes to its internal validity, that is, whether or not manipulation of the IV has really made a difference to the DV. External validity refers to the representativeness, or generalizability, of a study's results. The experimental study design's use of randomization, control groups, and experimental groups; manipulation of the IV; and pretests and posttests, or measures of the DV, are all remedies to ward off threats to internal and external validity.

Experimental designs are the only ones that can establish scientific causality. Causality requires three criteria: (1) A cause must precede an effect in time. (2) Evidence must indicate that the IV and DV are associated. (3) Evidence must as far as possible rule out other factors as determining conditions for the DV.

Quasi-experimental designs are used when the investigator cannot randomly assign subjects to control and experimental groups but instead uses some form of comparative group.

Ex post facto designs study something after the fact. Instead of introducing or manipulating an IV, the researcher selects subjects who have undergone some life experience and attempts to relate it to other variables. Such correlations, when they are found, should not be interpreted as cause and effect.

Methodological studies aim to develop tools, instruments, or methods appropriate for answering nursing research questions. Of particular interest are instruments that measure quality of nursing care in terms of patient outcomes.

References

Campbell DT & Stanley JC. *Experimental and Quasi-Experimental Designs for Research.* Chicago: Rand McNally;1963.

Christy TE. *Cornerstone for Nursing Education.* New York: Teachers' College Press, Columbia University;1969.

Christy TE. The methodology of historical research. *Nurs Res.* May/June 1975; 24:189–192.

Diers D. *Research in Nursing Practice.* Philadelphia: Lippincott;1979.

Duxbury ML et al. Measurement of the nurse organizational climate of neonatal intensive care units. *Nurs Res.* March/April 1982;31:83–88.

Fajemilehin RB. Factors influencing high rate of 'born-before-arrival' babies in Nigeria—A case control study in Ogbomosho. *Int J Nurs Stud.* 1991;28:13–18.

Gortner SR & Jenkins LS. Self-efficacy and activity level following cardiac surgery. *J Adv Nurs Stud.* 1990;15:1132–1138.

Hockett HC. *Critical Method in Historical Research and Writing.* New York: Macmillan; 1955.

Holm K. Single subject research. *Nurs Res.* July/August 1983;32:253–255.

Phaneuf MC. *The Nursing Audit: Profile for Excellence.* New York: Appleton-Century-Crofts;1972.

Roberson MHB. The meaning of compliance: Patient perspectives. *Qual Health Res.* 1992;2:7–26.

Sellitz C et al. *Research Method in Social Relations.* New York: Holt, Rinehart & Winston;1976.

Seymour E & Buscherhof JR. Sources and consequences of satisfaction and dissatisfaction in nursing: Findings from a national sample. *Int J Nurs Stud.* 1991; 28:109–124.

Toney L: The effects of holding the newborn at delivery on paternal bonding. *Nurs Res.* January/February 1983;32:16–19.

Waltz C & Bausell RB. *Nursing Research: Design, Statistics, and Computer Analysis.* Philadelphia: F. A. Davis;1981.

Wandelt MA & Ager JW. *Quality Patient Care Scale.* New York: Appleton-Century-Crofts;1974.

Wandelt MA & Steward DS. *The Slater Nursing Competencies Rating Scale.* New York: Appleton-Century-Crofts;1975.

Youngblut JM, Loveland-Cherry CJ & Horan M. Maternal employment effects on family and preterm infants at three months. *Nurs Res.* 1991;40:272–275.

QUANTITATIVE DATA COLLECTION: MEASUREMENT AND INSTRUMENTS

BRANDY M. BRITTON

SALLY AMBLER HUTCHINSON

HOLLY SKODOL WILSON

CHAPTER OUTLINE

In This Chapter . . .

Research in Nursing Second Edition by Diane La Rochelle, Ada M. Lindsey, and Nancy A. Stotts. *Research in Nursing* First Edition by Jane S. Norbeck, Ada M. Lindsey, and Nancy A. Stotts.

CHAPTER OBJECTIVES

After reading this chapter, you should be able to:

- Comprehend the concept of scientific scales of measurement
- Compare and contrast scales for nominal, ordinal, interval, and ratio data
- Discuss at least five psychological or social phenomena that can be measured by psychosocial instruments
- Classify psychosocial instruments as subjective or objective and as direct or proxy
- Describe the types of psychosocial measures most frequently used
- Discuss the concepts of reliability and validity and distinguish among the various types that can be established
- Evaluate a psychosocial instrument in relation to the four ideal qualities of measurement instruments, including various types of reliability and validity
- Compare and contrast the advantages and disadvantages of self-administered and face-to-face methods of data collection with psychosocial instruments
- Discuss factors that must be taken into account when scoring psychosocial instruments to measure variables
- Identify any biophysiologic instruments that have been used in a study
- Discuss factors that can affect the reliability and validity of physiologic measurement

8

Introducing Research in Nursing First Edition by Jane S. Norbeck, Ada M. Lindsey, and Nancy A. Stotts.

IN THIS CHAPTER . . .

After the study problem and design have been clearly developed, the researcher must make a series of decisions about how to collect data pertinent to the identified variables. **Data** are the information the investigator collects from the subjects or participants in the study. In nursing research, the great majority of studies involve **quantitative** data—test scores, rankings, ratings, temperature readings, laboratory findings, and the like. To read about research intelligently, and to understand quantitative data collection, you need to start with an understanding of the concept of *scientific measurement.* We all engage in informal measuring every day. The well-baby clinic was busy that day, or it wasn't. The operating room schedule was full or pretty full. A patient's wound is healing quickly or slowly. And we are all familiar with such nursing measurements as drug dosages, pulse rate, blood pressure, and blood counts. Measurement in research can be distinguished from day-to-day measuring by certain specific characteristics. Measurement processes in research should:

- be explicit enough that observers can use them to come up with the same measures

- be applicable to more than one individual

- occur according to a well-specified, reasonable set of rules for assigning numbers to represent the qualities or attributes being measured

- attempt to isolate one attribute at a time in complex concepts like *quality of care* or *creativity*

- correspond as precisely as possible to the reality being measured

- reflect the researcher's awareness that most of the time one can tap only a small percentage of the possible data relevant to the attribute being measured

- use the highest level of measurement scale possible given the phenomena being measured

Another important aspect of quantitative data collection is the use of instruments. **Instruments** are the devices used to record the data obtained from subjects. Many instruments are used in nursing studies, including interview transcripts, questionnaires, rating scales, performance checklists, pencil-and-paper tests, and biological measurement devices. Because psychosocial measures are by far the most commonly used data collection methods in nursing research, this chapter focuses primarily on psychosocial instruments. We have all filled out a variety of psychosocial instruments, ranging from highly structured intelligence tests to open-ended questionnaires about a course we have completed. Perhaps you were required to participate in research in

This chapter synthesizes material written by Jane S. Norbeck, Ada M. Lindsey, and Nancy A. Stotts for Wilson HS: *Research in Nursing* (1985) and by Diane LaRochelle for Wilson HS: *Research in Nursing,* 2d ed. (1989).

undergraduate psychology courses in which you completed large batteries of instruments. From these experiences you know that some instruments make sense and seem appropriate to the purpose; others may seem mystifying, irrelevant, or poorly developed. Some instruments are easy and even fun to complete; others may be confusing, repetitious, tedious, or annoying. Such reactions are important for researchers to consider, because they may affect the extent or quality of research subjects' responses.

Among the most important questions to evaluate when sizing up the worth of any instruments used to measure variables in a nursing study are their **reliability** and **validity.** A reliable instrument will produce consistent results, or data, on repeated use, usually because the investigator has standardized the procedure for administering it. Taking a blood pressure several times and obtaining the same readings given unchanged conditions is an example of a reliable measure. A valid instrument is one that measures what it is supposed to measure. A paper-and-pencil test of a client's knowledge about his or her diabetic diet may measure reading skill rather than grasp of nutritional information. Obviously this issue is a lot more complicated when you are measuring psychosocial variables such as professional commitment or social network than when you are measuring a more direct and concrete variable such as weight, height, or temperature.

This chapter examines both these important aspects of quantitative data collection, measurement and instruments. It presents the concept of scales of measurement and describes types of measurement scales used for various types of data. This chapter also examines the problems and challenges of measuring psychosocial concepts by exploring some of the many types of instruments used, discussing their reliability and validity, and describing how they are developed and used. The chapter briefly discusses the use of psychophysiologic measures in quantifying variables of nursing research.

MEASUREMENT SCALES

Measurement involves the process of assigning numerical values to concepts under investigation. **Statistics** allow us to analyze those numerical values. When an investigator spells out how something is to be quantitatively measured, he or she is in fact operationally defining and quantifying the study's key concepts or variables. Intelligence may be "a score" on a standard IQ test like the Stanford-Binet Intelligence Test. A patient's preoccupation with body diseases might be measured using his or her score on some of the 550 items of the Minnesota Multiphasic Personality Inventory (MMPI). Postoperative recovery rate might be measured by the number of hours that elapse before a child returns to preoperative eating, sleeping, playing, and communicating patterns.

Most authorities are quick to point out that it is not really possible to measure something itself. Rather, *one measures the attributes or qualities about something that vary.* You can't measure a female per se, but you can measure her height, weight, political attitudes, or self-esteem. These varying character-istics or attributes of something are the study's variables. The clearer and more credible a researcher's process of transforming concepts or variables into measurements, the more likely he or she is going to be convinced that the measurement reflects actual value rather than error.

Let's illustrate this process by imagining that we are interested in con-ducting a study of psychiatric nurses' beliefs about mental illness. We could collect data on this variable by interviewing a sample of nurses and using qualitative analysis methods. Or we could administer the *Beliefs About Mental Illness Inventory,* with a format like that depicted in Box 8–1. Our sub-jects' responses could then be transformed into scores or measures by devel-oping a system of assigning numbers to the responses. Interpretation of the results would then have to be done according to the proper uses of scales of measurement.

Defining a Scale of Measurement

A **scale of measurement** specifies all the possible values a given measurement might have. What really defines a scale of measurement is the complete set of potential measurement categories, not just the ones into which a study's sub-jects fall. Of course, measures can be crude or precise, ranging from only a few possible values to a larger number of them.

All measurement scales do have to have *at least two different possible measurement categories, or values.* In our example, for instance, we could score the psychiatric nurses who take our *Beliefs About Mental Illness Inventory* as simply "positive" or "negative." We could even score the inten-sity of the belief as "strong" or "weak." The actual system for scoring data generated using this particular instrument involves assigning numbers to responses. Totals for various items are then added to determine whether or not the subject's dominant beliefs reflect the following:

- authoritarianism
- benevolence
- a mental hygiene ideology
- social restrictiveness
- interpersonal etiology orientation

Whatever the scale of measurement, it should, in addition to having at least two possible values, *be exhaustive.* This means that the researcher must assign some number to each respondent in a study. For example, it would be inadequate to measure the clinical specialization backgrounds of registry nurses in a city by specifying only *OB-PEDS* and *MED-SURG* on a scale. The researcher would at least have to add the category *Other* to be exhaustive.

Finally, measures along any scale of measurement should be *mutually exclusive.* A researcher measuring the consciousness level of intensive care unit (ICU) patients could not put the same patient into both the "conscious" and the "unconscious" category at the same time. If a scale proves difficult to

---

Box 8–1 Beliefs about Mental Illness Inventory

Examples of a 2-Choice Scale
Beliefs about Mental Illness

Positive		Negative
(+)	.... or	(−)
Strong (1)	.... or	Weak (0)

---

use because neither category seems quite right, the scale may need to be made more precise and discriminating by providing, for example, a graded series of options between fully conscious and fully unconscious. Decisions about scaling must be made at a study's outset, however, so that all subjects will be measured with the same scale, using the same measurement rules. Knowing the scale to be used also influences what statistics one will be able to employ to analyze the data. This knowledge keeps the researcher straight about what kinds of question the study will and will not be able to address since statistical procedures must be appropriate for a study's purpose and level of data.

Types of Measurement Scales

Scales for Nominal Data   The most primitive and least precise measurement scale from a traditional scientific perspective is called a nominal scale—a scale for nominal data. **Nominal (or "naming") scales** arbitrarily assign some number to represent the categories into which an attribute or quality can be sorted. Measuring the sex of patients who develop lung cancer in the United States by labeling each as male or female and assigning numbers so that 1 = male and 2 = female is an example of a very simple nominal scale, or code, with two possible measurement categories. Sorting patients according to their blood type or nursing diagnosis is another example of creating a nominal scale. The numbers themselves have no real meaning except as *a convenient code.* There is no implication of equal-sized steps between the numbers or of any inherent ordering of the categories in relation to one another. All we can conclude from nominal scales is that data sorted into different categories are nonequivalent. Nominal scales are nevertheless considered examples of scientific measurement because two rules apply in the assignment of numbers: (1) all responses that are sorted into the same qualitative category are given the same number, and (2) no two categories can be assigned the same number.

Scales for Ordinal Data   **Ordinal scales,** or scales for ordinal data, are "ordering" scales. Numbers that are assigned to data according to ordinal scales have the characteristic of ordered categories. We can't assume, however, that the numbers along the scale represent the same amount or change in the variable from one point to the next. An ordinal scale allows us to rate or rank "low," "medium," and "high," but it doesn't tell us anything about the *distance between* low and medium or medium and high. In short, although we

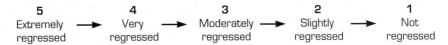

Figure 8–1   *Example of ordinal scale for regression where 5 > 4 > 3 > 2 > 1.*

can rate a variable on an ordinal scale, our measurement categories *cannot* be presented or treated as having equidistant intervals, even though the numbers we assign to the ratings might suggest it. Researchers could ask parents, for example, to rate their hospitalized children on a 5-point scale where 1 = *not at all regressed* while 5 = *extremely regressed*. Even though the raters use the numbers from 1 to 5 to make the ratings, there is no guarantee that the intervals between the numbers are equidistant in the same way that measures of weight or time are. It might take only a few behavioral changes to alter a rating from 2 (slightly regressed) to 3 (moderately regressed), yet a dramatic change in activity might be necessary to alter the rating from 4 (very regressed) to 5 (extremely regressed) (see Figure 8–1).

What we *can* assume with an ordinal scale like this one is that 5 is more regressed than 4, that 4 is more than 3, that 3 is more than 2, and that 2 is more than 1. Therefore, it's easy to see at least that ordinal scales are more precise quantitative tools than nominal scales. Obviously, being able to say that an attribute is *different in degree and direction* conveys more information than just saying that two attributes are in two different categories.

A Scale for Interval Data   An **interval scale,** or scale for interval data, consists of potential measurement categories that, as in an ordinal scale, have an inherent order; but in addition, the possible measures along an interval scale *are* equidistant from one another. This characteristic allows researchers to make statements about the *actual differences* between measures rather than just saying that something has more or less of an attribute than something else. Studies in the nursing literature concerned with the impact of preoperative care on postoperative patient outcomes might employ ordinal scales that simply rated a patient's overall postoperative course as having "more" or "fewer" complications. An interval scale that plots temperature elevations indicative of infection clearly offers more precise information on the study question. Investigators therefore prefer to use interval scales whenever possible, because they not only provide more precise information but also permit the adding and subtracting of measures and the use of more sophisticated statistics that require taking a mean of measures.

Most standardized psychological tests used in nursing research studies are based on interval scales. Blood pressure readings represent another example of an interval scale. A reading of $^{150}/_{90}$ is higher than a reading of $^{140}/_{90}$, and a reading of $^{140}/_{90}$ is higher than a reading of $^{120}/_{90}$. Furthermore, an interval scale assumes that the differences between systolic readings of 140 and 130 and 120 are essentially equivalent.

It's a good idea to point out, however, that even with interval scales where measurement rules indicate that differences have the same meaning, the meaning of a difference when it comes to clinical application may be a distinctively different one. For example, a hypertensive diet designed for two clients with blood pressure readings of $^{130}\!/_{90}$ and $^{120}\!/_{80}$ might be different, while a second plan for two other clients with blood pressures of $^{160}\!/_{100}$ and $^{150}\!/_{100}$ might be very similar. The first comparison reflects the difference between an elevated blood pressure and one that is clinically normal, while in the second case both readings are clinically hypertensive.

A final point on the subject of the interval scale is that, although it is considered to be a higher-level scale than either nominal or ordinal, it does not have what is called *an absolute zero point.* Zero on interval scales is arbitrary. Almost all authors on this subject use the Fahrenheit and Celsius thermometers for measuring temperature to illustrate this idea. Both are interval scales; the Celsius uses an arbitrary zero point of 0, and the Fahrenheit scale has an arbitrary zero point of 32. Neither point, however, really signifies the total lack of heat (see Figure 8–2). In sum, the interval scale has neither a real zero point nor the ability to provide information on the absolute magnitude of an attribute for any particular object.

A Scale for Ratio Data   A **ratio scale,** or scale for ratio level data, has rank ordering of measures, equal intervals between measures, and an absolute zero point. It is therefore considered to be the highest level of measurement scale for the purpose of applying statistical analysis procedures. These qualities allow the scale to communicate the maximum and most precise information and also make its data amenable to the most powerful and sophisticated statistical analyses. Examples of ratio scales used in nursing studies include time, length, and weight. Scores of zero on these measures really do represent the absence of the attribute being measured.

The important point to remember is that because ratio scales do have an absolute zero, all statistical procedures and arithmetic operations are appropriate with them. Ratio scales do tend, however, to dominate among the physical and biological measures and are rarely used when measuring more abstract psychosocial qualities. Most quantitative researchers prefer working at the highest level of measurement and tend to operationalize their study variables so as to increase their ability to do so.

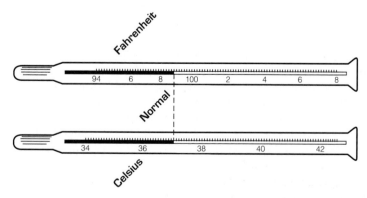

Figure 8–2   *Two types of thermometers.*

TABLE 8–1 *Phenomena Measured by Psychosocial Instruments*

Concept or Phenomenon	Examples
Abilities	Intelligence
Attitudes	Political, religious
Communication	Nonverbal
Coping	Style
Development	Infant, adolescent
Emotional states	Anxiety, depression
Family functioning	Cohesion, interaction
Individual functioning	Activities of daily living, adjustment
Interests	Vocational
Knowledge	Sex information
Mental functioning	Cognitive stage
Needs	Affiliation, achievement
Occupational functioning	Job stress
Personality	Traits
Role	Conflict
Self-concept	Ideal versus actual self
Sociometric standing	Social class, popularity
Social behavior	Social network, social skills
Social environment	Ward atmosphere
Stress	Recent life events
Values	Moral, interpersonal
Well-being	Life satisfaction

PSYCHOSOCIAL INSTRUMENTS

The range of phenomena included in psychological and social investigation is vast, and "new" concepts are continually being created along with the development of nursing theories and theories of human behavior. Thus, it probably isn't possible to compile an exhaustive list of topics in this field. Table 8–1 outlines major concepts or phenomena that are being measured with psychosocial instruments. In nursing many existing concepts are further refined to increase their specific relevance to nursing problems. For example, a measure of children's coping with new situations might be modified to measure children's coping with hospitalization, and the psychological variable *locus of control* has been adapted to measure health locus of control (Wallston et al 1978).

Many of the concepts in Table 8–1, such as well-being or coping, can be measured either objectively or subjectively. If you wanted an *objective measure* of patients' understanding of the teaching they had received about their diagnosis and treatment, you might administer a written or oral test with items about the material covered in the teaching. You would obtain a *subjective measure* if you asked them questions face to face or in a questionnaire about their perception of the adequacy of their knowledge of their diagnosis and treatment.

Certain of the psychosocial variables listed in Table 8–1 can be measured directly. For example, you can obtain a *direct measure* of a person's age, income, years of education, or number of children. The vast majority of psychosocial variables cannot be measured directly, however, and a **proxy measure**—a measure or count of something that stands for an object or quality—is developed to represent the construct. Thus, for example, the number of items describing anxious behaviors or feeling states that a person checks as applicable at a given time is taken as a proxy measure for the person's actual anxiety level. Most of the measurement of psychosocial variables is done with proxy measures. Extensive testing of such instruments should be done to validate that the items do indeed measure the intended construct. In the case of anxiety measures, testing to establish validity has included correlations between the questionnaire score and physiologic measures of anxiety, comparisons of scores between psychiatric patients and nonpatients, and anxiety-arousing experiments in which pretest and posttest scores are used to demonstrate that the score on the anxiety questionnaire does indeed increase after the anxiety-arousing experience. Different types of validity and ways to establish them will be discussed later in the chapter.

Standardized Instruments

Considering the great diversity of concepts or phenomena that might be measured in nursing and psychosocial research and the wide range of potential population groups that might be studied, it is likely that an instrument already exists to measure the variables the researcher has identified in the study problem and design. Instruments that have been developed, tested, and refined and are commonly used to measure a particular variable or construct are referred to as **standardized instruments**. A conservative estimate of the number of psychosocial instruments that have been developed and tested to some extent over the last several decades is between 5,000 and 8,000. These instruments vary widely in the soundness of their theoretical basis and the extent that reliability and validity have been established. Nonetheless, a great deal of unnecessary effort is expended in research because of the failure of investigators to search thoroughly for available instruments.

When the variable to be measured has been clearly delineated, the researcher can conduct a systematic search to locate an existing instrument by following these steps:

1. If the variable falls into a special category, compendia that feature specialized instruments, such as measures for use with children, should be consulted first.

2. The next resource to consult would generally be the current edition of *Tests in Print* or other compendia that index a wide variety of published

instruments. Two resources of particular relevance to nurse researchers are *Instruments for Measuring Nursing Practice and Other Health Care Variables* (Ward et al 1979) and *Instruments for Use in Nursing Education Research* (Ward & Fetler 1979).

3. Compendia that index unpublished instruments should be consulted next.

4. Recent instruments might be located by using citation abstracts for works that have not yet been compiled in compendia (for example, *Psychological Abstracts, Index to Nursing Literature*).

In addition to whole instruments that measure the variable, the search should include instruments that might measure the variable as a **subscale,** one of several specific measures that contribute to a broader measure. Personality tests such as the Minnesota Multiphasic Personality Inventory (MMPI), for example, often measure a number of elements in the construct of personality that are labeled as subscales, such as paranoia or depression. Tests that measure needs often have subscales for each of the needs postulated—for example, need for affiliation, need for control, and need for achievement. The subscales are usually imbedded in the instrument in such a way that the entire instrument must be administered in order to be valid. In these cases, though, only the subscale that measures the variable under study needs to be scored.

A common mistake in instrument selection is to assume that an instrument is sound because it is widely used. Certainly, many widely used instruments are excellent, but worth needs to be determined on a case-by-case basis. For example, the Edwards Personal Preference Schedule, which produces subscales for 15 needs, is consistently one of the most widely used instruments listed in the *Mental Measurements Yearbook* series. But the critical reviews over the years clearly state that the validity testing for this instrument is sketchy and inadequate.

Types of Measures Frequently Used

Several types of scales have been developed for psychosocial testing, particularly to assess attitudes, interests, and values. Commonly used scales are based on rank-ordering a list of stimuli, sorting stimuli into categories, making comparisons between pairs of objects or stimuli (paired comparisons), and rating techniques. Each of these scales will be described, along with examples of their use in nursing research.

Commonly Used Rating Scales   Several formats are used in creating scales for rating a set of items, but each involves selecting a step in a scale that can be assigned a numerical value. Figure 8–3 illustrates variations of graphic and numerical scales. Rating scales also vary in the number of steps provided for responses. Only two steps are used for bipolar adjectives (for example, *effective* or *ineffective*), whereas ten steps might be required for a rating scale based on percentages—for example, "for each item, estimate the percentage of time you spent in each activity." Whether an odd or even number of steps is preferable depends on dual considerations: Is the middle (neutral or uncer-

1. Graphic Scales without Numbers

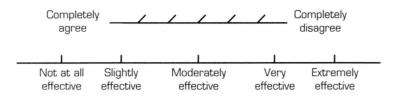

2. Graphic Scales with Numbers

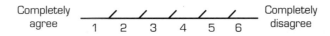

3. Numerical Scales

1. Completely agree
2. Mostly agree
3. Slightly agree
4. Slightly disagree
5. Mostly disagree
6. Completely disagree

a. Extremely well
b. Very well
c. Fairly well
d. Hardly at all
e. Not at all
   (numbers implied)

4. Numerical Scale Expressed in Percentages

Figure 8–3   *Types of rating scales.*

tain) step important to measure, or would this step encourage noncommittal responses and thereby reduce the discriminating power of the data? An even number of steps is usually preferable for scales that range across opposite dimensions (for example, from *agree* to *disagree*), thus forcing the respondent to select either *slightly agree* or *slightly disagree.*

Instruments based on scaling techniques usually have several items to be rated for each construct. (As you will recall, a *construct* is a concept used in a theory to account for relationships in observable events.) The ratings for each item are added to obtain a score for the construct. This method of measurement is referred to as a **Likert-type scale,** after the person who developed it for use in measuring attitudes. Likert scales are quite common in psychosocial research. Generally, when a Likert scale is used to measure a construct, statements are made and study participants are asked to rate their level of agreement or disagreement with each statement. There are customarily five choices on a Likert-type scale: strongly agree, agree, disagree, strongly disagree, and don't know or undecided. Figure 8–4 illustrates a Likert-type scale rating individuals' knowledge of the AIDS virus.

An example of a rating scale that is used frequently in nursing research is the State-Trait Anxiety Inventory (STAI), an instrument with 20 items to measure state anxiety (transitory responses) and 20 items to measure trait anxiety (stable individual differences in anxiety proneness) (Spielberger 1983). Each

	Strongly agree	Agree	Disagree	Strongly disagree	Don't know
1. Only gay men get AIDS.	[　]	[　]	[　]	[　]	[　]
2. You can contract AIDS from sharing utensils.	[　]	[　]	[　]	[　]	[　]
3. You can can tell by outward appearance if someone has AIDS.	[　]	[　]	[　]	[　]	[　]
4. You can contract AIDS by sharing a needle with someone.	[　]	[　]	[　]	[　]	[　]
5. One way that the AIDS virus is transmitted is through the exchange of blood.	[　]	[　]	[　]	[　]	[　]

Figure 8–4   *A Likert-type scale assessing AIDS knowledge.*

item describes a particular aspect of anxious behavior or feelings. This type of scale is also called a *summative* instrument, because the ratings for each item are added to obtain the score. Because some of the items may have been worded negatively to avoid creating a **response set**—that is, a tendency to respond to items in a consistent manner based on an irrelevant criterion, such as responding *true* to all items in a true-false test or agreeing with all the statements that appear to be more "socially desirable" than others—the scores for the negative items are reversed in scoring so that the scores for all of the items have the same meaning (high anxiety). After making this correction, the ratings from all 20 items are added to obtain the anxiety score. Because anxiety is an abstract concept with many defining features, it is important to have several items, including both anxious behaviors and conscious feelings, to increase the likelihood of measuring all of the variations that might occur among individual subjects.

Other Types of Scales   Another type of rating scale technique is the **semantic differential,** which is typically used to measure attitudes. The concept or object to be rated is written at the top of a page, followed by a list of bipolar adjectives (*responsible* and *irresponsible, bad* and *good*). The respondent rates the concept or object along a seven-point scale for each adjective pair. If more than one concept or object is subjected to the same list of adjective pairs, comparisons of attitudes can be made based on the ratings.

Sorting techniques involve giving respondents a stack of cards with one item per card and asking them to sort them into piles based on some specified dimension (for example, difficulty level or attractiveness). Respondents may be free to develop as many piles as they wish, with as many or few cards in each pile as they choose, or these decisions may be predetermined by the researcher. The **Q-sort** is an example of a constrained sorting technique, in which respondents are limited to a certain number of items at the extreme ends of the continuum of the piles but can place more items in the middle ranges. This method yields a normal distribution of responses, and the items that the respondent most strongly agrees or disagrees with are identified.

Similar to sorting techniques, **ranking techniques** involve considering a set of stimuli in relationship to other items in the set. Respondents are asked to rank-order the objects or stimuli on the basis of some property. Because only one item is assigned for each rank, however, a smaller number of stimuli can be accommodated than with sorting techniques. An example of a ranking task is to ask students to rank from one to ten the most important features of a course that should be retained if the course were to be revised. The list of ten stimuli to be ranked might include specific readings, films, lecture topics, or simulated experiences.

The method of **paired comparisons** involves asking people to choose between two objects or stimuli in each of a series of items. All possible pairs of the items are presented, to allow for comparisons of the relative values of each item in relation to each other item. This technique is often used in studying a person's values or interests.

A method that has emerged in recent reports of nursing research is the use of **patient logs** to record data on a daily (or more frequent) basis. These logs may vary from open-ended to highly structured checklists—for example, of symptoms, food choices, or moods.

Intelligence tests, achievement tests, skill tests, and many other types of **ability test** are used to study certain psychosocial variables. Some of these tests are developed for use in educational, vocational, or counseling settings. These tests are often highly developed measures that have normative data available for various population subgroups.

Tests of knowledge are probably most familiar to you because of your long history of taking examinations. When used in nursing research, tests of knowledge usually involve either the nursing knowledge required of practitioners or the knowledge of health behaviors required by patients.

IDEAL QUALITIES OF A PSYCHOSOCIAL INSTRUMENT

Decisions about the measurement of psychosocial variables should take into account four general considerations:

1. the congruence of the measurement instrument or approach with the variable to be measured
2. the validity and reliability of the instrument
3. the feasibility of using a particular instrument within the research plan
4. the acceptability of the measurement instrument or approach to the study respondents

Discussion of each of these considerations follows.

Congruence with Variable to Be Measured

Many psychosocial instruments are developed within the context of a theoretical framework for interpreting the meaning of the construct to be measured. Thus, an instrument to measure clinically significant indicators of depression in psychiatric practice might not be a valid measure of depressive mood states in nonpsychiatric populations. For example, many scales of depression include the "vegetative" symptoms of depression, including appetite and sleep disturbances. Because these symptoms are frequently associated with normal pregnancy, such items would spuriously increase the depression scores for pregnant women. An instrument that tested only depressive mood would be preferable for this clinical group.

Another problem in assessing the congruence of the construct with the variable identified in the study problem stems from the lack of agreement on the definitions or components of many psychosocial constructs. Depending on theoretical definitions, self-concept can be seen as distinct from or similar to self-esteem. Many instruments to measure self-concept or self-esteem exist, but they differ in what aspects of the larger construct they actually measure.

The State-Trait Anxiety Inventory is a good example of the refinement of measurement to keep pace with conceptual development in the field. Before the development of the STAI, anxiety measures combined transitory anxiety states and the more enduring anxiety-proneness trait in single measures of anxiety. Many research studies now specify one or the other form of anxiety from the STAI as the operationalized version of the concept of anxiety based on the theoretical model that was used to guide variable selection for the research.

Reliability and Validity

Any instrument used in research should have at least minimal levels of reliability and validity established. Box 8–2 outlines the usual types of reliability and validity that are tested in the development of an instrument. **Reliability** of measurement refers to the consistency, accuracy, and precision of the measures taken. **Validity** refers to relevance: Does the instrument really measure what it claims to measure? Because so much of the measurement of psychosocial variables involves proxy measures, considerations of reliability and validity are very important in nursing research. In fact, even well-designed research is unlikely to be published in scientific journals if the reliability and validity of the measurement strategies cannot be demonstrated.

Reliability   What constitutes a minimal level of reliability in an instrument? We want assurance that, as with a ruler, we will obtain the same reading each time the measurement is used (unless a "real" change in the value has occurred). Instruments that are reliable measure the construct or variable of interest in a consistent manner. Therefore, an instrument is reliable to the extent that it provides consistent measures across subjects and is stable over time. Reliability is often expressed as a coefficient of correlation. An instrument with perfect reliability has a coefficient of 1.00. If an instrument is com-

---

Box 8–2 Types of Reliability and Validity

I. *Reliability Estimates*

   A. test-retest reliability
   B. internal consistency reliability
   C. split-half reliability

II. *Validity Estimates*

   A. content validity
   B. face validity
   C. construct validity
   D. criterion-related validity
      1. predictive validity
      2. concurrent validity

Source: Adapted from Allen & Yen 1979. Reprinted with permission of Brooks/Cole Publishing Company, Monterey, Calif.

---

posed of several subscales, the reliability of each must be assessed (Gay 1985). Gay provides guidelines for coefficients of correlation for various instruments. Gay notes that a coefficient greater than .90 is acceptable for any instrument. A coefficient of at least .90 is recommended for achievement and aptitude tests, whereas a coefficient of .80–.89 is acceptable for personality measures. Gay points out that researchers using attitude scales usually report correlation coefficients in the range of .60–.80.

The major types of reliability tests used by researchers include test-retest reliability, internal consistency reliability, and split-half reliability. Researchers should obtain at least two reliability measures for each instrument because each method involves different sources of error (American Psychological Association 1974). **Test-retest reliability** is a measure of the stability of an instrument over time; thus, a high coefficient is desirable. This measurement is very easy to obtain. You simply administer the instrument to a representative sample of your target population; administer the instrument again after about a two-week lapse in time, and correlate the two sets of scores. There is no set standard for the interval of time between testings, but it should be long enough so that subjects are not able to recall their responses from the first administration.

The second type of reliability is internal consistency reliability. **Internal consistency reliability** is a measure of how well all of the items in the instrument relate to each other and of their ability to produce the same pattern of results in a similar population. To obtain this coefficient, you need to administer the instrument only once to a representative sample of subjects and then apply a statistical test. **Cronbach's alpha** is the most widely used measure of internal consistency. Waltz and colleagues (1984) claim that the alpha coefficient is the preferred measure of internal consistency because it provides one value for an entire set of data, and "is equal in value to the distribution of all possible split-half coefficients associated with a particular set of test data" (p. 136).

Split-half reliability is also an indicator of the internal consistency of an instrument, based on administration of the instrument to a representative sample of subjects from the target population. A split-half reliability co-efficient is computed by dividing the instrument in half (into even numbers and odd numbers), computing a score for every subject in each half, and correlating the two sets of scores.

Validity   Validity is an extremely important aspect of instrument development and assessment. A valid instrument measures the construct that it intends to measure. If an instrument does not measure what it intended to, the data that result are not very meaningful. For example, suppose an investigator sets out to study parents' anxiety about their children's surgical outcomes. The instrument of measurement consists of questions on parental food intake and alcohol consumption prior to the child's surgery. These are probably not valid measures of anxiety. Some parents' eating habits don't change when they are anxious, and some may not drink in response to anxiety. A better, or more valid, measure of parental anxiety might be to administer an instrument that asks parents specific questions about the surgery and their anxious feelings and behaviors related to the experience.

It is important to distinguish validity from reliability. An instrument may be reliable (that is, consistent) but not valid. In the example above, an investigator may consistently find certain eating or drinking habits in parents, but that finding does not mean the instrument is a valid measure of anxiety.

There are a number of different types of validity. **Content validity** is a systematic assessment of the content of an instrument to ensure that it adequately represents or includes the entire content area, or domain, specified. For example, if an instrument is designed to measure alcohol consumption among adolescents, but only includes questions about beer, it is not a valid measure of alcohol use. Wine and hard liquor are also alcoholic beverages, and must be included in order for the instrument to cover the entire domain of interest and provide a valid assessment of alcohol consumption. Content validity involves both quantitative and qualitative evaluation of an instrument. Generally, content validity is verified in a two-stage process, a developmental stage and a quantification stage. In the developmental stage, each content area is outlined, and representative behaviors or attitudes are identified. In the quantification stage, a number of expert judges (usually five to ten) employ rating scales to quantitatively verify that all relevant content is incorporated into, and measured by, the instrument.

Another type of validity is **face validity.** Face validity involves subjective judgments by experts or respondents about the degree to which the instrument appears to measure the relevant construct. This assessment is sometimes called "armchair validity," because it does not involve a quantitative assessment of the instrument as in content validity appraisal.

A third type of validity is **construct validity.** Construct validity is an estimate of how well a particular instrument measures a theoretical construct. It can be assessed in several ways but cannot be definitively established. Predictions of differences in scores for "known groups" can be compared to actual tested scores to validate an aspect of construct validity. For example, a test of developmental stages in the acquisition of certain cognitive structures can be administered to children of different ages. If the children in the younger age groups perform significantly worse than children in older age groups, some evidence of the validity of the developmental aspect of the construct has been established. Another aspect of construct validity is the degree to which it can differentiate between individuals who possess the trait under study and those who do not. For example, if an instrument is meant to measure anxiety, it should distinguish between anxious and nonanxious individuals.

Criterion-related validity is another type of validity important in the assessment of psychosocial instruments. There are two types of criterion-related validity, predictive validity and concurrent validity. **Predictive validity** assesses how well a score on an instrument can predict future performance. A classic example of predictive validity is the use of SAT and GRE tests to predict future performance in undergraduate or graduate school. These measures are consistently able to predict future performance; individuals who do well on SAT or GRE tests generally do well in college or graduate school. **Concurrent validity** indicates an individual's current standing on a criterion measure related to the construct of interest. For example, individuals who respond to an instrument on leadership style might also be asked to respond to an instrument on the management of people to determine if high scores on one are indicative of high scores on the other, more established instrument. For both predictive and concurrent validity, the correlation between the instrument and the criterion measure is used as the criterion-related validity coefficient.

Feasibility within the Research Plan

Practical considerations must also be taken into account in using a psychosocial instrument because the instrument is used in a larger context that may influence its appropriateness. The research plan specifies how subjects will be recruited and tested. The various methods of approaching subjects differ in the amount of face-to-face contact, the opportunity for explanation or clarification, the time and setting for completing the materials, and many other facets of the data-gathering process.

Consider the differences between receiving a questionnaire in the mail and sitting down with a researcher who is available to answer questions about the instrument. On the one hand, instruments with complex instructions may not be filled out appropriately or completely if the respondent cannot obtain help or is subject to frequent interruptions. On the other hand, the anonymity of the mails may increase the likelihood that the respondent will provide sensitive information such as income level, sexual orientation, or drug habits.

Another aspect of the research context to consider when selecting a measurement instrument is the overall data-gathering plan. Other variables are often measured at the same time. Not only must the overall time of the testing session be within reasonable limits, to prevent fatigue effects, but the researcher must take into account how the various instruments might influence one another. For example, if one of the instruments used measures attitudes toward disabled children and another measures attitudes toward public expenditures for health and welfare, the responses to the second instrument might be influenced by the feelings evoked by thinking about disabled children.

All instruments administered at the same time need to be compatible in their method of administration. For example, a Q-sort, which requires the presence of the research assistant, would not be possible in a mailed self-administered method. It is possible, however, to combine methods if more than one contact is planned with the respondents. Thus, a battery of self-administered questionnaires can be mailed to the respondent, followed (or preceded) by a face-to-face interview or testing session.

Acceptability to Respondents

Another practical issue for consideration is how the subjects are likely to respond to the measurement instrument that is selected for use in the study. Obviously, the instrument must be appropriate for the literacy and educational level of the respondents. Constructs that are likely to vary in specific content or expression for different cultural, ethnic, age, or sex groups should be measured with instruments that have been validated for the intended population in the study.

Less obvious, but equally important, is the fit between the implied values or sensitivities of the instrument and what would be considered acceptable to the respondents. For example, an attitude scale that seems to emphasize conservative attitudes might be regarded as irrelevant to college-age respondents who might refuse to answer parts or all of the questionnaire. This problem becomes particularly acute when the format of the questionnaire involves forced choices between pairs of alternatives, neither of which seems acceptable.

Some instruments have built-in devices to evaluate test-taking behavior. For example, consistency of responses is checked by presenting the same question more than once in the instrument and comparing the responses. Other devices attempt to assess the tendency for the respondent to "fake good" or "fake bad," as in psychological tests that assess personality or functioning. Respondents differ in their tolerance for these techniques, and they may refuse to complete the instrument if they find these features too annoying.

HOW PSYCHOSOCIAL INSTRUMENTS ARE ADMINISTERED

Once appropriate instruments have been selected for measurement of psychosocial variables, the researcher must select the most appropriate method of administration. Many psychosocial instruments can be self-administered, but there are situations in which it may be more appropriate to allow for more face-to-face contact. Depending on the characteristics of the respondents, the situation, and the design of the study, the same instrument might be administered through a self-administered mailing, through an interview, or through a combination of methods.

Factors that a researcher must consider when selecting the method of administering instruments are:

1. anticipated response rate

2. characteristics of the potential subjects

3. complexity of the instructions or task

4. quality of data required

Anticipated Response Rate

Generally, the response rate is higher when subjects are recruited through direct contact. This contact allows the researcher to "sell" the study and to answer questions. When study instruments are mailed to potential subjects, the response rate is much lower. Although there are no absolute rules, response rates of 50% for mailed administration of questionnaires are considered adequate, and rates of 70% are considered very good. Lower response rates are subject to question regarding **response bias;** that is, the sample might not be representative of the population in some systematic way—perhaps having a higher level of education than the nonrespondents. Thus, the validity of a study would be undermined if the researcher obtained too low a response rate. As is the case with any method of administration, the researcher must ensure that the sample is representative of the full population.

Another consideration regarding response rate is the projected sample size required to fulfill the design of the study. If the researcher has determined that at least 100 subjects are needed to conduct the appropriate statistical analyses but the pool of potential subjects is only 200, he or she may not have a sufficient margin to use a mailed administration.

There are techniques for increasing the response rates for mailed administration. These include an enticing cover letter, the promise to report the study findings, and follow-up mailings to remind or urge the person to participate. Similarly, strategies are used to increase the response rate in face-to-face recruitment. By imagining the point of view of potential subjects, the researcher can anticipate some barriers or inducements that influence a patient's decision about participating. Some respondent barriers are logistical, such as needing child care while participating in the study; others reflect the level of motivation to participate in research.

A variety of motivations exist for participating in research. For well-educated respondents, the promise of feedback of the study findings tends to be motivating. A small monetary reimbursement for the respondent's time and effort may facilitate recruiting patients who are highly stressed or overburdened. Patients who have experienced a particularly difficult illness or treatment frequently say that it is rewarding to think that their participation might help others in similar situations.

Characteristics of the Potential Subjects

The most appropriate method of administration depends in part on the subject's educational level, age, eyesight, hearing ability, language, and past experience (or lack of experience) with psychosocial instruments. Patients who have difficulties with any area of functioning that may be needed to complete the instrument would not be appropriate for self-administration methods. Because clinical populations in nursing often do not meet the "ideal" of being healthy, well-educated, and experienced research subjects, creative efforts are required to reach potential participants who are often excluded—for example, non-English speakers or hard-of-hearing patients—in order to increase the clinical relevance of the research.

Complexity of the Instructions or Task

Some methods of data gathering, such as the Q-sort, require direct contact with the subjects because the apparatus includes a large stack of cards to be sorted into piles. Other instruments require direct contact because the instructions are too complex for most individuals to understand without some assistance. Decisions about the complexity of the instructions or the task have to be made in relation to the characteristics of the potential respondents. If the study subjects are all expected to have advanced educational degrees, even instruments with very complex instructions or task requirements can safely be self-administered. Most samples are likely to have a range of individuals, however, and highly complex instruments are not likely to be filled out correctly by all respondents without some direct assistance.

Quality of the Data Required

Different methods of administering psychosocial instruments result in somewhat different responses from subjects. On the one hand, a research interview, as opposed to self-administered questionnaires, permits probing to obtain more detailed data, allows the establishment of rapport to facilitate less superficial responses, and provides for checking the completeness and the accuracy of the data. The quality of the data is usually better—for example, there are fewer "missing data"—when the researcher is available to answer questions and check on the completeness of the responses before the respondent leaves. On the other hand, self-administered instruments, if well constructed, allow for greater uniformity of responses; provide anonymity, which may encourage frankness and honesty; and may be more feasible and economical to reach a larger number, or more representative sample, of people.

HOW PSYCHOSOCIAL INSTRUMENTS ARE SCORED

Scoring instructions are usually provided for instruments, but they can be very complex. Investigators should check their interpretation of the instructions with others and should devise methods to reduce the likelihood of errors in the repetitive task of scoring raw data.

The instructions provided by the developer of the instrument assume that researchers will use methods to avoid introducing errors into the data. Special care must be taken in identifying the appropriate items for each subscale and in the handling of **reverse-scored items** (items worded in the opposite way to avoid response set bias). If the instrument will be hand-scored, templates must be developed for the various groupings of items (subscales, reverse-scored items) to prevent errors at the item level. **Templates** are cardboard or plastic overlays with holes that allow only certain items to be visible. For an instrument with several subscales, for example, there would be a separate template for each subscale. When a template is placed on the questionnaire, only the items for the one designated subscale are visible. The scores for this subscale are calculated according to the instructions on the template, and then the next subscale template is placed on the questionnaire.

Computer scoring not only reduces the time to score data but also greatly reduces the chance of errors. Program statements for scoring are developed to reverse the scores for the items indicated, to compile subscales from designated items, and to calculate any other weightings or transformations of the scores. Obviously, the instructions to the computer must be checked for accuracy or the entire data set will be scored incorrectly.

In dealing with actual data, researchers often encounter inconsistencies due to the respondents' interpretations of instructions, omitting of items, or other irregularities. In the case of the omission of a small number of items from a scale, the scoring instructions might call for substituting the mean score for the missing items or some other standardized method. For example, in a scale of 20 items the mean might be substituted for a small number of missing responses. If too many items have missing responses, however, the respondent's score is not calculated.

Patterns of unanticipated responses may appear in the data. To score these data, the research team develops **decision rules** to be used consistently whenever a similar response occurs. These decision rules ensure that such unusual responses will be scored in the same way for all respondents. For example, on a social support scale a few respondents listed entire families rather than individuals on some lines of their network list. In order to score all respondents in a similar way, the investigators established a uniform way to score the few occasions in which entire families appeared as a single entry on the list. This decision rule reduced the likelihood of experimenter bias in unconsciously manipulating scores for individual respondents. Thus, regardless of the size of the network for the respondent who listed an entire family, the scores for entire families were handled in the same way whenever they were encountered.

Normally, few unusual responses are found in scoring data. In some instances, however, many unusual responses occur. By keeping a log of these responses it is sometimes possible to discover a pattern after many instruments have been scored. In fact, it is sometimes found that a typographical error in some versions of the instrument accounted for the unusual responses.

BIOPHYSIOLOGIC INSTRUMENTS

Nursing research often includes variables that require physiologic instrumentation for their measurement. For example, if a researcher wanted to determine the effects of some specific nursing activity, such as turning, on the intracranial pressure of head-injured patients, instrumentation would be necessary to quantify changes in the dependent variable (intracranial pressure) as influenced by the independent variable (turning). If a researcher wanted to examine the effect of use of the bedside commode on oxygen consumption and heart rate in myocardial infarct patients, instrumentation also would be required to quantify those dependent variables.

An enormous array of biophysiologic phenomena and variables are of interest to nurse researchers. A considerable range of equipment has been used, and it varies widely in level of sophistication. In some situations the equipment is used to create the independent variable, such as equipment for administering oxygen, for suctioning, or for administering tube feedings. In other cases the equipment and instruments are used to measure the dependent variables of interest, such as a thermometer, a scale, a sound-level meter, or an electroencephalogram (EEG) tracing. Whether equipment is used for the independent or the dependent variable depends entirely on the research design and the research questions or hypotheses to be examined.

An example of equipment used to create and specify the independent variable is the treadmill, a platform covered with a moving walking surface. The speed of the moving surface and the angle of the platform can be altered to produce a known physiologic demand. The treadmill is used frequently in research. It is set at certain speeds and at certain gradients to establish different levels of activity as the independent variable; thus the effects of various levels of activity can be studied.

An example of equipment used to quantify changes in the dependent variable is the cardiac monitor (ECG tracing). It is used to determine changes in cardiac rhythm, rate, and conduction patterns in response to varying activity levels. These dependent-variable parameters could be used to assess the effects of drinking ice water on the myocardium in infarct patients. The independent variable, drinking ice water, could be varied by temperature (degree of coldness), amount given, and position assumed for ingestion of the water. In these two rather different studies, the same outcome measures could be used to show changes. The determination of what parameters to quantify is based on the operational definitions of the study variables.

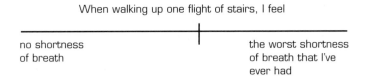

Figure 8–5 *Visual analog scale for measuring one dimension of the biophysiologic variable breathlessness. Using a ruler, the distance from the left end of the scale to the vertical cross line is the measurement.*

Paper-and-Pencil Instruments

Some biophysiologic phenomena are more subjective than objective in nature; pain, fatigue, and nausea are three examples. To quantify these phenomena, the investigator must rely on the subject's perception and evaluation of the magnitude or changes in the sensation experienced. In these instances paper-and-pencil instruments are often used to measure the sensation. The McGill-Melzack Pain Questionnaire (Melzack 1975), the Fatigue Symptom Checklist (Yoshitake 1971), and the Symptom Distress Scale (McCorkle & Young 1978) are classic examples of paper-and-pencil instruments for which some validity and reliability have been established. In addition, visual analog scales have been devised for subjects to rate the magnitude of the perceived sensation. These have a straight line with anchoring words placed at either end of the line. At one end the phrase could be "the worst I have ever had," and at the opposite end, "the least I have ever had." The subjects are given directions to place a mark along the line that best represents what they feel with respect to the phenomenon being assessed, for example, pain or nausea. An example is shown in Figure 8–5.

Some biophysiologic phenomena are assessed according to written criteria developed to quantify the status (or change in status) of individuals. The criteria were determined in respect to the accepted range of normal values. An example is the Glascow Coma Scale; it is used to evaluate an individual's responsiveness to specific graded stimuli (Teasdale & Jennett 1974). After the subject's responses to the listed items are evaluated, a composite score is determined by summing the ratings. Three areas in which the responses are rated are eye opening, best verbal response, and best motor response. The scale is short, and the responses are rated according to well-defined criteria such as eyes open spontaneously = 4, eyes open to speech = 3, to pain = 2, and none = 1. This scale is used clinically as well as for research to assess level of consciousness.

The guiding force for instrument selection, in all cases, must be appropriateness for the phenomena to be studied. There is no inherent value in using a sophisticated invasive measure, such as serum level of lactic acid, if it does not capture the real effect of the variables being studied. Paper-and-pencil instruments should not be ruled out in measuring phenomena just because the variable is physiologic. Remember the guideline of appropriateness: The instrument must measure the phenomena of concern sensitively, reliably, and validly.

Reliability and Validity

The issues of reliability and validity in physiologic measurement can be demonstrated by using the example of an interesting series of studies on the validity and reliability of thermometers as a measure of temperature. These studies illustrate the variability that a single instrument may show under different environmental conditions and when applied using different techniques. The research consumer must constantly read with a cautious eye to see what precautions the investigator has taken to minimize these threats to instrument validity and reliability.

Erickson (1980) examined the effect of sublingual site and type of thermometer on oral temperature. The three sublingual sites were the right and left sublingual pockets and the front sublingual area. The two types of thermometers were electronic and mercury in glass. A second purpose of the study was to examine the effect of insertion technique on temperature readings and thermometer response time. This researcher compared the thermometers to be used in the study against a bath of a known temperature to establish their validity. The electronic thermometers were then calibrated, and the amount of error of the mercury-in-glass thermometers was noted. This researcher used acceptable methods to ensure the validity of her measuring tool. Without this information the data would not be meaningful. The rigor in this approach is important.

Schiffman (1982), who examined the difference between axillary and rectal temperatures in neonates, used the same method to establish the validity of measurement by the thermometers. The researcher and three additional data collectors took the temperatures of the neonates, and the researcher noted that interrater reliability (to be discussed shortly) in reading the thermometers was established when the validity of the thermometers was evaluated. Description of the validity and reliability of instruments was critical to this study. The procedures used to establish validity and reliability make the data believable.

Hasler and Cohen (1982) examined the effects of various means of oxygen administration on oral temperature readings in healthy subjects. They compared subjects' temperatures before oxygen administration with those during oxygen administration. They built on the work of Erickson (1980) in selecting their thermometer placement. No check was made on the validity of measurement by the thermometer, although the investigators did standardize the thermometer used. Because of the failure to check the accuracy of the thermometer, the findings from this study must be questioned.

As a consumer of research, you must consider what role the establishment of validity of measures of physiologic variables has for drawing implications from the study for practice application. Appreciating the need to establish the validity of such a simple measure as taking a temperature suggests that in more sophisticated instruments validity procedures must also be undertaken.

Determining the reliability of an instrument is different from determining **interrater reliability.** Establishing interrater reliability is essential if more than one individual will be collecting the data. For instance, if a study requires collection of data using the calipers, all those who will be measuring the skinfold thickness should practice repeatedly on several different individuals with the calipers and record their measurements. Comparison of the values obtained will provide evidence of the similarity or dissimilarity in the measurements made by the raters. If the measurements obtained on the same individuals are statistically different between the raters, there is obviously a problem in ensuring interrater reliability. The point is that both reliability of the instrument in measuring and reliability across raters in obtaining the measurements must be established. Both of these kinds of reliability issues influence data collection. This kind of information should be included in research reports and clearly must be part of the research plan.

ANNOTATED RESEARCH EXAMPLE

Citation

Weiss SJ. Measurement of the sensory qualities in tactile interaction. *Nurs Res.* 1992;41(2):82–85.

Study Problem/Purpose

A good deal of nursing practice and caregiving to patients depends upon touch. Research has found that touch may influence a number of important patient outcomes. However, there is little agreement among existing studies concerning the meaning and measurement of touch. The purpose of this study was to evaluate the validity and reliability of a measure of interpersonal touch: the Tactile Interaction Index (TII).

The investigator moves toward the development of a standard measure of touch (the TII).

Methods

The TII a measure touch.

Based on an extensive literature review of studies of touch, the investigator defined (operationalized) four aspects or qualities of touch: location, action, intensity, and duration. These dimensions were incorporated into a broader measure or index of touch, the TII. The content validity of the TII was evaluated in the area of nonverbal communication by five experts. Construct validity of the TII was tested by comparing self-report touch experiences in the daily lives of 16 individuals with their scores on the TII. Stability of the TII was evaluated by readministering the index to the 16 individuals a second time, a month after the first administration.

Expert evaluation is one way to measure content validity.

Findings

The five experts evaluating the content validity of the TII achieved 100% agreement on each of the four qualities of touch. The results of the construct validity tests suggested that the TII does measure the construct it purports to measure—touch. The investigator found that individuals who had engaged in

Test-retest reliability demonstrates the stability of the TII over time.

frequent touching in their daily lives and who reported positive experiences related to this touching also participated in varied and extensive touching during a TII evaluation of their touching interaction. Consistency across the two sets of scores for the 16 individuals was moderate to high, suggesting that the TII is a reliable measure of touch.

Guidelines for Critique

What methods of measurement were used for quantifying the study's variables? Does the researcher explain why these measures were chosen?

If a scale has been used, does it meet the criteria of having at least two possible values, being exhaustive, and containing mutually exclusive items?

Has the highest level of scale available (interval or ratio) been used? If not, why not?

What instruments were used in collecting quantitative data? Were they existing or self-developed? What reasons are given for choosing these instruments?

If the instrument was self-developed, has the researcher included a description of the processes used for developing it and methods used to establish its validity and reliability? Has the investigator included a copy of the instrument?

Were measures objective or subjective? Direct or indirect (proxy)?

Were these instruments logical and practical ways of gathering evidence on the study's variables?

Was the data-collection method used appropriate to the study problem and the research purpose?

Did the researcher include checks to guard against possible errors in collecting and recording data?

Was the data-gathering approach appropriate to the particular subjects being studied?

What were the attitudes of the respondents toward the instrument? Could these attitudes have affected their responses?

How was the instrument administered? Why was this method chosen?

What measures were taken to reduce the likelihood of error in scoring the instruments and tabulating raw data?

If the research used biophysiologic instruments, were they used to create independent variables or to quantify changes in dependent variables? What methods were used to ensure the validity and reliability of the instruments?

Summary of Key Ideas and Terms

Scientific measurement involves measuring the attributes or qualities of a phenomenon, referred to as a variable.

Measurement is the process of assigning numerical values to attributes of subjects under investigation.

A *measurement scale* specifies all the potential measurement divisions into which a variable might fall and includes at least two categories that are exhaustive and mutually exclusive.

Psychosocial measures are the most commonly used quantitative data collection methods in nursing research. The range of phenomena included in psychosocial investigation is vast.

Psychosocial variables can be measured subjectively or objectively, directly or indirectly (by *proxy measure*).

A wide variety of instruments are available for measuring psychosocial variables. A researcher should conduct a systematic search for an existing measure before going to the effort of trying to develop a new instrument.

Among the most commonly used psychosocial instruments are rating scales, the semantic differential, sorting techniques, ranking techniques, paired comparisons, patient logs, ability tests, and tests of knowledge.

Ideally, a psychosocial instrument should (1) be congruent with the variable to be studied, (2) demonstrate *reliability* (test-retest reliability, internal consistency, or split-half reliability) and *validity* (content validity, face validity, construct validity, or criterion-related validity), (3) be feasible in the context of the particular study, and (4) be acceptable to respondents.

Factors that a researcher must take into consideration when administering a psychosocial instrument include (1) anticipated response rate, (2) characteristics of the potential subjects, (3) complexity of the instructions or task, and (4) quality of data required.

Scoring of psychosocial instruments employs a variety of methods to reduce the likelihood of errors in the data. Any *reverse-scored items* must be carefully identified, missing responses must be accounted for, and decision rules must be developed for handling unanticipated responses.

Biophysiologic variables are measured with a considerable variety of instruments. These instruments can be used to create independent variables or to measure dependent variables. Some biophysiologic phenomena are subjective and are best measured through paper-and-pencil instruments.

As with any type of instrument, the investigator measuring physiologic variables must take precautions to minimize threats to instrument validity and reliability.

References

Allen MJ & Yen WM. *Introduction to Measurement Theory*. Belmont, Calif: Wadsworth;1979.

American Psychological Association. *Standards for Education and Psychological Tests.* Rev ed. Washington DC;1974.

Erikson R. Oral temperature differences in relation to thermometer technique. *Nurs Res.* 1980;29:157–164.

Gay LR. *Educational Evaluation and Measurement.* 2nd ed. Columbus, Ohio: Charles E. Merrill;1985.

Hasler ME & Cohen JA. The effect of oxygen administration on oral temperature assessment. *Nurs Res.* 1982;31:265–268.

Layton JM & Wykle MH. A validity study of four empathy instruments. *Res in Nurs & Health.* 1990;13:319–325.

McCorkle R & Young K. Development of a symptom distress scale. *Can Nurs.* 1978; 1:373–378.

Melzack R. The McGill Pain Questionnaire: Major properties and scoring methods. *Pain.* 1975;1:277–299.

Schiffman RF. Temperature monitoring in the neonate: A comparison of axillary and rectal temperatures. *Nurs Res.* 1982;31:274–277.

Sitzman J et al. Biofeedback training for reduced respiratory rate in chronic obstructive pulmonary disease: A preliminary study. *Nurs Res.* July/August 1983;32:218–223.

Spielberger CD. *Manual for the State-Trait Anxiety Inventory.* Rev. ed. Palo Alto, Calif: Consulting Psychologists Press;1983.

Teasdale G & Jennett B. Assessment of coma and impaired consciousness: A practical scale. *Lancet.* 1974;2:81–83.

Wallston KA et al. Development of the Multidimensional Health Locus of Control (MHLC) Scales. *Health Education Monographs.* 1978;6:160–170.

Waltz CF, Strickland OL, & Lenz E. *Measurement in Nursing Research.* Philadelphia: F. A. Davis;1984.

Ward MJ & Fetler ME. *Instruments for Use in Nursing Education Research.* Boulder, Colo: Western Interstate Commission for Higher Education;1979.

Ward MJ & Lindeman C, eds. *Instruments for Measuring Nursing Practice and Other Health Care Variables.* Vols 1 and 2. Washington, DC: U.S. Department of Health, Education, and Welfare;1978.

Ward MJ et al, eds. *Instruments for Measuring Nursing Practice and Other Health Care Variables.* Vols 1 and 2. DHEW Publication No. HRA 78-53. Washington, DC: U.S. Government Printing Office;1979.

Yoshitake H. Relations between the symptoms and the feelings of fatigue. *Ergonomics.* 1971;14:175–196.

SAMPLING

BRANDY M. BRITTON

SALLY AMBLER HUTCHINSON

HOLLY SKODOL WILSON

CHAPTER OUTLINE

In This Chapter . . .

CHAPTER OBJECTIVES

After reading this chapter, you should be able to:

- Comprehend the difference between a sample and a population

- Discuss why samples are studied rather than populations

- Discuss the importance of a representative sample

- Classify sampling methods according to probability and nonprobability methods

- Discuss the relevant issues related to sample size

- Discuss sampling with special population groups

- Discuss the relationship of sampling to external validity

9

IN THIS CHAPTER . . .

Intelligent evaluation of research studies requires an understanding of sampling principles. The **population** for a study is the total possible membership of the group being studied. Because it is not always feasible to study everybody in a particular population (such as pregnant teenagers or all psychiatric nurses), a microcosm of the population, called a **sample** of participants or respondents, is usually selected. When a sample is representative, the investigator is in a better position to conclude that the study results are generalizable to the entire population and settings being studied.

This chapter discusses the importance of sampling and explores such key issues as probability versus nonprobability sampling, sample size, and external validity.

SAMPLING

Assume that you have just been selected to be a taster for the nutrition department of your small community hospital. Your job is to taste 30 low-calorie desserts and rate them according to specific criteria. Eating the entire 30 desserts is probably impossible and unnecessary. Rather, you will take a small bite—a sample—of each, which you will assume to be representative of the entire dessert. Sampling is a vital part of the research process, and the strategies for choosing a sample will influence both the results and the researcher's interpretation of them.

A **sample** is a group (of people, records, organizations) drawn from the population. The **population** is the total group being studied, and is often referred to as the *universe* or the *target population*. Figures 9–1 and 9–2 illustrate the difference between the larger population and a sample taken from that population. If a researcher plans to study quadriplegic patients with decubitus ulcers, all such patients are the target population. Because finding and contacting all of these people is impossible, you will choose a sample of quadriplegics with decubitus ulcers. The sample will come from the **accessible population,** the population that is feasible. Perhaps the researcher has access to two large rehabilitation hospitals, to five general hospitals, or to a home health service, all of which care for quadriplegic patients with ulcers. Any of the patients available as subjects would constitute the accessible population.

All researchers use sampling because it is a feasible and logical way of making statements about a larger group based on a smaller group. Studying a sample is much less expensive and much less time-consuming than studying an entire population, or universe. For example, even if a researcher interested in knowing about pregnant women's attitudes toward prenatal care in the United States were able to locate all such women, it would be expensive and time-consuming to talk to every one of them. Rather than attempting to talk to

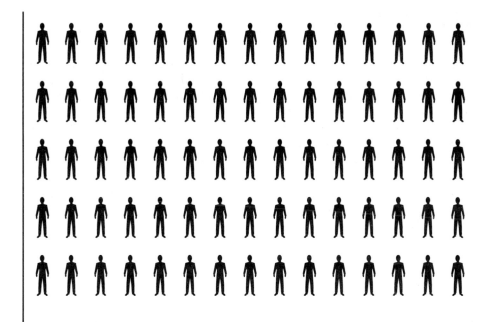

Figure 9–1 *A population from which a sample is drawn.*

every pregnant woman, the researcher studies a sample of these women. If the sampling procedures are carefully thought through and carried out, one can find out about the larger group of pregnant women by talking to only a few of them.

There are two major types of sampling procedures: probability and nonprobability. Each of these types of sampling is further broken down into specific techniques. **Probability sampling** includes the techniques of simple random sampling, systematic sampling, stratified random sampling, and cluster sampling. The techniques of **nonprobability sampling** include convenience sampling, snowball sampling, purposive, or judgment, sampling, expert sampling, and quota sampling. Probability sampling requires that every element in the population have an equal chance—that is, a *random* chance—of being selected for inclusion in the sample. Nonprobability sampling, in contrast, provides no way of estimating the probability that each element will be included in the sample. With the nonprobability approach, the results may not be representative of the larger population. Therefore, generalizing study findings is difficult.

PROBABILITY SAMPLING

Probability sampling procedures are employed to ensure sample representativeness and to avoid sampling bias. A **representative sample** is one that is

---

TABLE 9–1   *Random Numbers*

09 18 82 00 97	32 82 53 95 27	04 22 08 63 04	83 38 98 73 74	64 27 85 80 44
90 04 58 54 97	51 98 15 06 54	94 93 88 19 97	91 87 07 61 50	68 47 66 46 59
73 18 95 02 07	47 67 72 62 69	62 29 06 44 64	27 12 46 70 18	41 36 18 27 60
75 76 87 64 90	20 97 18 17 49	90 42 91 22 72	95 37 50 58 71	93 82 34 31 78
54 01 64 40 56	66 28 13 10 03	00 68 22 73 98	20 71 45 32 95	07 70 61 78 13
08 35 86 99 10	78 54 24 27 85	13 66 15 88 73	04 61 89 75 53	31 22 30 84 20
28 30 60 32 64	81 33 31 05 91	40 51 00 78 93	32 60 46 04 75	94 11 90 18 40
53 84 08 62 33	81 59 41 36 28	51 21 59 02 90	28 46 66 87 95	77 76 22 07 91
91 75 75 37 41	61 61 36 22 69	50 26 39 02 12	55 78 17 65 14	83 48 34 70 55
89 41 59 26 94	00 39 75 83 91	12 60 71 76 46	48 94 97 23 06	94 54 13 74 08
77 51 30 38 20	86 83 42 99 01	68 41 48 27 74	51 90 81 39 80	72 89 35 55 07
19 50 23 71 74	69 97 92 02 88	55 21 02 97 73	74 28 77 52 51	65 34 46 74 15
21 81 85 93 13	93 27 88 17 57	05 68 67 31 56	07 08 28 50 46	31 85 33 84 52
51 47 46 64 99	68 10 72 36 21	94 04 99 13 45	42 83 60 91 91	08 00 74 54 49
99 55 96 83 31	62 53 52 41 70	69 77 71 28 30	74 81 97 81 42	43 86 07 28 34

---

similar to the larger population from which it was drawn with regard to the distribution of major characteristics. In order for research to use sample results to make valid statements or generalizations about the larger unmeasured population, the sample must be representative. Representativeness is enhanced by the use of probability sampling. Probability sampling techniques help prevent collecting a sample that is biased in any particular way. A **biased sample** is one that is not representative of the population it aspires to represent. For example, a researcher wants to find out about attitudes toward drug use among adolescents in a particular city. She or he goes to a local high school cafeteria during lunch hour to recruit participants into the study. The investigator may be more likely to approach individuals of the same gender, or individuals that look approachable and friendly, or she or he may be more likely to talk to people who are sitting by themselves rather than in a group. Further, the investigator will only be exposed to students who eat lunch in the cafeteria and will miss students who go home for lunch or who have cars and leave school during the lunch hour. And what about the choice of the school where she or he is recruiting participants? Is it public or private? What about the ethnic makeup of the school? When nonprobability procedures are used, the sample is likely to be biased in some way, and may include some groups while excluding others. Biased samples make generalizing research findings difficult.

Simple Random Sampling

The best-known probability sampling approach is simple random sampling. Each individual in the **sampling frame** (all subjects in the population) has an equal chance of being chosen. If a researcher plans to study patients with

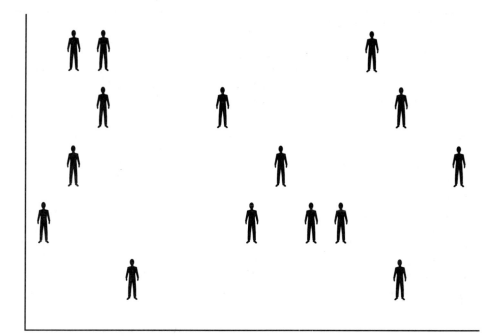

Figure 9–2   *A sample: a subset of the larger population.*

acquired immune deficiency syndrome (AIDS), for example, he or she will need a list of all of the patients who make up this population. To select the sample, the researcher can:

- assign a number to each member of the population, and utilize a table of random numbers, such as Table 9–1.

- with eyes closed, use a pencil to point to a number on the table.

- move in a systematic way—up, down, or diagonally—choosing the sample by picking those subjects whose numbers correspond to the table of random numbers.

- stop when the desired sample size is obtained.

Other methods of random selection may be used as long as they ensure that each subject has an equal chance of selection. Such methods include putting well-mixed names in a hat or shuffling name cards thoroughly and then selecting the required number from a deck. Today it is common for computers to randomly select cases for a study. Once the sampling frame is entered into the computer, the computer program numbers the elements in the sampling frame and generates its own series of random numbers.

Systematic Sampling

Systematic sampling involves drawing every *n*th element from a population. If a researcher wanted to do a survey of nurses who subscribe to the *American*

Journal of Nursing, he or she could begin as with the random sample, by (with closed eyes) pointing to a number and then choosing every *n*th number that follows. This method is technically called a systematic sample with a random start. The **sampling interval** is the distance between elements or subjects selected in the sample. The sampling interval is decided by dividing the entire sampling frame by the number of subjects needed for the study. For example, if the sampling frame contains 300 individuals, and 30 subjects are needed for the study, the sampling interval is ten. If the randomly selected start number is 11, every tenth element after 11 is picked. Numbers 21, 31, 41, 51, and so on are drawn until all subjects are selected. It is important that the sampling interval be calculated based on the entire sampling frame and the number of subjects needed for the study, so that every element has an equal chance of being selected. For example, suppose a study is being conducted in which only five subjects are needed, the sampling frame is still 300, the sampling interval is still ten, and the random start number is again 11. Every element in the sampling frame will not have an equal chance of being selected. Five subjects will be chosen rather quickly, and the numbers at the end of the list will not have a chance to be included. This biases the sample toward individuals at the beginning of the list.

Systematic sampling results in a representative sample if the sampling frame doesn't have any built-in bias. For example, bias would result if *AJN*'s circulation lists were arranged in such a way that nurse subscribers were listed by state or by year of beginning subscription. Instead of getting a sample representative of subscribers, the researcher might get a sample that included only nurses in the Northeast or only nurses who had subscribed for ten or more years. Systematic sampling is generally used when a list of the sampling frame is available because it is more efficient and less time-consuming than simple random sampling.

Stratified Random Sampling

A **stratum** is a subpopulation, and **strata** are two or more homogeneous subpopulations. Examples of strata of interest to nursing include patients who have certain diseases, patients who live in specified areas, or patients who require certain treatments. Major political polls use stratified random sampling, assessing different strata of the population. To use this method, a researcher:

1. selects a population and determines the relevant strata.
2. samples a number of people in each stratum. The number in a sample should be the same as the proportion of the group in the total population. For example, if the population is patients with collagen diseases and the strata are patients with lupus (3% of the population), patients with arthritis (95% of the population), and patients with scleroderma (2% of the population), the same proportions should be used in the sample—3% lupus patients, 95% arthritis patients, and 2% scleroderma patients.

3. chooses the subjects within each of the categories according to random sampling methods.

Cluster Sampling

Cluster sampling requires that the population be divided into groups, or clusters. If a researcher is studying associate degree nursing students, he or she may not have the time, money, or ability to get all the individuals' names, but may have a list of the associate degree schools in the area. The sample is therefore randomly derived from this list of clusters (schools). The researcher can sample all students in each chosen cluster or only randomly selected students from each cluster.

Most large-scale surveys use cluster sampling because simple or stratified random sampling involves too many subjects from too many places, resulting in much wasted time, money, and energy.

A Critique of Probability Sampling

Probability sampling is based on probability theory, which focuses on the possibility of events occurring by chance (Kerlinger 1973, Winer 1962). Probability sampling is less likely to result in a biased sample that is not representative of the population because it insists that each element in the population have an equal chance of being selected. Ensuring a representative sample avoids bias, making it possible to generalize research results to the accessible population.

Sampling error can be estimated with probability sampling. *Sampling error* refers to the differences between sample values and population values. Some amount of sampling error is inevitable in any research study, but probability sampling does allow estimates of the degree of expected error. (For more about this, see Cohen 1977.)

Probability sampling with small populations (for example, patients with liver transplants) may be efficient and effective. If the group is homogeneous, however, sophisticated sampling is not necessary. In nursing, because we deal with human beings and thus many variables, it is unlikely that our population is ever homogeneous. Most people are different psychologically, culturally, or socioeconomically, bringing homogeneity into question.

In life, it is said, death and taxes are the only certainties. In sampling, there is no certainty that a probability sample ensures everyone's participation. If a group is underrepresented or refuses to participate for whatever reasons, a biased sample may result.

NONPROBABILITY SAMPLING

Nonprobability sampling is nonrandom sampling of subjects. Therefore, it offers less chance of obtaining a representative sample. Most nursing research involves nonprobability sampling.

Convenience Sampling

Convenience sampling allows the use of any available group of research subjects. For example, to study children in well-baby clinics, a researcher might pick a public clinic because of its geographical proximity and because of its ready accessibility. These children are relevant subjects, and they are available. Because of a lack of randomization in sampling, however, they may be atypical of well babies in some unidentified ways. The investigator has no control over the sampling process—the sample, the sampling representativeness, or the possible biases.

Snowball Sampling

Snowball sampling is a kind of convenience sampling. It involves subjects' suggesting other subjects to the researcher, so that the sampling process gains momentum, like a snowball rolling down a hill. A nurse was studying women prisoners with an in-depth interview technique. Because only certain women were willing to be involved, the researcher asked each prisoner after the interview to suggest one or two other prisoners who might be interested in participating. This was a convenient and effective way of soliciting subjects. Of course, sampling bias was likely to be present, because women who agreed to participate might have been different from those who did not agree.

Snowball sampling is used if subjects are difficult to identify because they are hidden in the population (transsexuals, faith healers, women who have had abortions), but who may be part of an informal network. Brink and Wood (1983) use the term *network sampling* and say it is useful in finding "socially devalued urban populations such as addicts, alcoholics, child abusers, and criminals," because these people are usually hidden from outsiders.

Purposive, or Judgment, Sampling

In **purposive sampling** the researcher selects a particular group or groups based on certain criteria. In this subjective sampling method the researcher uses his or her judgment to decide who is representative of the population. Because objectivity is lacking, this method is not recommended except in certain circumstances. For example, if a researcher wanted to test an instrument to measure stress in patients who have just been admitted to the hospital, she or he could use a purposive sample of patients from surgical units, CCU units, labor and delivery units, medical units, and outpatient units. A pretest with such heterogeneous groups might offer interesting information. Or a researcher who wanted to validate an instrument measuring self-concept or locus of control might give it to normal adults, normal teenagers, depressed adults, and depressed teenagers. The researcher would expect group differences to be evidenced in the test scores. If there were no group differences, the validity of the instrument would be called into question.

Expert Sampling

Expert sampling is a type of purposive sampling that involves choosing experts in a given area because of their access to the information of relevance to a study. The **Delphi technique** uses expert sampling. Several rounds of questionnaires focusing on a specific topic are sent to experts, with the aim of eliciting their opinions. After data analysis the questions are reformulated and sent out again. The aim is for fairly rapid group consensus.

Quota Sampling

In **quota sampling** the researcher makes a decision, based on judgment, about the best type. of sample for the study. For example, a researcher studying nurses' attitudes toward nurses who have problems with chemical abuse might want to get a representative quota of male and female nurses from different age groups and with different educational preparation. The researcher decides what the strata are, based on the variables that might affect the dependent variable being investigated. The gender and age of nurses probably affect their attitudes toward nurses with chemical abuse problems (dependent variable). Their educational preparation might also be a meaningful stratum. Since 3% of nurses are male and 97% are female, similar percentages can be drawn for the study. Since W% of nurses are ages 20 up to 30, X% are 30 up to 40, Y% are 40 up to 50, and Z% are 50 and up, the sample can reflect these same proportions.

With quota sampling a researcher can also sample *matched pairs*. This means selecting the sample based on predetermined important characteristics. For example, a researcher comparing how preoperative education affects cardiac bypass and angioplasty patients' behavior postoperatively might match the patients according to risk factors, such as age, weight, exercise, and smoking.

Quota sampling is used when an investigator cannot select a random sample but aims for more control than is possible with accidental, or convenience, sampling. Subjects are selected if they fit the criteria for each stratum as set by the researcher. The aim is to reduce bias or sampling error.

A Critique of Nonprobability Sampling

Most nursing researchers settle for nonprobability sampling because the population is too unknown to obtain a random sample or because the expense in time and money of a random sample is too great. Also, informed consent is vital in research, and this requirement decreases the possibility of a random sample. Instead, subjects are willing, informed participants who have the freedom to withdraw from a study at any time.

Because nursing research studies regularly use nonprobability samples, researchers need to be knowledgeable about the strengths and limitations of each type and attempt to make the sample as representative as possible.

Caution in generalizing findings of studies with nonprobability samples beyond what is warranted is important.

As the previous discussion demonstrates, there are a number of different sampling techniques within probability and nonprobability sampling. Decisions about which sampling technique to use in a particular study depend on the study's aims, the research questions, the target population, and the resources available to the investigator. Table 9–2 provides a general overview of conditions under which each sampling procedure is commonly used.

SAMPLE SIZE

Of vital importance in every researcher's mind is the question, "How many subjects do I need?" As is true of much of the research process, there are no hard and fast rules for sample size. Rather, the investigator must consider the research purpose, the design, and the size of the population. Generally, with the exception of case studies, the larger the sample, the more valid and accurate the study, because a larger sample is more likely to be representative of the population. Depending on circumstances, however, a large or small number of subjects may be appropriate.

If the population being studied is homogeneous, the researcher can use a smaller sample than if it is heterogeneous. For instance, a study examining the experiences of breast-feeding mothers will involve much variability, because mothers of all ages, of all socioeconomic groups, and of all ethnic groups breast-feed. A study of the health habits of eighth-grade girls in a private school, on the other hand, will have less variability. The girls are approximately the same age and come from the same socioeconomic group, so a smaller sample will be more likely to yield "typical" subjects.

Investigators who use a research design that requires numerous treatment groups (experimental design) must determine the number of subjects needed for the smaller groups (called cells) and not just for the entire study. For example, if an investigator were to study the use of Orem's self-care model by chronically ill geriatric patients, she or he would not base decisions about sample size exclusively on the entire group of geriatric patients needed. Perhaps the design requires that a comparison be made between patients in a private hospital and patients in a public hospital, or between cardiac patients and cancer and kidney patients. Because of all these subgroups of interest, more subjects would be required than if the study merely examined a single group of chronically ill patients. In order to compare the groups with one another on dependent variables (or outcomes) of interest, it is necessary to decide the cell size for each subsample and then add these together to get the total number of subjects, or *n*. If the cell size is too small (ten or fewer), the treatment mean, or average, is more likely to be changed dramatically by one atypical number. A cell size of 20 or more generally yields more accurate

TABLE 9–2   *Commonly Used Sampling Techniques*

Sampling Procedure	Conditions under Which the Procedure Is Typically Used
Probability Sampling Procedures	
Simple random sampling	Survey research in which the investigator wants to avoid sample bias and ensure that every element has an equal chance of being in the study
Systematic sampling	Survey research when a list of the sampling frame is available
Stratified random sampling	Survey research in which the investigator wants to study particular homogeneous strata or subpopulations
Cluster sampling	Survey research when it is difficult and/or expensive to obtain an exhaustive list of the population
Nonprobability Sampling Procedures	
Convenience sampling	Surveys or experiments in which an easily accessible group is required
Snowball sampling	Surveys or experiments in which study participants are difficult to identify, hard to locate, or socially devalued
Purposive, or judgment, sampling	Surveys or experiments in which the researcher wants to study a group or groups based on particular characteristics or circumstances
Expert sampling	Surveys in which experts on a particular subject are necessary
Quota sampling	Surveys or experiments in which the investigator has hypotheses about different strata or subpopulations

results and allows more options during statistical analysis. However, in nursing, because of all the variables we must control, getting even a cell size of 10 is often very difficult, at times impossible. Case studies and case histories require even fewer subjects, usually between one and ten.

Survey designs frequently use many more subjects than observational or experimental designs, because telephoning or mailing questionnaires to a large number of people is feasible, whereas observing large numbers of people may not be. However, survey research has a different problem associated with it, that of low response rate. Often people are not willing or able to take the time to fill out a questionnaire and mail it back to an investigator. In deciding on the sample size for survey research, an investigator must keep the possibility of a low response rate in mind.

Power analysis is another important issue to consider when deciding on sample size. **Power** refers to the probability that an inferential statistical test will reject the null hypothesis and allow an investigator to declare that the research hypothesis is supported. Generally speaking, power is related to sample size and **effect size** (the frequency of the phenomenon under study in the population being investigated). The larger the sample size, the more power a researcher has, or the more able he or she is to detect group differences. The larger the effect size, the more power the researcher has. Cohen (1977) has written extensively on power analysis. A statistical consultant can also be helpful in determining the required sample size for a study by making a power analysis.

A thorough review of the literature will reveal size samples typical for certain types of research questions and designs used in nursing research. However, be aware that in many studies the sample size is too small and therefore should be viewed with a critical eye.

SAMPLING FROM SPECIAL POPULATION GROUPS

Special population groups present practical and ethical problems to researchers. Access to certain patient groups may be difficult or require extra effort by the researcher. According to Sexton (1983), some problems confronting researchers who study the chronically ill (COPD patients) include:

- identification of subjects and their reluctance to participate in studies—a problem of sufficient sample size.

- implementation of certain designs (a panel study, longitudinal, experimental, or correlational) due to the exacerbations, remissions, and mortality of the illness—a problem of limited study designs.

- consideration of the feasibility of the energy and the abilities required of the patient for each type of data collection—a problem of data collection.

Nurses should not be reluctant to pursue research with chronically ill patients but must focus energy on working toward the best and most feasible approach, taking into account the typical problems these patients present.

Children, the mentally ill, the mentally retarded, and the elderly are also people who require special consideration by the nurse researcher. Although informed consent aims to protect patients' rights, it sometimes is less than effective. General agreement seems to exist on two points (Hayter 1979):

1. Persons who are unable to give their own informed consent should not be research subjects if other subjects can be used.

2. The less able people are to protect themselves, the more vigilant the investigator must be in protecting them.

SAMPLING AND EXTERNAL VALIDITY

Research purpose and design affect how important representativeness, which yields external validity, is. Different types of research questions require, to a greater or lesser degree, representative samples. In descriptive research, which aims to describe behaviors or attitudes of a group, representativeness is very important, because the researcher is aiming for descriptive accuracy (external validity). If the sample is biased or not representative, the description will be inaccurate and invalid.

Investigators conducting methodological studies will need to be concerned with all types of reliability, internal validity—content, construct, and criterion-based validity—and external validity. Those conducting case studies or case histories may be more concerned with illustrating or generating theory; for them the issue of representativeness is not critical. In contrast, representativeness and external validity are of great significance in experimental studies. Because obtaining representative samples in experimental nursing studies is often impossible, however, replication studies are useful in establishing external validity.

Sampling is a complex but essential stage in the research process. Some authors have devoted entire books to the various sampling procedures. For more information, review the References.

ANNOTATED RESEARCH EXAMPLE

Citation

Geritz MA. Saline versus heparin in intermittent infuser patency maintenance. *West J Nurs Res.* 1992;14(2):131–137.

Study Problem/Purpose

The use of venous access devices for intermittent therapies is a routine nursing practice. While the patency of these devices is often maintained by regular flushing with heparin-sodium chloride solutions, the concentration of the irrigating solution has not been uniformly established. The purpose of this study was to determine the most appropriate ratio of heparin to saline in solutions used to flush and maintain venous access devices. A second goal of the study was to recommend and develop a standardized mix for these solutions for use in hospitals across the United States.

Methods

sample size = 90.

A double-blind and quasi-experimental study of 90 subjects with 150 intravenous access devices was conducted in a 200-bed general hospital in the Southwest. A convenience sampling procedure was employed to recruit patients admitted to five different units within the hospital. Subjects were

the sample may not be representative of all individuals with intravenous access devices in the larger population.

convenience sampling is a nonprobability sampling technique.

[handwritten margin note, left:] The non-non-random, non-representative sample may pose a threat to external validity.

[handwritten margin note, right:] The study sample was drawn from the feasible or accessible population of a southwestern hospital. Because convenience sampling was used (a non-random technique) to recruit subjects, the study finding may not be valid.

randomly assigned to receive one of two different irrigating solutions to flush their venous access devices. The first solution tested was 0.9% sodium chloride; the second was 0.9% sodium chloride with ten units of heparin added. Subjects were monitored over a 60-day time period for evidence of phlebitis at the access site or loss of patency of the intravenous device.

Findings

There were no significant differences between the saline-only solution and the heparin-saline solution with respect to phlebitis and device patency. Normal saline, which is less expensive and has less potential for interfering with the administration of a number of medications, was found to be as effective in maintaining the patency of intravenous devices as heparin solutions.

Guidelines for Critique

What type of sampling procedure did the investigator employ?

Did the investigator choose a probability or nonprobability sample? Is a rationale given for the choice?

Is the sample representative of the population to which the findings are being generalized?

What strategies were used to avoid collecting a biased sample?

Is the sample size large enough to allow for meaningful statistical analysis?

How were the rights of subjects protected?

Summary of Key Ideas and Terms

Sampling is the process of selecting observations, elements, or individuals to be studied. A sample is drawn from the larger population about which the researcher wishes to make conclusions or generalizations.

A sample is drawn and studied because studying it is more feasible and much less expensive than studying an entire population, or universe.

In order for a researcher to make inferences about a population, a sample must be representative of that population.

A *biased sample* is one in which certain groups important to the study have been excluded.

The research purpose should lead an investigator to appropriate subjects for the sample.

There are two major types of sampling: *probability sampling* and *nonprobability sampling.*

Probability sampling, the most rigorous sampling approach, requires that every element in the population have an equal (random) chance of being included in the study. Types of probability sampling include simple random sampling, systematic sampling, stratified random sampling, and cluster sampling.

With *nonprobability sampling* the results are representative of the sample only and cannot be generalized to a larger population. Types of nonprobability sampling include convenience sampling, snowball sampling, purposive (judgment) sampling, expert sampling, and quota sampling.

Most nursing studies use nonprobability sampling, because the population is too unknown to obtain a random sample, or because the expense of time and money for a random sample is too great.

Sample size is very important and is dependent on the research purpose, the design, and the size of the population. Generally, the larger the sample, the more valid and accurate the study.

Special population groups, such as the chronically ill, children, the elderly, the mentally ill, and the mentally retarded, present practical and ethical problems to researchers.

References

Brink P & Wood M. *Basic Steps in Planning Nursing Research, from Question to Proposal.* Belmont, Calif: Wadsworth;1983.

Cohen J. *Statistical Power Analysis for the Behavioral Sciences.* New York: Academic Press;1977.

Cranley M et al. Women's perceptions of vaginal and cesarean deliveries. *Nurs Res.* 1983;32:10–15.

Hayter J. Issues related to human subjects. In *Issues in Nursing Research.* Downs F & Fleming J (editors). New York: Appleton-Century-Crofts;1979.

Holm K. Single subject research. *Nurs Res.* 1983;32:253–255.

Kerlinger F. *Foundations of Behavioral Research.* New York: Holt, Rinehart & Winston;1973.

Muhlenkamp A et al. Attitudes toward women in menopause: A vignette approach. *Nurs Res.* 1983;32:20–23.

Scott D. Anxiety, critical thinking and information processing during and after breast biopsy. *Nurs Res.* 1983;32:24–28.

Sexton D. Some methodological issues in chronic illness research. *Nurs Res.* 1983; 32:378–380.

Toney L. The effects of holding the newborn at delivery on paternal bonding. *Nurs Res.* 1983;32:16–19.

Weaver R H. An exploration of paternal-fetal attachment behavior. *Nurs Res.* 1983; 32:68–72.

Winer B J. *Statistical Principles in Experimental Design.* New York: McGraw-Hill;1962.

QUANTITATIVE DATA ANALYSIS: STATISTICAL

SECOND EDITION
REVISION BY

BRANDY M. BRITTON

CHAPTER OUTLINE

In This Chapter . . .

- Descriptive Statistics
    - Frequency Distributions
    - Measures of Central Tendency
    - Measures of Variability
    - Measuring the Relationship between Two Variables
- Inferential Statistics
    - Inferring from a Sample to a Population
    - Estimation
    - The General Logic of Hypothesis Tests
    - Statistical Tests
- Use of Computers in Statistical Analysis

Research in Nursing Second Edition by Joyce A. Verran and Sandra Ferketich

CHAPTER OBJECTIVES

After reading this chapter, you should be able to:

- Differentiate between descriptive and inferential statistics

- Explain the processes for calculating frequency distributions; measures of central tendency, including the mode, median, and mean; and measures of variability, including the range, the interquartile range, the variance, and the standard deviation

- Interpret descriptive statistics from graphic presentations in research articles

- Explain the logic and language associated with inferential statistics

- Identify whether parametric or nonparametric statistics have been used in a nursing study

- Compare and contrast appropriate use and interpretations of *t*-tests and analyses of variance (ANOVA)

- Discuss nonparametric statistical procedures

- Recognize when advanced multivariate statistics are required

- Describe the use of computers in performing statistical analyses

10

IN THIS CHAPTER . . .

Once data have been collected, statistical analysis procedures constitute the initial tools that are used to interpret or make meaning out of the findings in relation to the study's theoretical framework and its specific research problem. This chapter presents the information you'll need as a consumer of nursing research to interpret, evaluate, and base decisions on the growing body of statistical data applicable to improving nursing practice.

Studying statistics in relation to nursing research should not become a matter of calculated tedium, fear, or trepidation. Nor should you shy away from this topic because you think of statistics as inappropriate for nurses who are dedicated to discovering the truth through case studies and field research. Unless you can interpret statistics and know the worth of the data and conclusions, you risk basing your practice decisions, and the health care decisions of patients who consult with you, on poor information.

In this era of pocket calculators and personal computers a reasonable degree of competence in the field of statistics need not involve complete mastery of all complex derivation computations. Once you know what statistics are appropriate, can interpret their meaning, can translate them into words, and can arrive at logical conclusions based on them, you probably need not become involved in elaborate mathematical calculations.

This chapter introduces you to the statistical concepts and operations used in much of contemporary nursing research. They are presented in the hope that being able to think statistically will sharpen your ability to think critically about nursing research. The kind of statistical knowledge that this chapter emphasizes will help you sustain a healthy attitude of skepticism when you read in the local newspaper that "a high proportion of women who take birth control pills have strokes" or that "compulsive jogging is just like anorexia nervosa." Furthermore, it will instruct you in the various considerations necessary to avoid inadvertently using statistics yourself that mislead others. If you, as a reader of research, are able to detect the misuse of statistics, you have gained important knowledge with which to decide if an investigator's conclusions are justified.

Some say that the element of *uncertainty* sets statistics apart from other areas of applied mathematics. In arithmetic, algebra, and geometry, conclusions can actually be proven. In statistics, the ultimate aim is only to show that something is either *more* or *less likely* to occur. While it would be advantageous to know for certain that a specific treatment will be effective, in many situations this isn't possible. In some of those situations, however, a treatment is *likely* to be effective. Systematically knowing even that much about the outcome of a particular nursing intervention is an advance in the scientific basis for a practice far beyond trial and error or the authority of tradition. Statistics are valuable tools for analyzing numerical data to answer certain research questions relevant to nursing practice and building the knowledge base for the discipline.

In the pages that follow, statistics are covered as both a collection of numerical facts expressed in terms that describe and summarize quantitative data, and as tools for going beyond description to use results as a basis for speculation and prediction. Thus, both *descriptive statistics,* which organize, summarize, and present information in a usable, understandable form, and *inferential statistics,* which are concerned with making inferences about populations based on samples taken from them, get full treatment.

DESCRIPTIVE STATISTICS

Descriptive statistics are summary statistics and visual displays that illustrate the characteristics of a study's sample. Descriptive statistics include measures of central tendency, dispersion, and association. The term may also apply to tables and graphs used to display the results of these procedures.

Descriptive analysis includes a range of possible statistical operations, from crude to precise methods of summarizing an entire data set. The choice depends first, of course, on the study question and then on the level of measurement at which data were collected. Imagine that a school nurse has administered a number of assessment tests (visual, hearing, intelligence, personality inventories, health histories, and physical exams) to a group of elementary schoolchildren. What are some of the strategies available for transforming this vast array of data into some useful and meaningful form? She or he could:

1. rearrange the various scores according to how often they occurred to get an overall picture of the data set

2. construct tables, graphs, and figures to permit visualization of the data

3. convert raw scores to other types of score such as percentile ranks or standard scores

4. calculate averages on each important variable to learn something about the typical status of the group

5. figure out the ranges or dispersion of scores and ratings in relation to the central point

6. look for relationships or correlations between two or more different measurements

All of the procedures in this list represent various kinds of descriptive statistics. Let's look at some methods that will accomplish summarizations such as this.

Frequency Distributions

A **frequency distribution** represents one way of organizing a mass of what might appear at first to be overwhelming and chaotic information. It involves systematically arranging numerical values from the lowest to the highest, or

Table 10–1   *Frequency Distribution of Test Scores ($\underline{n} = 55$)*

Raw Score (a)	Frequency (b)	Percent (c)*
28	1	2
27	1	2
26	2	4
25	5	9
24	5	9
23	9	16
22	10	18
21	5	9
20	6	11
19	4	7
18	3	5
17	3	5
16	0	0
15	1	2

*Rounding causes a slight variation from 100%.

from highest to lowest, and then counting the number of times each value appears in the data. A frequency distribution lets the researcher quickly see what the lowest and highest scores are, where most of the scores tend to cluster, and, in fact, what the most commonly obtained score is (see Table 10–1). The construction of frequency distributions and frequency tables is really a rather simple process. If you are working with an extremely large number of measures, a computer program can construct frequency tables for you automatically. The steps for constructing a frequency distribution manually are:

1. Find the lowest and highest scores or numbers in the data set.

2. Decide what the class interval will be to group scores together and how many classes of grouped scores you will have.* Arrange them from lowest to highest value. Be sure that the classes of observation are mutually exclusive and exhaustive.

3. A simplified table has columns for (a) each class, (b) the frequency, or count, of how often the class appeared in the data, and (c) the percentage of the total for each class.

4. Read through the raw data sequentially and make a mark in the count column using the familiar method of four vertical lines and then a slash for the fifth occurrence (卌).

5. Add up all the frequencies, called the *f*s, and put the total number for each class in the *frequency* column. The sum of the numbers in that column ought to equal the total size of the sample ($\Sigma f = n$).

*Generally fewer than 5 or more than 15 classes are not helpful. Too few classes mask smaller variations in the data whereas too many classes are difficult to read. Since few categories were needed to describe the data in this example, raw scores were used.

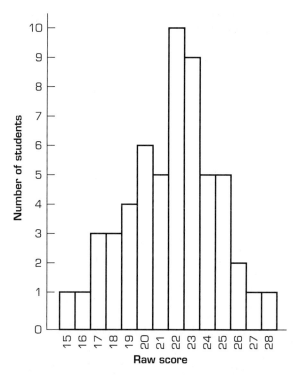

Figure 10–1   *Histogram based on test scores from Table 10–1.*

6. Complete the percentage column by dividing each frequency by the total number of data items and multiplying by 100 (% = 100 × f/n).

Many research studies that you read may display frequency data in **histograms** or **frequency polygons.** These are simply ways of displaying in graphic form the same information contained in a frequency table. In the histogram in Figure 10–1 you can see that the vertical axis contains the frequency totals, with a zero at the bottom and the highest frequency at the top. The horizontal axis contains the classes of totals, with the lowest value on the left and the highest value on the right. Next, bars are drawn in the shape of rectangles over each class of score with a height equal to the frequency of that particular class. In the case of frequency polygons, dots connected by straight lines are used instead of bars to show the number of times that a class occurs. Figure 10–2 shows a frequency polygon. Some researchers and consumers believe that such visual depictions of frequency information are easier and quicker to read than a table.

A set of measures of the same thing are called a **distribution,** which is characterized by shape. Shape is either symmetrical or nonsymmetrical (also called skewed). **Symmetrical distributions** are shaped so that if divided into halves, the halves could be folded over on each other and fit almost exactly (see Figure 10–3). **Skewed distributions** have off-center peaks or humps and longer tails in one direction or another. If the longer tail points to the right, it

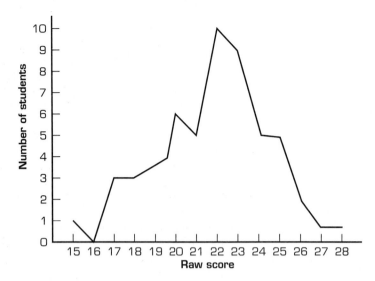

Figure 10–2   *Frequency polygon based on test scores from Table 10–1.*

is called *positively skewed;* if the longer tail points to the left, it is called *negatively skewed.* An example of data that would appear as a skewed frequency distribution is the age at which American women complete menopause, because the majority of subjects would be located in the later half of life. (See Figure 10–4 for examples of skewed distributions.)

Distributions are also characterized by the modality of their shape. A **unimodal distribution** has only one high point, while a **bimodal** or **multimodal** shape has two or more (see Figure 10–5). The most common type of symmetrical, unimodal curve is called a normal curve. A normal curve is bell shaped, with the greatest frequency at the center. As you move away from the center, the frequencies become smaller and smaller.

Measures of Central Tendency

Comparing frequency distributions is one way to make some sense of an array of numerical data. But it can also be somewhat awkward when several groups or conditions must be taken into account. In many cases a group pattern is of less importance than some statistic that can summarize some aspect of a distribution in a single number. Whenever a researcher is interested in questions like "What is the APGAR score of most babies born at home birth centers?" or "What is the average length of hospital stay for open heart surgery patients?" the researcher is raising questions of **central tendency.** *Central* refers to a middle value, and *tendency* refers to the general trend of the numbers. The three main measures of central tendency are the mode, the median, and the mean.

The Mode   The **mode** is the most frequent or common score in a set of data. It is most often used as a measure of central tendency for nominal data. For a

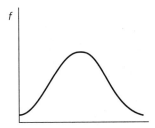

Figure 10–3 *Symmetrical distribution.*

frequency distribution of data from a nominal scale, in which the data are assigned arbitrary numerical labels, the mode is the only measure of central tendency that makes sense. Calculations of the mean and median, discussed in the sections that follow, require equidistant categories, or ordered categories. Neither of these is possible with a nominal scale.

Data may have more than one mode. Data with a single mode are called unimodal; data with two modes are bimodal. If data have several modes, the mode is not a very useful measure of central tendency. In the extreme case, each value in a data set occurs only once, and such data have no mode. Researchers figure out the mode by inspecting the frequency distributions of their data. Computers can also do this task. In the case of a symmetrical distribution with a single peak, the mode will be the same value as the median or the mean (if you can calculate them). The mode identifies the most "popular score." Uses of modes in further statistical analyses are, however, limited.

The Median   The **median** is the measure that corresponds to the middle score because it lies at the midpoint of the distribution and divides the scores into halves. The median is calculated by arranging the scores in increasing order and finding the score that divides the sample in half. The median cannot be calculated for nominal data, but is appropriate for ordinal, interval, and ratio level data. One major characteristic of the median is its insensitivity to extreme scores. While the mean, discussed in the following section, is excessively influenced by extreme values, the median is not. This can work as a limitation or an advantage, depending on a study's objectives. For example, if

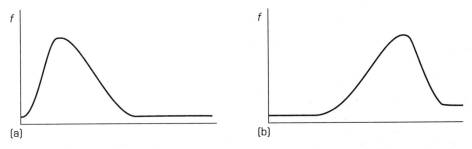

Figure 10–4 *Examples of skewed distributions. (a) Positive skew; (b) negative skew.*

a set of scores on an AIDS knowledge test administered to five patients is 12, 15, 22, 31, and 35, the median score is 22, and the mean is 23. However, if one value changes and the set of scores is 12, 15, 22, 31, and *125,* for example, the median is still 22, while the mean is now 41.

The Mean   The **mean** (*arithmetic mean*) of a set of measurements is simply the sum of the values divided by the total number of subjects. This measure of central tendency, also called the *average,* is the most widely used one in statistical tests of significance. Most researchers attest that of all the measures of central tendency, the mean is the most stable and the most reliable. If you calculate means of different samples drawn from the same population, they will fluctuate or vary less than modes or medians. However, the mean is also excessively influenced by extreme values and can be "pulled" in the direction of those extreme values.

Because calculating the mean involves the addition of different values, the mean can only be properly calculated for intervally scaled data, as categories must be ordered and equidistant. Whether the mean is necessarily the best statistic to describe the center of intervally scaled measures depends on whether the frequency distribution is *symmetrical* and *unimodal.* Skewed distributions will have means that lie below the distribution's peak, and the mean for a bimodal distribution may fall between the two humps and not be very representative of actual values.

The basis for a decision to use the mode, median, or mean as a measure of central tendency is the nature of the study question and the shape of the distribution. If a researcher wants to know what a typical well baby weighs at a certain age, but there are extremes at one end of the distribution, the median is the best statistic. If the problem is to determine whether two groups of patients receiving different nursing care for decubiti are different on an attribute, the researcher will need to use the mean. If an investigator wants to know what the self-care ability of the majority of a nursing home population is, he or she will go for the mode. Figure 10–6 provides illustrations of measures of central tendency in normal and skewed distributions.

Measures of Variability

The purpose of describing the central tendencies of data is to describe the ways subjects group together. The **variability,** in contrast, examines the dispersion, or how the measures are spread out. If the scores in a data set are very similar, there is little variability. Two sets of data with the same sample size and same mean could, however, be very different in terms of the set spread or distribution of the measurements (see Figure 10–6a). A measure of central tendency without a corresponding measure of variability provides limited information about the distribution.

The most common descriptions of variability are the range, the interquartile range, and the standard deviation. Let's start with the range.

The Range   The **range** is the simplest measure of dispersion. It defines the difference between the smallest and largest numbers in the distribution. It is

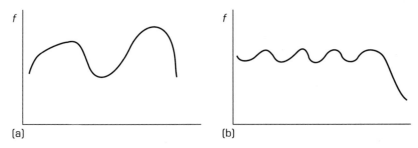

Figure 10–5 *Examples of bimodal and multimodal distributions. (a) Bimodal curve; (b) multimodal curve.*

computed by subtracting the lowest score from the highest. One of the obvious advantages of reporting the range is that it is easy to compute, but its disadvantages tend to outweigh this advantage. For one thing, it is considered a comparatively unstable statistic because one extreme score can change it. The range also doesn't take into account variations in scores between extremes and thus is customarily reported along with other measures of variability.

If a researcher relied exclusively on the range, a change in one individual score, the lowest or the highest, could alter the entire range figure drastically. To correct for this last problem the interquartile range or semiquartile range is often used as the measure of variability.

The Interquartile Range   The interquartile range is based on middle cases rather than extreme scores. It is more stable than just the range. It is found by

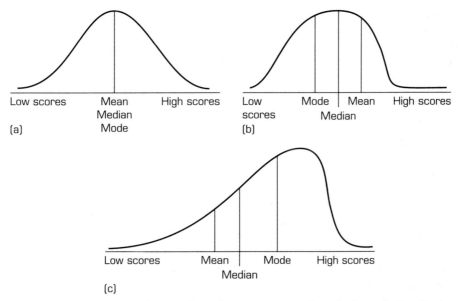

Figure 10–6 *Measures of central tendency in normal and skewed distributions. (a) Normal distribution; (b) positive skew; (c) negative skew.*

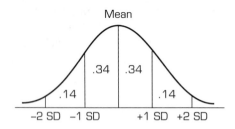

Figure 10–7   *Bell-shaped curve and standard deviations. The numbers in the areas under the curve represent the probability that the mean will fall within the interval.*

lining up the measurements in order of size and then dividing the array into quarters. The range of scores that includes the middle 50% of the scores is the interquartile range.

The semiquartile range is one-half of the range of scores within which 50% of the scores lie and is obtained by dividing the interquartile range by 2. The addition of deviant cases at either extreme leaves the interquartile (and semiquartile) range virtually unchanged. If the median is the appropriate measure of central tendency, then usually the interquartile range or semiquartile range is the appropriate measure of variability. The interquartile range is rarely reported in nursing research.

The Standard Deviation   The **standard deviation** is an average of the deviations from the mean. Standard refers to the fact that the deviation indicates a group's average spread of scores or values around their mean. Deviation indicates how much each score is scattered from the mean. In reporting standard deviations for the sample, authors may use the abbreviation *sd* or *s*. When reporting the standard deviation for the total population, the Greek symbol σ is used. If the mean is the appropriate measure of central tendency, then the standard deviation is the appropriate measure of variability.

The Normal Distribution   Many random variables of interest to nursing research have normal distributions. Normal distributions are continuous bell-shaped frequency curves. First called the Gaussian curve, after its originator Carl Friedrich Gauss, the normal curve forms an important base for most statistical procedures.

Four important characteristics about the shape of this curve are worth noting:

- The terms tend to cluster around the main vertical axis.

- The curve is symmetrical about the vertical axis.

- The size of the distribution is not limited, and positive and negative numbers can extend without limit toward infinity.

- The mean, median, and mode all have the same value.

These characteristics are a bit easier to graph if we consider them in terms of the normal curve that has been transformed to a standard normal curve by changing all values to *z* scores (discussed later in this chapter). Now the central value in this distribution is zero and positive scores extend to the right of the zero line and negative scores extend to the left.

With a normal curve, deviations for each individual score from the mean fall one-half on the positive side of the curve and one-half on the negative side, resulting in a summated score of 0 (see Figure 10–7).

The standard deviation of a set of scores is found by the formula

$$SD = \sqrt{\frac{\Sigma(x_i - \bar{x})^2}{n-1}}$$

> *where x_i = individual score*
> $\bar{x}$ *= group mean*
> n *= the number of scores*

The standard deviation can be thought of as the amount a "typical" score varies from the mean. Like the mean, the standard deviation takes into consideration all the scores or values in a distribution. It tells how variable the scores in a data set are. If, for example, we compared anxiety-scale scores for two samples of patients, each from a different culture, we might find that both distributions had a mean of 35. But when we calculated the standard deviation, we would discover that one had a standard deviation of 4 and the other a standard deviation of 9. We could immediately conclude that although the means were the same, the first sample was more homogeneous on the variable measured by the anxiety score. Figure 10–8 illustrates how samples with the same mean may vary in terms of how far each score falls from the mean.

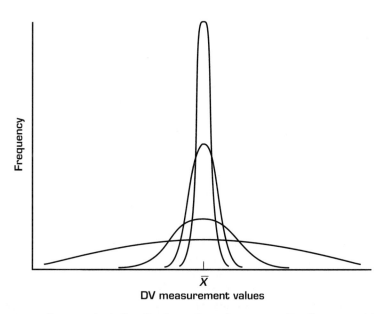

Figure 10–8 *Symmetrical distributions. Four frequency distributions with the same mean and the same total sample size but different variabilities.*

Standard scores, represented by the small letter *z*, tell us how many standard deviations away from the mean a particular raw score is. Many intelligence and achievement tests use standard scores with a preestablished mean and standard deviation. The formula for computing the standard score is

$$z = \frac{(x_i - \bar{x})}{sd}$$

Where *z* = *standard score*
x_i = *an individual score*
x̄ = *mean score*
sd = *standard deviation*

If the distribution is normal, the *z* score can be looked up in a standard normal table to find out how much of the distribution would lie below and above the corresponding raw score. In this way the *z* score can be used to determine the percentile of any particular raw score (for example, the percentage of values equal to or less than that score). When a researcher reports an individual test score, it is sometimes more meaningful to give a *z* score or a percentile than to give just the raw score. From a *z* score it is possible to express one person's test performance in relation to the whole group. Another value of the *z* score is its ability to compare scores on two different tests.

Measuring the Relationship between Two Variables

Many nursing studies are not just *factor-isolating,* or one-variable, studies. Most of the time researchers are asking more complicated questions about the relationships, or correlations, between variables. A **correlation** addresses the question of to what extent two variables are related to each other in a linear fashion. For example: "To what extent is cigarette smoking related to the incidence of lung cancer or emphysema?" "To what extent is a diet high in saturated fat related to gall bladder disease?" "To what extent is a positive attitude toward labor and delivery related to the presence of one's mate in the labor and delivery rooms?" These questions are answered by calculating a statistic, or index, that expresses the magnitude or degree of relationship.

Statistics of correlation, **correlation coefficients,** vary between +1 and −1. A correlation of 0 indicates no relationship, while those correlations approaching ±1 indicate strong relationships or perfect correlations. The plus or minus sign indicates whether the correlation is positive or negative. A positive relationship, or direct relationship, indicates that as the values of one variable become larger or smaller, so do the values of the other variable. A negative, or inverse relationship, indicates that as the values of one variable tend to become large the values of the other variable tend to become small.

It is important to remember that correlation coefficients reflect relationship and do not mean that one variable caused the other variable to change. There are many controversies about causation but they are not solved with simple correlation statistics. For example, if a nurse weighed and measured all patients on an inpatient psychiatric unit and found that the people who

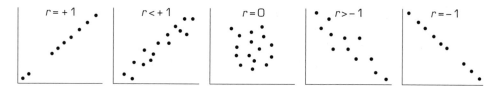

Figure 10–9 *Sample scatter diagrams for different degrees of linear correlation between two variables.*

weighed the most also tended to be the tallest and the people who weighed the least also tended to be the shortest, it could be said that a positive correlation existed between height and weight for this sample. It would not be statistically correct to say that a person's weight caused a change in his or her height.

The graphic, or visual, presentation of the relationship between two variables is called a scatter diagram, or **scatter plot.** Each point represents the position of a subject on the x and y axes. For these graphs x and y are convenient notations for the horizontal and vertical axes respectively. A scatter diagram can reflect both the direction (positive or negative) and the approximate magnitude of a correlation. The more the dots resemble a straight line at a 45 degree angle to the axes, the higher the correlation (see Figure 10–9). A perfect correlation (negative or positive) is depicted on a scatter diagram by a sloped straight line.

Perfect correlations are rarely found in research, including nursing research. If you read the results of a study involving psychosocial variables, correlations between +.50 and +.70 or between −.50 and −.70 may be considered quite strong. On the other hand, in studies with physiologic variables rather than psychosocial ones, correlations of less than +.85 or −.85 may be considered weak. Researchers frequently report a quantity called the coefficient of determination to help interpret the strength of the correlation. The correlation coefficient is squared and the resulting quantity expresses the amount of shared variance between the two variables. In other words, how much would one know about variable x if one knew about variable y? For example, if a researcher knows that the correlation between two variables is −.70, then the coefficient of determination is .49 or 49%. Therefore, if the correlation between self-esteem and depression is −.70, then 49% of the difference among people in the sample in terms of depression is accounted for by the differences in their self-esteem scores.

INFERENTIAL STATISTICS

In the previous section, descriptive statistics—numeric or graphic summaries of data—were discussed. While descriptive statistics are useful, they are limited in that they simply provide information about the *sample* they are describing. Many nursing studies are conducted for purposes that go beyond merely reporting characteristics of a particular sample. The investigators want to report something about the characteristics of the *population* from which the sample was drawn. **Inferential statistics** are the statistical techniques that researchers use to generalize from the *sample* to the larger, unmeasured population. In inferential statistics, sample statistics can be used to estimate corresponding population parameters, which are population characteristics of interest such as the mean and standard deviation. A *statistic* is always derived from a *sample* and used to make inferences about population parameters or to test hypotheses about populations.

Inferring from a Sample to a Population

Suppose researchers wanted to know the average length of hospital stay for organ transplant patients in the United States. On the one hand, they could track every single patient admitted to an American hospital for this procedure—an approach that would be costly and time-consuming. On the other hand, they could use the principles and procedures of inferential statistics to select a representative random sample from the population, calculate its mean length of hospital stay, and then make an inference about the mean length of hospital stay for the entire population.

Even when researchers infer characteristics of a population from a properly selected random and representative sample, there is always some chance that the actual mean of the population will be different from the means suggested in samples drawn from it. There is a strong chance that the population mean will be slightly different from the sample mean, and there is a small chance it will be quite different. The fluctuation of a statistic from one sample to another is called **sampling error.** Hypothetically, if we plotted a frequency polygon of the means of all the possible samples that could be drawn from the population, we would end up with what is called a *sampling distribution of the mean* and we would then be able to determine the mean of the population by taking the mean of the distribution of sample means in that frequency polygon. This notion, however, is really a theoretical one, because it requires us to draw an infinite number of samples. Theoretically, though, statisticians tell us that the sampling distributions of means tend to follow a normal, or bell-shaped, curve if the *n,* or sample size, is large enough. "Large enough" depends on the shape of the population distribution. For many population distributions an *n* of 5 is large enough, and for almost all population distributions an *n* of 25 is large enough. Therefore, we can calculate the standard deviation of a sampling distribution and reasonably assume that 68% of all the sample means fall between +1 and −1 standard deviations from the population's actual mean. The standard deviation of a theoretical frequency distribution of means of samples is called the **standard error of the mean.** As the *n* gets larger, the standard error of the mean gets smaller, and as the *n* gets smaller, the standard error of the mean gets larger. Obviously, the smaller the standard error, the more accurate a sample mean is as a reflection of a population mean.

Estimation

Estimating the parameters of a population from a sample is one of the major uses for inferential statistics. In estimation we are trying to find out the value of the population parameter by using information contained in the sample. One of the most common procedures is estimation of the population mean *u*. There are two types of estimation procedures, a point estimate and an interval estimate. In **point estimation** a single number is calculated from the sample data, such as the sample mean *x,* and is used to infer that this number is the population mean *u*. It is not likely that the population mean is *exactly* the same as the sample mean. Rather, it is likely that the population mean is close to the sample mean. Therefore, it is much more common to calculate an interval estimate. An **interval estimate** is a range of numbers likely to include the population parameter of interest. For an interval estimate, two numbers, called the *endpoints* of the interval, are calculated, and inferences are made about the likelihood that the population parameter falls within this interval.

The General Logic of Hypothesis Tests

All inferential statistical tests are built on the fact that chance can produce variation among samples even if the populations from which the samples are drawn are identical. Using a mathematical model, statisticians can calculate the probability that such chance variations will occur between identical populations. Most tests are designed so that the larger the statistic, the lower the probability that data could have been produced by chance if the populations are really the same. So that researchers do not have to keep recalculating the probabilities of different test statistics over and over again, these values are available in tables. Most test statistics and tables are set up so that the claim that the populations are the same is rejected if the test statistic exceeds some value (called the **critical value**) on the table.

Usually a researcher uses inferential statistics to determine whether two or more groups differ with respect to some outcome or dependent variable. Hathaway and Geden (1983), in a study of energy expenditure during three types of exercise programs, used an inferential statistical procedure called *analysis of variance* (ANOVA) to demonstrate that for oxygen consumption and heart rate the sample groups *were not similar.* Further statistical analysis showed that for these two dependent variables, the isometric and active exercise programs were significantly more demanding than the passive or rest programs. Statistical procedures provide investigators with the means for deciding whether a study's outcomes reflect true population difference or an apparent difference is due only to chance and is not likely to happen again.

Understanding the Hypotheses   The **null hypothesis** is a statement that no difference exists between the populations being compared. The **alternative,** or **research, hypothesis** is a statement that there is a difference between these populations. (Sometimes a one-sided alternative hypothesis is used; for example, population A has a smaller mean than population B.) Hypotheses are always about *populations,* not about samples. The data, of course, will almost certainly have different values for the summary statistics for two samples. Does that mean that the two populations are really different? Only if the different values from the samples are far enough apart for us to be convinced that the difference is not due to chance alone. How far is far enough? Statisticians calculate the probability of chance causing this large a difference in the sample data of identical populations (null hypothesis). If this probability is small, they conclude that the populations are not really the same, and they reject the null hypothesis. If this probability is not small, they conclude that the difference in the sample data is probably due to chance, and accept the null hypothesis.

How small is a small probability in this context? Different answers are possible. Some studies will define .05 as the appropriate cutoff point. We say that the test is at the .05 **level of significance.** Other studies use .10, .01, or .001. Some researchers choose to simply report the probability and leave it to the reader to decide whether it is small or not. When they report the probability, they call it a p-value.

Example

Using a stratified random sample of 130 patients from three hospital units, Nichols, Barstow, and Cooper (1983) tested the relationship between frequency of changing IV tubing and percutaneous sites and the incidence of phlebitis. They found that there were no significant differences in rates of phlebitis whether tubings were changed every 24 or 48 hours or whether sites were changed every 48 or 72 hours. Their null hypothesis was stated as follows:

Null Hypothesis:

There will be no difference in the incidence of phlebitis between the three treatment groups.

Group 1: IV tubing changed every 24 hours, percutaneous site changed every 48 hours.

Group 2: IV tubing changed every 24 hours, percutaneous site changed every 72 hours.

Group 3: IV tubing changed every 48 hours, percutaneous site changed every 72 hours.

Choosing a Significance Level   How do researchers choose an appropriate level of significance for a study? To understand that, we must first understand the two types of error that can be made in a hypothesis test. Figure 10–10 shows the four possibilities for the conclusion of a hypothesis test. Notice that two of them are correct. We anticipate that one of these will occur most of the time. But the other two are errors. Consider an example in which the null

REALITY

	Hypothesis true	Hypothesis false

Figure showing a 2×2 table. Row labels on left under **RESEARCHER'S DECISION**: "Reject hypothesis" and "Do not reject hypothesis". Column headers under REALITY: "Hypothesis true" and "Hypothesis false". Cells: top-left = Type I error; top-right = correct decision; bottom-left = correct decision; bottom-right = Type II error.

Figure 10–10 *The four possibilities for the conclusion of a hypothesis test.*

hypothesis is that a new, more costly treatment for diabetes is equally effective as the old treatment. The alternative hypothesis is that the new, more costly treatment is more effective. A **Type I,** or alpha, error would be to decide that the new treatment is more effective when it really isn't. If a Type I error is made, money may be needlessly spent on the more expensive treatment. A **Type II,** or **beta,** error would be to decide that the new treatment is not more effective when it actually is. The consequence of a Type II error is passing over a more effective treatment. Of course, in most cases, the results of the study will be to make one of the two correct decisions, not to make either a Type I or a Type II error.

How can we reduce the probability of making a Type I (alpha) error? A Type I error is rejecting the null hypothesis when it is really true. We can reduce the probability of a Type I error by making it very difficult to reject the null hypothesis. That is, we only reject the null hypothesis if the probability we calculated (the probability that the difference in the sample data is due to chance) is very small, perhaps .001. That is, we choose a very low significance level. However, if we require data this clearly different to reject the null hypothesis, then we are more likely to make a Type II (beta) error, failing to reject a false null hypothesis. So there is a trade-off. We choose a very low significance level if the consequences of a Type I error are worse, and we choose a relatively high (.05 or .10) significance level if the consequences of a Type II error are worse. In some situations the two types of error are about equally undesirable, so we choose a medium significance level.

Statistical Tests

Most statistical tests used in hypothesis testing by nurse researchers are classified into two types: **parametric** statistics and **nonparametric** statistics. Parametric tests have three important requirements:

1. They involve the estimation of at least one parameter.

2. They require measurements on at least an interval-level measurement scale.

3. They assume that the sampling distribution of the statistic is close to normally distributed, or that the n is large enough (20 or more) that the sampling distribution is approximately normal.

Parametric tests are more powerful and therefore are preferred by most nurse researchers who are analyzing numerical data. If the assumptions for parametric tests cannot be met, the second type of statistic is used. The nonparametric statistic is based on weaker assumptions:

1. It can be used with nominal and ordinal measurements.

2. It can be used when the sample size is small and there is no way to assume that the scores follow a bell-shaped curve or normal distribution.

Commonly used parametric tests are the t-test and analyses of variance (ANOVA). A commonly used nonparametric test is the chi-squared test.

The *t*-Test   The ***t*-test** is a statistical test used to determine whether means of two groups are significantly different. For example, in either a *within-subjects design* or a *matched-groups design,* a score in one situation can be paired with a score in another. In a within-subjects pretest and posttest design, there is a prescore and postscore for each respondent. From the scores, the researcher can figure out the effect of a nursing intervention by testing whether there are statistically significant differences between the pretest and posttest mean scores. In a matched-groups design, a score in one situation can be paired with a score in another, and the researcher can figure out the effect of intervention by calculating the difference for each pair and using that to test whether the difference between the two groups is significantly different from zero. In each case here, the researcher can use corresponding estimation techniques to estimate the difference in scores between the two groups.

The t-test is often used in studies that don't have control or experimental groups but rely instead on comparing values or scores of a sample from before an intervention (biofeedback training, for instance) with scores from after the intervention. The procedure involves comparing the pretest and posttest measures using an equation for paired-measure t-tests and then comparing the computed value of t with the t values in a table.

Analysis of Variance   A one-way **analysis of variance** (abbreviated ANOVA) is an inferential statistical procedure that has about the same purpose as a t-test—that is, to compare the mean scores of two groups. The difference between an ANOVA and a t-test is that the t-test is used for comparing two groups or two sets of scores, whereas a one-way ANOVA can be used to compare two or more groups. Because the ANOVA can be used with a greater number of groups, it is considered to be a more versatile statistical procedure.

Using an ANOVA involves calculating what is called the *F* ratio and then checking the value of that statistic against a table of **F values** for its statistical significance. Calculating an analysis of variance consists of obtaining two independent estimates of variance. One is based on the variability between groups and the other is based on the variability within groups. If the between-group variance is large relative to the within-group variance, then the scores in the different groups are far apart and we can conclude the group means are different. If the between-group variance is about the same as, or smaller than, the within-group variance, then the scores in the different groups are not far apart, and we conclude that the group means are not different. Since the *F* ratio is the between-group variance divided by the within-group variance, a large value of *F* leads to rejecting the null hypothesis and a small value of *F* leads to accepting the null hypothesis.

Nonparametric Statistical Tests   The statistical tests of inference that we have discussed thus far all rely on two important assumptions: (1) that the sampling distribution is close to normally distributed, or that the *n* is large enough that the sampling distribution is approximately normal, and (2) that the data collected are interval- or ratio-level scales of measurement. Many nursing studies, however, focus on variables that don't conform to these two assumptions. A study that ranked patients in terms of their cooperativeness with a health care regimen would be an example. The data would be ordinal, not interval or ratio, data and would not necessarily be distributed according to a bell-shaped curve. Clearly, parametric statistics would not apply, and the investigator would have to choose a statistical test appropriate to the data.

Nonparametric tests are those statistical tests that make no assumptions about the shape of the population distribution, and they are therefore called distribution-free tests. Different nonparametric statistical tests have been devised for few-category and many-category situations as well as for different designs. Some of the tests for ordinal data have one version for small samples (fewer than 20) and another for large samples. For analysis of data involving nominal, ordinal, or nonnormally distributed interval level scales, you'll need to refer to a good nonparametric statistics book, such as Conover's (1980) *Practical Nonparametric Statistics*. Remember, using parametric statistics when they don't apply can lead to mistaken conclusions. Using nonparametric statistics, however, when parametric statistics are appropriate can mean that a less powerful test has been used, and the significance of differences in the sample data can easily be underestimated.

The Chi-square   The **chi-square** (χ^2) is one of the most frequently used nonparametric statistics reported in the nursing research literature. This test can be used when data are nominally scaled and the researcher is interested in whether the number of responses, objects, or people that fall in two or more categories follow some expected pattern. The chi-square is calculated from the differences between observed frequencies and the frequencies expected under the conditions of the null hypothesis (based on some expected pattern). Sometimes it has been called the "goodness of fit" test. When the discrepancy is large between what turns up in the data and what would be expected to occur according to the null hypothesis, the chi-square statistic will be large. If it exceeds the critical value in a chi-square table, the researcher can reject the null hypothesis and accept the alternative hypothesis, concluding that the data do not fit the expected pattern.

Other Statistical Tests   When a study is intended to untangle relationships among three or more variables, an investigator must sometimes consider using multivariate or more advanced and complex statistical procedures. These procedures include multiple correlations, multiple regression (simultaneous, stepwise, and hierarchical), analysis of covariance, factor analysis, and discriminant analysis (Cohen & Cohen 1983, Keppel 1991). The purpose and conditions for some of these tests are presented in Table 10–2. When research requires such advanced procedures, computers become invaluable.

USE OF COMPUTERS IN STATISTICAL ANALYSIS

Computers are used by nurse researchers to clean data (that is, to find data entry errors, implausible responses, and missing data), to explore data, and to compute the statistical procedures discussed in this chapter. Operations a computer can perform on data include:

- *calculations.* A computer can add, subtract, divide, multiply 1 million problems in a second! These calculations are commonly called "number crunching."

- *rearrangements.* A computer can put data into alphabetical or numerical order.

- *reading input.* A computer can read 100,000 characters each minute.

- *writing data onto an output unit.* A computer can print out 260,000 characters each minute.

- *storage.* A computer can store data in its own temporary memory or transfer it to an external storage device.

Before using a computer program to analyze quantitative data, a researcher must be sure that his or her data are "clean." **Data cleaning,** or finding the errors in data, is one of the most unpopular parts of data analysis, because most people find it tedious and boring. But it can mean the difference between an otherwise fine study and disaster. Poor-quality data yield poor-quality results—thus the expression "garbage in, garbage out," or GIGO. The usual method for data cleaning is to run frequencies for all the scores on each item and then inspect them for the appearance of anything that is not plausible. For instance, if the possible range of scores is 1 to 5 and two cases have a 6, a data entry error has probably been made.

Once data are clean, the investigator usually asks the computer to obtain descriptive statistics or marginals on it, including measures of central tendency (mean, mode, and median) and measures of distribution (standard deviations, variance, and range). If relationships between variables are to be

---

Table 10–2   *Multivariate (Advanced) Statistical Procedures*

Name of Procedure	What Is It?	When Is It Used?
Multiple regression	A way of making predictions by understanding the effects of two or more independent variables (IV) on a dependent variable (DV)	When the DV is interval level data, there are two or more IVs, and the researcher wants to know the magnitude of the association between the IVs and DV
Stepwise multiple regression	A method in which potential predictors can be considered to see which combination has the greatest predictive power	When there are many IVs and the researcher wants to know which set is most powerful in predicting the DV
Repeat measures ANOVA	Extends the ANOVA procedure when the same measurement is taken several times on the subject	Answers the question of whether the effects of a treatment/experiment are the same over time
Analysis of covariance (ANCOVA)	A combination of analysis of variance and regression that tests the significance of group means after first adjusting scores on the DV to eliminate effects of covariance	If an experimental design is not possible and the researcher wants to adjust or control statistically for differences between treatment and comparative groups
Factor analysis	A statistical means for condensing or combining many variables into smaller numbers that are interrelated	Used to reduce a large set of variables into a smaller set of unified concepts
Discriminant analysis	An alternative to multiple regression when the criterion variable (DV) is at the nominal rather than interval level of measurement	Used to predict membership in a category or group based on measure of the IVs
Canonical correlation	A test that analyzes the relationship of a set of variables with another set of variables	Answers the same questions that a correlation coefficient does except there are multiple variables
Multivariate analysis of variance (MANOVA)	A test that extends ANOVA to two or more DVs	Lets the researcher answer ANOVA questions when there are multiple DVs

explored, various plots of the data are helpful at this stage. In addition to descriptive statistics, most researchers ask for a printout of all the data elements for each subject to be used for reference in the future.

Once data are cleaned, the researcher makes use of a special computer program to analyze the data. A popular approach in nursing research is the **Statistical Analysis System** (SAS), a package of programs for analyzing research data. SAS can:

- create an SAS data set (that is, all the scores obtained by all the subjects in a sample) and print it out

- do statistical operations or procedures (PROCS) on that data set

Although scientists agree that SAS is a most powerful statistical package, it does not have a very complete selection of nonparametric statistics, nor does it have good capacity for doing scale reliability. The Statistical Package for the Social Sciences (SPSS) and the Biomedical Statistical Software Package (BMDP) are other statistical application packages. SPSS can do reliability analysis of scales including Cronbach's Alpha. Some of the programs that are available with SPSS include:

1. descriptive statistics
2. frequency distributions
3. cross-tabulations
4. *t*-test
5. correlations
6. scatter diagrams
7. analysis of variance
8. multiple regression
9. multivariate analysis of variance

Use of computer programs has enabled researchers to eliminate a great deal of the drudgery in quantitative data analysis and to instead focus on the actual statistical findings of their studies. However, there are dangers in becoming too dependent on computers. It is often easy to use a computer program to carry out a statistical procedure on data even when you do not understand what the statistical procedure does, what assumptions must be met for it to be valid, how to check those assumptions, or how to interpret the output. Beware of carrying out procedures you don't understand. If you want to use a statistical procedure, look up an explanation of it in a reference book and be sure you understand when and how to use it and how to interpret the results before you carry it out.

In the methodology corner of *Nursing Research*'s July/August 1981 issue, Dr. Barbara S. Jacobsen wrote a guest essay titled "Know Thy Data." She commented that inferential and confirmatory data analyses were rapidly becoming more widespread in nursing studies, perhaps because nurse researchers have greater access to and skill in using computers to analyze

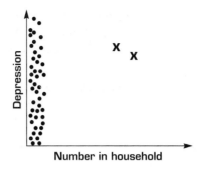

Figure 10–11   *Scatter diagram.*

their data. An unfortunate side effect, according to the author, is that "researchers know their F ratio and p values (statistics), but do not know their data. . . . Confirmatory design and analyses may be easier to teach and computerize, but all too often it is learned in a mechanistic way and performed as a ritual" (p. 254).

The consequence of computer dependence without full understanding of data is that researchers may make false interpretations of statistics. Jacobsen reports an incident in which an excited researcher raved that the computer had isolated a "key variable" in her questionnaire that correlated with everything! Often these correlations were difficult to explain, such as that the number of people living in a household correlated with a measure of depression. It took a scatter diagram printout that looked like Figure 10–11 to illuminate the mystery. The two outliers (subjects who were very different from the rest of the group) simply lived in large institutions and also happened coincidentally to be depressed. When their scores were removed, the positive correlations between numbers of people in the household and depression score changed to reveal the *absence* of any correlation. The visual diagram of score frequencies solved the mystery.

Extreme scores in a data set can likewise make it appear that no relationship exists between two variables. A single **outlier** (extreme score) can invalidate means, standard deviations, regression coefficients, and *t*-tests as appropriate summaries of the information in the data. Jacobsen maintains that visual presentations can help a researcher know when to question the validity of statistical analyses. They can help researchers uncover patterns in the data that offer suggestions and cues for future research and enable them to better "know their data."

ANNOTATED RESEARCH EXAMPLE

Citation

Troumbley PF & Lenz ER. Application of Cox's interaction model of client health behavior in a weight control program for military personnel: A preintervention baseline. *Adv Nurs Sci*. 1992;14(4):65–78.

Study Problem/Purpose

Increasing employers' recognition of how life-style influences health and illness among employees has led to the expansion of occupational health programs that emphasize diet and exercise. Nurses often play a key role in such programs. Research and evaluation of these programs has not kept pace with their growth, and many programs are based on untested assumptions about the population they serve or on misinformation about the efficacy of interventions. This study's goal was to test the applicability of a middle-range nursing theory, Cox's Interaction Model of Client Health Behavior, in explaining client behavior and outcomes in a weight control program.

the investigators use inferential statistics to test a number of research hypotheses.

Methods

Secondary analyses of data collected to explore the assumptions underlying the U.S. Army's Weight Control Program were employed to test the applicability of Cox's model. Multiple regression techniques were used to test a number of hypotheses concerning predictors of client motivation, success in the program, and health status. The data were analyzed using the Statistical Package for the Social Sciences (SPSS-X).

Multiple regression is a type of parametric statistical test.

multiple regression is a technique for measuring the degree of association or the relationship between a number of independent variables and a dependent variable.

Findings

The investigator's hypothesis concerning the relationship between client motivation and demographic characteristics was supported. Both education and marital status were significant predictors of client motivation ($p = .04$). The investigators also found that health status was related to demographic or background variables of the subjects. Clients who were married, younger, and of normal weight were at lower risk for future health problems than were single, older, overweight clients.

age, marital status, and weight are the independent variables in this regression model, and health status is the dependent variable, or outcome measure.

Level of significance

the p value is statistically significant; therefore, the analysis supports the investigator's hypothesis.

Guidelines for Critique

Does the researcher clearly state the types of statistical analyses performed on quantitative data?

Are the statistical procedures the right ones to answer the research question?

What descriptive statistics are reported? Do data reported in the text match those presented in tables and figures?

What correlational findings are reported? Are the researcher's conclusions warranted on the basis of these correlations?

How has sampling error been controlled for?

QUALITATIVE RESEARCH METHODS

HOLLY SKODOL WILSON

CHAPTER OUTLINE

In This Chapter . . .

CHAPTER OBJECTIVES

After reading this chapter, you should be able to:

- Identify purposes of qualitative research.

- Enumerate three characteristics of field research

- Describe the stages of fieldwork: locating the field, gaining entree, collecting and recording data, and leaving the field

- Recognize the advantages and disadvantages of the role of complete participant as opposed to observer as participant or complete observer

- Comprehend the characteristics of partially structured and unstructured interviews

- List the advantages and disadvantages of interviews

- Describe unobtrusive means of collecting qualitative data

- Relate the major purposes of qualitative analysis

- Explain the procedures for four types of qualitative analysis

- Discuss the relevance of qualitative research to nursing practice and knowledge development in the discipline

11

IN THIS CHAPTER . . .

Qualitative analysis is something that you probably do every day in your clinical practice. Each time that you collect information about a patient that is not numerical—not a blood pressure, a temperature, or a laboratory test value— you have to conceptualize, compare, combine, and categorize in order to come up with a clinical interpretation of it. Whenever you use the nursing process to arrive at a nursing diagnosis, you have to make some meaning out of qualitative data. After all, a patient's lived experience with AIDS, adaptive functioning, self-care abilities, support systems, attitude toward health, and so on usually involve more than scores or measurements that can be plotted on a scale and subjected to statistical procedures. One expectant father whom you meet in the labor room is "involved," and a second is "detached." One recovery room patient is "stable," and another is "unstable." One family uses "open" communication, and another engages in "disturbed" communication patterns. Nurses are experts in grasping the significance of data acquired through observing and listening to patients' stories about their subjective, lived experiences. We may be inclined to call this skill sensitivity, insight, intuition, or perceptiveness, but in fact it involves a form of qualitative analysis.

Qualitative research methods and qualitative analysis aspire to capture what other people and their lives are about without preconceiving the categories into which information will fit. In order to understand others, the qualitative analyst and field researcher try to put themselves in others' shoes to discern, and sometimes interpret, how they think, feel, act, and behave. Qualitative methods of collecting data include observation, interviews, case studies, case histories, and document review, which rely on "firsthand knowing" under natural conditions.

This chapter presents an overview of **field research** (a term that encompasses the various methods of qualitative research), its advantages and its disadvantages. The chapter also discusses **qualitative analysis**—the *non*numerical organization and interpretation of data in order to discover patterns, themes, forms, and qualities found in field notes, interview transcripts, open-ended questionnaires, journals, diaries, documents, case studies, and the like. By thinking analytically, researchers impose order on a large body of data to answer a study's questions and avoid overwhelming a research consumer with detail when reporting the findings.

PURPOSES OF QUALITATIVE RESEARCH

The purposes of qualitative research are as diverse and wide-ranging as the types of qualitative research. In general, however, qualitative research methods are used "when the research context is poorly understood, the boundaries of the domain are ill-defined, and the nature of the problem murky" (Morse

1991 p. 147). Qualitative research employs nonnumerical data, usually collected through interviews, observations, and document analysis (called narrative text or stories by some experts). Qualitative research methods are useful when a study has purposes like the following:

- to explore, describe, and explain social psychological processes, themes, and patterns, or a social world, culture, or setting
- to interpret lived experiences in their natural context
- to analyze case studies or historical data to grasp the flow of events
- to analyze communication patterns
- to account for and illustrate quantitative study findings

CHARACTERISTICS OF FIELD RESEARCH: DATA COLLECTION IN QUALITATIVE RESEARCH

Fieldwork (also called naturalistic inquiry by some) as a mode of scientific inquiry immerses the researcher in processes of day-to-day life that may be as novel as living with vanishing forest people, or as tense as spending many months in the desert during a war in the Middle East. Fieldwork is the major data-collection strategy for qualitative research. "The field" is the social-psychological arena where the investigator gathers qualitative data to find answers in the central area of inquiry. In a pain study the field might be hospital wards; in a study of face-to-face interaction with disfigured or handicapped persons it might be bureaus or agencies. Field studies have been conducted by nurses in prenatal classes, labor rooms, nursing homes, self-help-group meetings, herbal pharmacies, ICUs, and rock concerts. The features that characterize such studies, whatever their location, are these:

1. The researcher, through face-to-face interviewing or participant observation, is the primary "instrument" for data collection.

2. Data collection and analysis go on in the natural setting. The investigator tries to learn about how variables vary under usual and unusual conditions rather than trying to control all variables except for the few under scrutiny.

3. The logical progression of field research contrasts with more traditional research in the ways summarized in Table 11–1.

4. Field researchers must make particular accommodations to the ethical principles discussed in chapter 12. They usually conduct their work in close association with the people and situations they study. The potential for conflicts of interest, deception, exploitation, invasion of privacy, inconvenience to the subjects, and loss of confidentiality are all particularly intense. If I learn in a study of prior child abusers and their children that a new incident has occurred, should I report it? Should I make my

field notes accessible to the police? What should I tell subjects about such matters from the start? No matter how unobtrusive, field research always pries into the lives of informants, usually with little personal gain to them. It can be used, however, to affirm their rights, interests, and sensitivities, and all informants have the right to know the researcher's aims, to remain anonymous, to refuse to participate, and to withdraw at any time without penalty.

The heart of the fieldwork enterprise, according to sociologist Herbert Blumer, is "getting close to the people involved in it, seeing it in a variety of situations they meet, noting their problems and observing how they handle them, being party to their conversations and watching their way of life as it flows along" (1969 p. 37). As you can surmise, fieldwork commits the researcher to learning to define the world from the perspective of those being studied and requires that he or she gain as intimate an understanding as possible of their way of life. Methodological techniques in field research include observation, informal interviews, life histories, document analysis, and other nonintrusive, nonstructured methods.

STAGES OF FIELDWORK

Appraising the suitability of the setting or field is the first stage in doing fieldwork. Researchers examine the setting to determine whether it will yield data bearing on the purpose or research question of their study. The success of a field study often depends on the attention paid to this preresearch phase. Familiarity with the routines, realities, and structure of the proposed setting facilitate not only the negotiations that follow but also the qualitative data that can be collected.

Gaining Entree

Field research proceeds by clearing the initial hurdle of gaining entree, or being admitted into the selected setting or situation so that one can observe and talk to people about the research question. Then one must build rapport and trust so that subjects will willingly serve as informants and respondents. Barriers to gaining entree abound, and success depends on the researcher's ability to determine the wisest approach to the situation and cultivate the various "gatekeepers."

Problems and strategies for gaining entree are influenced in part by the decision of whether to engage in covert or overt field research. The complete participant role obviously eliminates the need to explain and justify the research or the researcher's presence. Here the investigator becomes an authentic participant in the setting to get a look at the social life of the subjects without influencing them with the knowledge that they are under study.

Table 11–1 *Comparison of Quantitative Research with Qualitative Research*

Traditional Deductive Research	*Field Research*
Start with hypotheses derived from reading existing literature—for example, independent variable yields dependent variable (x → y).	Look at the data first. Then come up with your own multiple tentative hypotheses.
Study a few propositions. Proceed through a linear process.	Study many propositions. Proceed through a multidimensional process resembling a Rubik's cube or a spiral.
Comply with precise steps for correct data collection and analysis.	Gather data and analyze it simultaneously based on the general principle of being pragmatic and evolving the analytic scheme.
Test, confirm, or refute hypotheses.	Develop concepts, propositions, and middle-range theories.

Complete participant research carries with it three potential problems:

1. The investigator may become so self-conscious about revealing his or her identity that both the participant and observer role performances are hampered.

2. The researcher may "go native," lose the intellectual distance required to analyze the how and why of study data, and instead begin thinking in terms of should or shouldn't, right or wrong.

3. The demands of participation on the investigator may use time, energy, and flexibility needed for data collection.

Many experts now agree that the combination of these scientific problems along with important ethical questions about the propriety of doing "undercover" research outweigh the potential benefit of learning about aspects of behavior that otherwise might not be accessible to the field-worker. The exception, of course, might be in the case of research conducted in a free-access setting such as a subway station or supermarket. Most human subjects committees and institutional review boards (IRBs), as well as this author, discourage the covert observer role except in public places.

A preferred alternative to covert research is for both the researcher and the informants to be aware of the observation process as the researcher participates in the situation. The advantage of the role of participant as observer is that the researcher not only watches what others do but also learns from doing it. The major problem is that participants may come to expect the field-worker to become more of a colleague and participant than he or she is capable of being without jeopardizing the research. Nurses are particularly vulnerable to these conflicting demands when conducting research in a health care setting where they possess the skills to actively intervene in situations and, in fact, are accustomed to doing so.

The observer may also take a more detached position. This role, called observer as participant, involves more formal observation and entails less risk of getting overly involved in the work of the setting. The researcher limits his or her interaction to seeking clarification of events going on. This approach diminishes intrusion, conveys interest, and gets at meaningful data. In some cases, however, brief relations with a greater variety of people over shorter periods of time lead to fundamental misperceptions and misunderstandings of the social worlds under investigation.

At the opposite end of the spectrum from complete participation is complete observation. In the role of complete observer, the field researcher attempts to observe people in ways that make it unnecessary for them to take him or her into account. Examples include systematic eavesdropping, loitering, bystanding, and spectating in free-access public places. This role also can involve analysis of cultural artifacts and secondary sources such as patients' charts, case histories, or diaries. Obviously, this approach decreases the chances of losing intellectual distance as well as the impact of the investigator's presence on natural conditions in the field. But its drawbacks include the inability of the researcher to collect focused data from informants by interacting with them and the risk of never coming to understand their point of view. Complete observers watching the world go by risk less and are probably less anxious about rejection from others. But they also often wish that they could interrupt and ask questions about the meaning of what is going on. Many studies that begin with a completely passive observer role—for example, observing from outside the window of a hospital nursery to see how nurses hold infants and how long they allow them to cry—move on to a more active form of involvement by the researcher.

Collecting and Recording Data

The objective of field research is to spend an intense period of time in an arena of social interaction and record the ongoing experiences of its participants. This requires that the field researcher gain an understanding about others' ways of perceiving life. Data collection is shaped by the emerging themes and hypotheses that develop in the course of doing qualitative analyses; thus, in most field studies data collection and analysis go on simultaneously.

Data collection begins with the question "What shall I look at?" Douglas (1976) suggests that we begin by "casting a wide net." This means talking to all kinds of people and investigating all kinds of settings associated with the phenomenon in question. Polsky (1969) says that the initial rule for field researchers is "keep your eyes and ears open but keep your mouth shut." In Box 11–1 Hutchinson (1986) gives us a sense of the breadth of data-collection strategies by listing those she used to develop her analyses of chemical dependency among nurses.

Clearly, the initial data-collection principle in a field study is to record everything that might be vaguely or remotely relevant to the researcher's

---

Box 11–1 Qualitative Data Sources in a Study of Chemically Dependent Nurses.

1. Case histories of ten nurses who had appeared before the board of nursing because of a problem with chemical dependency

2. In-depth interviews with 20 nurses who acknowledged problems with drugs and or alcohol and who were in the process of recovery

3. Semistructured interviews with representatives of the board of nursing's department of professional regulation and nurse investigators

4. Field observation at board of nursing hearings and meetings concerning nurses who had violated the nurse practice act.

5. Participant observation with a nurse investigator on her rounds to do urine checks on chemically dependent nurses who were on probation

6. Field observation of meetings of a chemical dependence self-help group for a period of one year

   Source: Hutchinson 1986.

---

unfolding analyses, because at first he or she doesn't know what might be useful. This process historically was called "hanging around." In contemporary times, data collection in a qualitative naturalistic field study includes all types of interviewing, observation, and document analysis. As the study progresses, observations and interviews become more purposeful and focused.

Leaving the Field

Although the fieldwork experience is viewed by many as more of a continuous process than a series of separate stages, all agree that a wise field researcher attends to closure and leaving the field at some point in the process. Ultimately, the investigator must gracefully withdraw from the study setting and from most, if not all, of the personal relationships that have for a time been relatively intense. Clearly, if one researcher is insensitive or is viewed unfavorably upon departure from the field, future investigators' efforts to gain access will be handicapped.

SOURCES OF QUALITATIVE DATA

The major sources of qualitative data are (1) participant observation, (2) interviewing of informants, and (3) analysis of documents, case studies, case histories, and other such "unobtrusive" measures. We will examine each of these methods more closely.

Participant Observation

Whether a researcher opts for full participation or a more detached role, he or she will need to begin by gathering information about the persons and activities that constitute the "site" (Schatzman & Strauss 1982). Initial visits to the site and introduction to subjects help the observer decide on locations from which to observe, times to observe, special occasions or events to observe and whom to interview.

A qualitative researcher needs a system for remembering observations and, even more importantly, retrieving and analyzing them. If the observer's identity and general purposes are known, he or she may take notes on a notepad or small clipboard in the presence of participants. Most of the time, field researchers jot a key word, phrase, or cue down and periodically leave the scene briefly to fill in full notes. Some field researchers dictate their observations into a tape recorder and later rely on a transcriber to type them. The danger of the latter approach is that weeks and months of observing and interviewing can yield a veritable ocean of disorganized data, and its continuous flow can be as overwhelming to a researcher as the original experience of entering the field.

Types of Field Notes   There are many different types of field notes. **Observational notes (ONs)** are descriptions of events experienced through watching and listening. They contain the who, what, where, and how of a situation and contain as little interpretation as possible. An example of an ON from a classic field study of a burn unit follows:

ON: *The burn unit is laid out with a central nursing station that faces three glassed-in wards. Male and female patients are in the same ward. The treatment room has a big tub shaped so that arms and legs can be spread out. The tub has a whirlpool mechanism. The ratio of staff to patients seems to be one staff member to three patients. Staff members seem to work in groups of twos and threes, and the atmosphere is one of tremendous hustle and bustle.**

Methodological notes (MNs) are instructions to oneself, critiques of one's tactics, and reminders about methodological approaches that might be fruitful. See the following example.

MN: *I decided to spend one day observing the varieties of painful treatments. There seem to be plenty of them! I decide to look for situations in which staff members actually talk about the god-awful pain these people are experiencing instead of the technical matters related to burn management.*

---

*This and other quotations from Fagerhaugh & Strauss 1977.

Personal notes (PNs) are notes about one's own reactions and reflections and experiences. Fieldwork relies on the investigator's ability to "take the role of the other" and be introspective. See the following example.

PN: *I had a somewhat unnerving morning. There's so much pain and misery on the unit yet the lightheartedness of the staff and the lack of pain expression among the patients except during treatments creates in me a sense of horror and awe! My friends and husband don't want to hear about working with burn patients. It's too horrible! I feel isolated and wonder if other nurses avoid the nurses on the burn unit or keep shop talk to superficial social "chit-chat."*

After field notes are recorded, they are customarily entered into a computer, paginated, labeled and dated, duplicated, and stored and become the basis for analytical memos. The development of a good set of field notes not only relieves the investigator of some of the burdens of remembering events but also constitutes a written record of the development of observations and ideas to be used in future publications of the research findings and method.

Interviewing

Interviews depend on the respondents' verbal reports about experiences, perceptions, preferences, problems, feelings, attitudes, or whatever other phenomena may be relevant to the study question. Some interviews may be highly structured, in the sense that the wording of questions, the sequence in which they are asked, and the possible responses are planned by developing an interview schedule (a lot like a script). Interviewers are trained to use this schedule. Structured interviews are akin to questionnaires, with the exception that the interviewer and the respondent are in each other's presence when the interview is used.

Semistructured Interviews   A **semistructured,** or focused, **interview** begins with at least an outline of topics the investigator intends to cover with each subject; but both the interviewer and the subject are free to deviate from the prepared agenda and introduce thoughts or observations that are particularly relevant to their personal perspective as the conversation unfolds. (See Box 11–2 for a progression of questions from a study of lesbian self-disclosure of sexual orientation to health care providers [Hitchcock & Wilson 1992].) Semistructured interviews offer the interviewer more latitude to move from content area to content area, to follow up on cues suggested by the respondent, and to spend various amounts of time interviewing one subject or another. Focused interviews, however, require that by the end of the interview all of the predetermined topics or questions have indeed been covered in some sequence, in some form with each interviewee (Hutchinson & Wilson 1992). Most researchers who use semistructured interviews believe that they are effective for exploration and hypotheses formulation but not appropriate or practical for hypothesis testing.

Box 11–2 Guide to Interview Questions for a Study of Lesbians

Examples of questions:

1. When you go to see a health care professional, what factors influence your decision whether or not to tell her/him about your sexual orientation?

2. How do you make the decision as to whether or not you should indicate your sexual orientation to your health care provider?

3. In your experience, how is disclosure to a health professional similar to or different from disclosure to others?

4. What kinds of behavior or attitudes would you need from health care providers for you to be comfortable disclosing sexual orientation to them?

Unstructured Interviews   The **unstructured interview** may be either spontaneous or scheduled, but its identifying characteristic is that respondents are encouraged to talk about whatever they wish that is relevant to the researcher's interest. Many such interviews begin with open-ended questions such as: "What was it like when you and your husband first learned that Michael was retarded?" or "What concerns you most when you think about managing your life, knowing what you do about your illness?" Some unstructured interviews begin by just inviting the interviewee to talk about whatever he or she wishes. The intent of the unstructured interview is to get to the subject's perception of the meanings in his or her world without introducing the investigator's conception of it. In fact, it is the method of choice among field researchers, and most researchers intentionally *avoid* structuring their interviews. Structure limits in advance what topics are important to ask about and often what the possible categories of response from interviewees might be. Unstructured interviews, in contrast, allow the interviewer a great deal of freedom in exploring whatever seems important to the respondent and promote the likelihood that responses will be spontaneous, self-revealing, and personal. Many interviews in phenomenologic studies begin with open-ended, unstructured questions.

Advantages of Interviewing   Listening to people talk about their perceptions and experiences has a number of important advantages as a data-collection strategy.

1. Inviting subjects to tell their story face to face to an empathic person usually gets a better response rate than mailing them an impersonal questionnaire or structured data form.

2. Interviews allow researchers to collect data from people who, either because of their literacy level or some other communication barrier such as paralysis following a stroke, bandages after burns, or immobilizing tubes or traction, simply can't write.

3. Interviews are usually more effective in getting at people's complex feelings or perceptions.

4. Interviews allow researchers to clarify responses that they don't understand fully, to probe certain responses in more depth, and to reword and rephrase questions so that they are more easily grasped by the interviewee.

5. Unstructured interviews, particularly, allow researchers to discover the unexpected.

Disadvantages of Interviewing   As you might imagine, such free-response, unstructured interviews also have disadvantages, according to their critics.

1. In nursing studies particularly, interviewees often expect some sort of direct help as a result of participating in the interview—a solution to their problems or even a complete change in their life. They may assume that the nurse interviewer can put them in touch with some special resources or benefits, unless he or she is careful in addressing with all candor the personal benefits section of the consent process.

2. Open-ended, nonstructured, or semistructured interviews are time-consuming procedures for collecting data and are similarly time-consuming to analyze word by word, phrase by phrase.

3. It is difficult to make conventional quantitative comparisons across interviews in the absence of an interview schedule that assures that all interviewees are asked the same set of questions with the same terminology.

4. If a substantial number of interviews are to be conducted, interviewers must be trained, particularly in the use of clear, nonleading language, the ability to expand or clarify a respondent's initial response, and listening skills.

5. Subjects may be self-conscious about being recorded on tape or about notes being taken about their replies. Thus, they may omit comments that they would include on an anonymous questionnaire.

Analysis of Documents, Case Studies, and Case Histories

Documents such as diaries, books, letters, newspapers, meeting minutes, legal documents, nursing notes, procedure manuals, and reports, as well as photographs, films, and drawings, are all used as sources of data.

Case studies and case histories have a long and valued history in the sphere of clinical practice research. Here the clinician or researcher conducts an in-depth investigation of a patient, a community group or aggregate, or an institution such as a hospital or clinic. Some clinicians have used literature, studying Tennessee Williams's *Glass Menagerie* to learn more about a physical handicap or Eugene O'Neill's *Long Day's Journey Into Night* to learn about destructive family dynamics. Sylvia Plath's poignant novel *The Bell Jar* may be of great value in learning to understand severe depression.

Whether fictional or not, case studies offer information that is rich and sometimes difficult to come by. Obviously, Freud developed his psychoanalytic theory and methods primarily from careful case studies conducted in turn-of-the-century Vienna. Critics of sole reliance on case-study data underscore their lack of generalizability. The methodology for compiling such data is not as rigorously prescribed as that for collecting survey or even participant observation field notes. Some say there is considerable freedom, if not outright ambiguity, in devising the data-collection strategies. The main principle is once again pragmatism in addressing the study question.

Example of a Case History

In 1970 two medical sociologists in collaboration with a team of nurses involved in field research published a classic book entitled Anguish: A Case History of a Dying Trajectory. *It was the story of a woman's protracted death in the hospital. According to its authors, the case demonstrated two major features; it was of long duration and it moved slowly but steadily downward. In presenting the case history of this lingering trajectory, Glaser and Strauss (1970) told the life story, or biography, of the patient; the story of how a hospital's staff reacted to her slow decline on their turf; the case history of the two nursing students who served as informants for the study; and, finally, the story of a final stage of a research project that had addressed the topic of dying and lasted more than five years.*

The interweaving of these four substories illustrates the rich fabric, detail, and complex information that a case history can produce. Its authors remind us, however, that case history is not a novel or merely exciting informative description. It is deliberately intended to highlight and explicate theoretical principles that can be more broadly generalizable.

QUALITATIVE ANALYSIS

When a study involves open-ended, nonnumerical data, collected through formal or informal interviewing, participant observation, documents, diaries, and case studies, the researcher is faced sooner or later with the challenge of making sense of this mass of heterogeneous data in relationship to the study's central questions. You as an intelligent reader of this kind of research must similarly be prepared to evaluate the credibility of a study's findings when they are based on qualitative data. If a study purports to test hypotheses, establish causal relations, summarize numerical patterns, or demonstrate statistical significance according to the laws of probability, the quantitative methods discussed in chapter 10 should be used. If a study has different purposes and raises different questions, however, particularly questions about people's experiences under natural conditions, qualitative methods will be used to analyze the data.

Purposes of Qualitative Analysis

The major purposes that can be served by using qualitative techniques are exploration and description, accounting for and illustrating quantitative findings, discovery and explanation, and extension of theory.

Exploration and Description   Sometimes a research study is designed to look for answers to questions in a field where a great deal of scientific work has already been done. A nurse conducting a study about early childhood development and the differential responses to hospitalization based on a child's developmental level would be one example. In this instance the investigator would build his or her study on prior research and theory in the area, perhaps by measuring variables that others have reported as important or using instruments or findings developed by others. If a researcher is tackling a study question about which very little is known, however, and the study is intended to gain insight about a particular group of patients or health conditions, data that are collected may be analyzed to present descriptive and exploratory findings. In this second kind of research the investigator tries to collect and present rich and diverse accounts of findings so that any promising leads and ideas can be developed. Questions would include "What is going on?" "How does something work?" "What is important here?" "What variations exist?"

Analyzing qualitative data for the purpose of description allows researchers to characterize an event, a patient population, a process, or a setting. Dickoff and James (1968) call this factor-isolating research.

According to Schatzman and Strauss (1982), description can be done in one of two ways. First, the analyst may use categories or organizational schemes that already exist in the literature of a discipline and simply find classes or cases in the data that correspond to the classification scheme taken from the literature. This is called straight description. Describing a unit's patient population by diagnosis or social class would be an example. In the second instance, the analyst attempts to think up new classes or categories suggested by an active inspection of the data. This is called analytic description. May's (1980) typology of detachment and involvement styles of first-time fathers is an example of the originality that characterizes analytic description.

Accounting for and Illustrating Quantitative Findings   Qualitative anecdotes are often used to answer "why" and "how" questions associated with quantitative study findings. For example, Mosher and Menn (1978) conducted a longitudinal comparative-outcome study of two modes of residential treatment for first-break schizophrenics. They relied on standardized scales like the Ward Atmosphere Scale and a global psychopathology rating before and after treatment to collect data about the settings and patients. Their two-year follow-up study findings supported the effectiveness of the experimental setting (Soteria House). My own qualitative field study was used by them to explain *how the Soteria approach worked (Wilson 1982).*

Discovery and Explanation   Sometimes a researcher wants to go beyond even abstract analytic description to discover in the data core patterns, variables, and categories that provide the basis for developing and then validating hypotheses about relationships. Some call this work *concept specification.* The concept may be "caring," "comfort," "empathy," or "advocacy," to name a few. Once relationships are discovered, the analyst attempts to weave what Schatzman and Strauss (1982) call "these key linkages" into an explanatory scheme, such as a model or a theory.

The value of describing and explaining nursing phenomena is illustrated in the following classic example:

Example of a Concept Discovery Study

Norris (1975), in a clinical study titled "Restlessness: A Nursing Phenomenon in Search of Meaning," traced the behavioral manifestations of restlessness and related her observations to a theory of rhythmicity. She began with questions like "Who is restless?" "When does it occur?" "How do people experience restlessness?" "How does it differ from rest?" She concluded her study with what she described as a sense of urgency "for all nurses who are at the bedside to observe and describe nursing events until nurses wherever and however they work have the data they need to recognize and assign meaning to the phenomena of nursing."

Extension of Theory   Sometimes a researcher has developed a theoretical explanation under one set of conditions and wants to extend it, refine it, or even move it from a middle-range **substantive theory** that explains something under a specific set of conditions to a **grand,** or formal, **theory** that explains how something occurs under a great variety of conditions. In such a study, questions might include: "Is the original substantive theory correct?" "Does it fit other circumstances?" "Are there additional categories or relationships?" Glaser and Strauss's (1971) theory of *status passages* to explain transitions that dying patients experience has been extended to explain a wide variety of situations.

Table 11–2 summarizes the four major purposes of qualitative analysis.

How Qualitative Data Are Analyzed

Data gathered through fieldwork methods can occasionally be collected in a standardized form and transformed into statistical data. An observational checklist of a psychiatric unit's dominant philosophy might be an example. But usually the qualitative data we have been discussing are not collected in a form that meets the assumptions of statistical tests. Consequently, some critics of this kind of research question the scientific merit of conclusions drawn from qualitative data because they are often presented to readers with the comment, "We have gone over our data and find that they support this conclusion." Consumers of this excuse for methodology find it difficult to accept the findings without being told what exactly that "going over" consisted of. They feel uncomfortable in the position of having to accept research conclusions on faith.

This section considers five major procedures for systematically making sense out of transcriptions of open-ended interviews, field notes, and documents. These procedures include (1) converting qualitative data to quantitative data, (2) doing a content analysis, (3) analytic induction, (4) discovering grounded theory, and (5) phenomenologic-interpretive analysis.

Converting Qualitative Data to Quantitative Data In some studies, particularly those whose purpose is exclusively descriptive, an investigator elects to report the frequency and distribution of categories assigned to the data or to

Table 11–2 *Purposes of Qualitative Analysis*

Purpose	Research Questions	Methods	Outcomes
1. *Exploration and description*	1. What is going on? 2. How does it work? 3. What is important here? 4. What variations exist?	1. Straight description using categories from existing literature 2. Analytic description generating novel categories from data 3. Content analysis 4. Quasi-statistics	1. Case studies 2. Ethnographies 3. Frequency reports 4. Descriptive narrative 5. Typologies 6. Cross-tabulations
2. *Accounting for and illustrating quantitative findings*	1. How did something occur? 2. Why did something occur? 3. What are the characteristics, conditions, and consequences involved?	1. Analytic induction	1. Anecdotes 2. Grounded substantive theory
3. *Discovery and explanation*	1. What is the basic social-psychological process here?	1. Constant comparison	1. Grounded substantive theory 2. Paradigms 3. Conceptual maps
4. *Extension of theory*	1. Is the original substantive theory correct? 2. Does it fit other circumstances? 3. Are there additional categories or relationships?	1. Comparative analysis 2. Content analysis	1. Formal theory

correlate their frequency or distribution with some other variables. In these cases the study reports some numerical conclusions but not with the precision evident in most statistical studies. For this reason Becker (1958) calls such an attempt an application of quasi-statistics. The essential objective of quasi-statistics is to decide whether the concepts or categories in the analysis represent typical and widespread patterns distributed in the data, thereby giving the analytic scheme more credibility. The analysts who blend quantitative methods with qualitative work usually engage in three processes in order to conclude that their final analysis is likely to be an accurate representation of the data or to descriptively depict the frequency and distribution of analytic categories. These processes are:

1. searching for **negative cases** in order to reformulate propositions that don't account for them (**negative cases** are bits of data that run counter to the researcher's propositions)

2. counting numbers of cases (not necessarily subjects) in each category and, where possible, running descriptive statistics that yield information about the frequency with which certain themes are supported in the data

3. constructing scales for nominal data

The limitations of basing an analysis of qualitative data exclusively on converting the data to some quantified form are probably obvious to you.

- Although searching for negative cases might force revisions in the analysis, there are no hard-and-fast rules to guide the researcher in answering questions such as "How long should I look?" "How many negative cases are too many?"

- The generation of analytic descriptions depends in part on the theoretical sensitivity of the analyst. Field research is designed to allow for the flexibility and creativity required to develop classes, categories, and propositions that are grounded in observational data. There is no guarantee that two analysts working independently with the same data will necessarily achieve the same results.

- Scales for nominal data are sorting devices that might help an analyst group subjects into pigeonholes. But because there is no underlying continuum for the scale that links the categories together, they may be more confining than helpful to the rich portrayal of findings that a qualitative analyst seeks.

Doing a Content Analysis   One of the earliest specific procedures for analyzing unstructured qualitative data is the **content analysis.** It is one way of categorizing verbal or behavioral data, and it shares with the other procedures in this section a requirement for analytic thinking and creativity in the researcher. The first studies that used the method of content analysis simply counted words or their synonyms when analyzing an interview or a document. If, for example, you were studying sexist stereotypes in journal recruitment advertisements for nursing positions you would do the following:

1. Make a list of all the relevant terms that reflect sexist stereotypes.

2. Read a randomly selected sample of recruitment ads from journals.

3. Count the frequency with which each of the key indicators (terms) appear in the data.

Later content analysis studies assigned codes for latent feeling tone (akin to connotation) as well as for the actual appearance of the terms themselves. Both of these types of content analysis were the prototypes for the two types used in contemporary nursing research: (1) *semantic content analysis* and (2) *feeling tone, or inferred, content analysis.* Some authorities differentiate these two types by making a distinction between content analysis done at the obvious, or manifest, level and content analysis at the implication, or latent, level. Semantic content analysis—simply coding and counting responses in a transcription—is an example of manifest content analysis. Feeling content analysis is an example of latent content analysis. Because in the latter the researcher goes beyond what was said directly to infer the meaning of something, research consumers usually require more evidence of a study's validity. Some studies involve both manifest and latent analyses.

A careful reading of the example on page 232 not only gives you a sense of how content analysis is presented in published research reports, but also allows you to tease out the indicators that were used to code a response into one of the four categories of orientation.

Content analysis, although ostensibly rigorous in its procedure and certainly arduous in its conduct, is still accused by critics of being prone to problems of validity and reliability. Some of the critical questions directed toward studies that use content analysis include:

1. How personal and idiosyncratic are the categories?

2. Would another researcher independently come up with the same ones?

3. How clear are the instructions for placing a response into a code?

4. How reliable is the coding?

5. What checks did the researcher include on the reliability and thoroughness of the coding?

6. Do the categories have at least face validity?

7. What kind of evidence is presented to establish face validity?

8. Do the content analysis categories meet other necessary criteria such as homogeneity, inclusiveness, usefulness, mutual exclusiveness, and clarity and specificity?

Analytic Induction **Analytic induction** and a cluster of approaches resembling it depart from the two previous methods in that reliance on frequency and the hope of quantifying qualitative data, even using scales for nominal data, is no longer the key to discovering the truth. Instead, the analyst attempts to search for concepts and propositions in the data that apply to all cases of a question under analysis. This approach assumes the careful consideration of all analytical evidence, the intensive analysis of individual cases, and the comparison of cases to one another. According to Norman Denzin (1989), a sociologist whose name has become linked with this method in the social science literature, analytic induction involves the following steps:

1. Formulate a rough definition of the phenomenon to be explained. What is the study problem?

2. Based on files of qualitative data, formulate concepts and hypothetical explanations about what is going on (that is, identify general categories).

3. Examine cases in the data to see if emerging propositions fit the facts.

4. Search for negative cases and reformulate hypotheses based on them.

5. Continue this process until a universal pattern of relationships or set of propositions is identified, explained, and supported with data.

6. Compare with other groups or conditions to develop an even more abstract and generalizable explanatory scheme.

Example Evaluation of a Nursing Program: An Illustration of Content Analysis

In the late 1970s a team of educational and nursing researchers completed an evaluation study of the first bachelor of science program for RNs accredited by the National League for Nursing, at Sonoma State University in California. This program and the research it generated are now considered classics in educational evaluation research. The task required that the team analyze qualitative responses to some open-ended questions collected during entry interviews with successive classes of students. In this case data were coded into four categories that reflected the students' attitudes toward their intended role vis-à-vis the profession of nursing. The four concepts or categories were (1) traditional, (2) academic, (3) leadership, and (4) frontiering. The findings were reported in the following way in the study's final report, giving you an idea of how the results of content analyses appear in a published document.

Frequency of cases

More than one-third (35%) of the students were categorized as predominantly traditional in their outlook, seeking to maintain or to further their positions in nursing but without volunteering any particular dissatisfactions with the hospital as a practice setting. One responded, "My husband and I separated and I began to think of my profession as a life-term career." Another said, "The handwriting is on the wall; if you want to work in nursing, you need that degree!"

Traditional orientation was one category

Academic orientation was one category

Far fewer entering students indicated an academic orientation, but those that did (11%) were so categorized because they spoke of scholastic aspirations, usually including plans for graduate school and a career in teaching and/or research. For example: "At the age of thirty-two and with family responsibilities, I couldn't pursue my interests. Now my children are no longer dependent on me and I want variety, mobility, and intellectual stimulation. I'd like to prepare myself to teach and do research in nursing."

A somewhat larger group (24%) had a clear leadership *orientation and came back to school seeking avenues to power and status. One respondent whose long-range objective was the presidency of the American Nurses' Association stated, "I'm convinced that change evolves from the top. To elicit change, you have to be involved at the top!"*

Leadership orientation was one category

The most intriguing of the orientations is the one that earned the label frontiering. *More than 4 out of every 16 entering students were so categorized. Their responses in the interviews reflected an interest in nontraditional positions and careers, a questioning of established health care delivery, and a willingness to pioneer or even create new and autonomous nursing roles. Many looked forward to functioning as independent practitioners, particularly in remote rural areas. Others hoped to "set up new programs, develop new ideas for health care in the community, participate in the management of an out-patient health service organization, set up programs for mental health and nutrition; to improve the current system; to be creative, innovative, and constructive." One respondent characterized his intended role as "to joust with the system."*

Frontiering orientation was one category

Indicators for coding data into the frontiering category

Just as quantifying qualitative data and doing a content analysis can be questioned for their reliability and validity, so can analytic induction. Critics ask: "Can the observations made in one setting with one population be generalized to others?" "Do observations represent real differences, or are they merely a product of the observer's biases?" "How honest and reliable are informants and respondents?"

When it comes to answering the first question about generalizability, the researcher must demonstrate that the case or cases studied are representative of the class of units to which he or she wants to generalize the findings. This is accomplished by carefully specifying the conceptual conditions under which observations were made and propositions were advanced. In answering the second objection, the investigator must introspectively examine his or her own perspective and any indications in the data that it colored either what was seen or how data were interpreted. Anecdotes about personal notes (PNs) in the research report often emphasize these efforts. Finally, when evaluating the credibility of informants, the researcher must ask:

1. Do the informants have reason to lie or conceal what they think is the truth?

2. Does vanity or expediency lead them to misstate the facts?

3. Are they firsthand witnesses to the occurrence?

4. Are feelings about issues likely to lead to an alteration in the story line?

Discovering Grounded Theory   One of the most highly evolved and carefully systematized methods for developing categories and propositions about their relationships from qualitative data is called the *discovery of grounded theory.* According to Glaser (1978), one of the method's originators, "The **grounded theory method** offers a rigorous, orderly guide to theory development that at each stage is closely integrated with a method of social research. Generating theory and doing social research are two parts of the same process" (p. 2).

Developing theory from qualitative data using Glaser and Strauss's discovery method (1967) rests on a set of basic assumptions:

1. *One goal of a theory or analytic explanation is that it must have "grab."* "Grab" means that a theory is interesting and useful. To achieve this, theories must fit, be relevant to, and work to explain, predict, and be modified by the social phenomena under study. Therefore, data are not forced or selected to fit preconceived theories. Instead of testing a few hypotheses deduced from existing theory, data are used to develop a rich, dense, complex explanatory or analytic scheme.

2. *Unlike verificational research, in which data collection and analysis are viewed in a linear way—that is, as separate, consecutive steps—data collection and analysis go on simultaneously.* The concepts and propositions that emerge from the data direct subsequent data collection. Although this process is sometimes called "an inductive approach" because it starts with the more specific and moves to the more abstract, it actually reflects both inductive and deductive thinking at various points.

3. *The grounded theory method is transcending.* Substantive theory developed in one area of study always has the potential for transcending a particular setting and being extended to a wide variety of circumstances. It is also transcending of other theories. It does not confirm or refute existing theories but incorporates them as part of the data base for the analysis. It also transcends scholarly disciplines and can be as useful to nursing as to sociology. The possibilities, according to Glaser, are limited only by the analyst's capabilities.

4. *Despite the diversity that characterizes qualitative data, the grounded theory approach presumes the possibility of discovering fundamental patterns in all of social life.* These patterns are called core variables, or **basic social processes** (BSPs), and they account for most of the variations characterizing an interaction under study. After spending months on three neonatal intensive care units, Hutchinson found that the nurses had to cope with the social-psychological problem of dealing with the horror associated with the deformities, the deaths, and even some of the treatments of the newborns. The BSP, or core variable, she explicated in her theory was called *creating meaning.* It explained how, given the conditions and problems in an NICU, the nurses created meaning and obtained satisfaction from their work. When nurses failed to make some kind of meaning of their work world, they experienced burnout, depression, and low morale (Hutchinson 1984).

5. *Generating grounded theory takes time and the ability to think conceptually.* It takes time for ideas to develop about the data, and the analyst must be sensitive to pacing the study to provide for the creativity and energy it requires.

The final product of a grounded approach to qualitative analysis is a theoretical explanation that

- fits the substantive area under study
- is sufficiently *dense* (accounts for a great deal of variation) and abstract to generalize to diverse situations
- allows for partial control over structures and processes in daily situations such as nursing practice

A good grounded theory, according to nurse scientists who work to develop them,

- results from formulating and discarding hypotheses if they are not supported by data
- has included a look for contradictory occurrences
- is based on a variety of *slices of data,* direct observations, interviews, and document analysis
- can transcend the substantive area and have broader relevance
- specifies the conditions under which it was developed and to which it can be generalized
- fits the data
- works to explain the variations in behavior in a given area and to predict what can occur when conditions change
- is relevant and comprehensible to people in the study setting
- is modifiable, dense, and integrated into a tight analytic framework

May (1985) suggests that the consumer ask the following questions when evaluating the credibility of a grounded theory.

1. *The research question.* Is it too narrow? Has the original question been supplanted with one grounded in data? Does it focus on exclusively psychological variables or social-interactional ones?

2. *Data sources.* Are multiple slices of data from a variety of sources (field notes, interviews, documents) used as the basis for analysis? Is the data base sufficient to capture all the range and variation in codes and categories?

3. *The literature.* Does the study include correspondence with, but not over-reliance on, related literature?

4. *The analytic scheme.* Is it clear, plausible, and well integrated?

5. *Relevance to the real world of practice.* Will it make a difference?

Phenomenologic-Interpretive Research   The terms phenomenology and **hermeneutics** are often used interchangeably. They refer to the study of human meanings and practices, with an emphasis on interpreting lived experience from narrative text, or "stories." The term hermeneutics can be traced to the Greek word meaning "to interpret." This word was derived from the messenger Hermes, who was responsible for changing the unknowable messages from the Delphic oracle to a form humans could understand through language and writing. The aim of phenomenology is to understand how people experience the world without classifying it or taking it out of context. The goal of interpretive research is to discover meaning and achieve understanding, not to generate theoretical constructs.

Research questions in phenomenologic research are designed to grasp lived human experiences and meanings connected to them. In a study of family caregivers of young schizophrenics, Chesla (1991) posed the following questions:

1.   What are parents' explanatory models of schizophrenia?

2.   What adaptive demands do schizophrenic illness behaviors place on parents and the family unit? Are there themes across families?

3.   How do personal backgrounds and interpersonal concerns shape day-to-day stress and coping?

Interpretive analysis relies on text or narrative data to discover meanings and unveil common practices. Interpretive analysis is committed to understanding, not to generalizing or preparing for subsequent quantitative research. Interpretive research is a writing and thinking activity that results in (1) paradigm cases, (2) exemplars, and (3) thematic analyses that are useful in presenting the meaning of the text.

Paradigm cases are whole cases that stand out vividly, revealing particular patterns of meaning. Chesla (1991) used paradigm cases to formulate particular forms of care, such as "engaged care," "self-care in tension with care of the other," "care as specialized management," and "care from a distance."

Exemplars are both interpretive and presentation strategies. They share the characteristics of paradigm cases, except they are shorter stories or vignettes that capture similar meanings in objectively different contexts (Benner 1985).

Thematic analysis involves recognizing common themes that appear in the textual data. Themes in Chesla's study of family care for young schizophrenics included "impact of illness on work," "social life of caregivers," and "personal meaning changes."

Ultimately it falls to the reader to judge whether the product of an interpretive study has succeeded in transforming a lived experience into a textual expression that reflects something meaningful. Validation from study participants themselves is viewed as a powerful indicator of credibility in this type of research.

APPLICATIONS TO NURSING PRACTICE

Clinical nurses have only recently begun to rely significantly on reports of research findings to answer their questions. Heretofore they tended to turn to authority, tradition, and trial and error when deciding whether to warm an infant's formula or to oxygenate before, in between, or after suctioning. Much of nursing practice was a combination of folk healing traditions and technology. As nursing's unique perspective has become clearer, Goldman's challenge has become more compelling: "It is up to us to accept strange and difficult ideas and to abandon the complacency of converting all that is novel into clichés of the familiar" (1980 p. 14).

The methods of qualitative analysis discussed in this chapter offer nursing one approach for developing much-needed middle-range theories for practice while capitalizing on the observational sensitivity of practicing nurses. Nursing needs modes of inquiry and analysis that offer the freedom to explore on a conceptual level the richness of human experience, with all its variation. Nursing care requires an understanding of people in complex, changing social contexts. Its scope of practice encompasses people of all ages, social classes, developmental levels, and degrees of wellness and illness who are engaged in all sorts of psychological, physical, and social processes. Nurses apply and synthesize knowledge from physical, social, and medical sciences as well as from the humanities to form their knowledge base. They recognize that theirs is a complex and diversified professional domain. They need research methods that are rigorous and that allow them to predict causes and outcomes. But they also need analytic methods that allow them to define, describe, and explain the real practice world of nursing to themselves and others.

Various research and analytic approaches need not compete with one another. No one entrenched philosophical stance or pet method in and of itself will lead to theoretical advances in nursing. True discoveries in nursing will probably come only from the use of many methods of analysis. The qualitative methods and procedures described in this chapter represent one set of legitimate approaches for understanding certain kinds of research questions about everyday nursing practice—one way of moving from observations to explanations and from practice to theory.

RESEARCH EXAMPLE

Hutchinson SA. Responsible subversion: A study of rule-bending among nurses. *Scholarly Inquiry for Nursing Practice: An International Journal.* 1990;4(1):3–17.

Study Problem/Purpose

The purpose of this qualitative field study was to explore and describe how nurses bend the rules for the sake of patients.

Purpose is theory generating

Methods:

Three hundred hours of participant observation on several clinical units, including neonatal intensive care, labor and delivery, and psychiatry, along with in-depth informal interviews with nurses on these units and a purposive sample of 21 additional nurses from coronary care, midwifery, medical-surgical, and pediatrics units, served as the data base for this research. The methods associated with discovering grounded theory were employed to analyze this data.

Findings

Responsible subversion emerged as the core variable, or key construct, to describe nurses bending the rules for the sake of their patients. Nurses who engage in the responsible subversion process have knowledge, an ideology, and experience. The process has four phases: (1) evaluating, (2) predicting, (3) rule-bending, and (4) covering. Strategies for rule-bending include pretending, stalling, critically evaluating timing, contouring information, exaggerating, encouraging patients to refuse medication, interpreting orders flexibly, and collusion.

Implications

Responsible subversion may result in positive or negative consequences. In both cases, actions taken by nurses reveal caring behaviors and demonstrate nurses' belief in the self-determination of the patient and the ethical notion of beneficence. This study explains how nurses make decisions about what is professionally right and wrong in a context of ambiguity, conflict, and frustration.

Guidelines for Critique

Does the researcher fully describe the way in which field research was conducted?

What data collection strategies were used? Why were they chosen?

If the data were collected by a participant observer, was the observer able to maintain intellectual distance from the subjects and events?

Were interviews semistructured or unstructured? What procedures were used to record responses?

What methods of qualitative analysis were applied to the data? Why were these methods chosen?

If a content analysis was performed, what efforts were made to establish validity and reliability of content categories?

If analytic induction was used, has the investigator demonstrated that the results are generalizable? Have observer biases been taken into account? Was the credibility of respondents carefully evaluated?

If the researcher has used a grounded theory approach, does it meet the standards for credibility outlined in the chapter?

If phenomenologic-interpretive methods were used, has the investigator used textual data to uncover themes, exemplars, and paradigm cases?

Summary of Key Ideas and Terms

Qualitative research relies on firsthand knowing under natural conditions and on unstructured data-collection methods in which the investigator is the primary instrument or tool.

The major characteristics of *field studies* are:

- face-to-face interviewing or observation by the investigator
- data collection and analysis of complex sets of variables that go on simultaneously and in the natural setting
- a combination of inductive and deductive thinking to yield multiple, complex concepts, propositions, and middle-range theories

Appraising the suitability of the setting or field is the first stage in doing research. Any place or set of activities can be considered "the field" for a study.

Problems and strategies for gaining entree to the field vary according to whether your research is overt or covert and to the general degree of accessibility of the study setting itself. The role of observer can range along a continuum from complete participant to complete observer. Each role has advantages and disadvantages.

Data collection in field research begins with an initial mapping of the setting to orient oneself to its various social, spatial, and temporal dimensions. Then it is guided by categories and ideas that emerge during the course of observation.

Methods of field research include participant observation, interviewing, and analysis of documents, case studies, and case histories, and other unobtrusive measures.

One model for recording field notes is to use a system that organizes them into *observational notes* (ONs), *methodological notes* (MNs), and *personal notes* (PNs).

Semistructured and unstructured interviews are preferred by field researchers, because they emphasize freedom in exploring whatever is important to the interviewee and stimulating responses that are spontaneous and revealing.

Documents such as diaries, books, letters, meeting minutes, legal papers, reports, films, photographs, and nursing notes are all excellent sources of data in field studies. *Case studies* and *case histories* are also valuable sources of data.

Qualitative analysis is the nonnumerical organization and interpretation of data in order to discover patterns, themes, forms, and qualities found in unstructured data.

Four major purposes of qualitative analysis are exploration and description, accounting for and illustrating quantitative findings, discovery and explanation, and extension of theory.

The major procedures for analyzing qualitative data are converting to quantitative data, doing a content analysis, analytic induction, discovering grounded theory, and the phenomenologic-interpretive approach.

References

Becker HS. Problems of inference and proof in participant observation. *Am Soc Rev.* December 1958;23:652–660.

Benner P. Quality of life: A phenomenological perspective on explanation, prediction, and understanding in nursing science. *Adv Nurs Sci.* 1985;8(1):1–4.

Blumer H. *Symbolic Interactionism.* Englewood Cliffs, NJ: Prentice-Hall;1969.

Chesla CA. Parents' caring practices with schizophrenic offspring. *Qual Health Res.* 1991;1:446–468.

Denzin NK. *Interpretive Interactionism.* Newbury Park, Calif: Sage;1989.

Dickoff J & James P. A theory of theories. *Nurs Res.* September/October 1968;17: 197–203.

Douglas JD. *Investigative Social Research: Individual and Team Field Research.* Beverly Hills, Calif: Sage;1976.

Fagerhaugh S & Strauss A. *Politics of Pain Management.* Menlo Park, Calif: Addison-Wesley;1977.

Glaser BG. *Theoretical Sensitivity.* Mill Valley, Calif: Sociology Press;1978.

Glaser BG & Strauss A. *The Discovery of Grounded Theory: Strategies for Qualitative Research.* Chicago: Aldine;1967.

Glaser BG & Strauss A. *Anguish: A Case History of a Dying Trajectory.* Mill Valley, Calif: Sociology Press;1970.

Glaser BG & Strauss AL. *Status Passage.* Chicago: Aldine;1971.

Goldman I. Boas on the Kuskiutl: The ethnographic tradition. *Sarah Lawrence College: Essays from the Faculty.* 1980;4:5–23.

Hitchcock J & Wilson HS. Personal risking: Lesbian self-disclosure to health professionals. *Nurs Res.* May/June 1992;41(3):178–183.

Hutchinson S. Chemically dependent nurses: The trajectory toward self-annihilation. *Nurs Res.* July/August 1986;35(4):196–201.

Hutchinson SA. Responsible subversion: A study of rule-bending among nurses. *Scholarly Inquiry for Nursing Practice: An International Journal.* 1990;4(1):3–17.

Hutchinson SA & Wilson HS. Validity threats in scheduled semi-structured research interviews. *Nurs Res.* March/April 1992;41(3):117–119.

Hutchinson S. Creating meaning out of horror. *Nurs Outlook.* 1984;32:86–90.

May KA. A typology of detachment and involvement styles adopted during pregnancy by first time expectant fathers. *West J Nurs Res.* 1980;2:445–461.

May KA. Writing the grounded theory study. In: *Qualitative Research in Nursing: From Practice to Grounded Theory.* Chenitz WC & Swanson J (editors). Menlo Park, Calif: Addison-Wesley;1985.

Morse JM. *Qualitative Nursing Research: A Contemporary Dialogue.* Newbury Park, Calif: Sage;1991.

Mosher LR & Menn A. Community residential treatment for schizophrenia: Two year follow-up. *Hosp Comm Psych.* 1978;29:715–723.

Norris CM. Restlessness: A nursing phenomenon in search of meaning. *Nurs Outlook.* February 1975;23:103–107.

Polsky N. *Hustlers, Beats, and Others.* Garden City, NY: Doubleday;1969.

Schatzman L & Strauss A. *Field Research: Strategies for a Natural Sociology.* 2nd ed. Englewood Cliffs, NJ: Prentice-Hall;1982.

Wilson HS. *Deinstitutionalized Residential Care for the Mentally Disordered: The Soteria House Approach.* New York: Grune & Stratton;1982.

ETHICS AND THE RIGHTS OF RESEARCH SUBJECTS

HOLLY SKODOL WILSON

CHAPTER OUTLINE

In This Chapter . . .

CHAPTER OBJECTIVES

After reading this chapter, you should be able to:

- Demonstrate awareness of the characteristics of ethical scientific research

- Compare the similarities between existing codes of research ethics

- Recognize human subjects who are particularly vulnerable to risk in nursing research

- Evaluate a research study's provisions for the protection of the rights of research subjects: (1) freedom from harm, (2) full disclosure, (3) self-determination, and (4) privacy, anonymity, and confidentiality

- Define **ethics, debriefing, risk-benefit ratio, minimal risk, informed consent,** and **institutional review board**

- Appreciate the complexity involved in balancing individual rights with society's rights to the development of scientific knowledge

- Advocate the protection of human rights and the principles of ethical research in clinical and scientific activities according to a personal and professional ethical framework

12

IN THIS CHAPTER . . .

Ethics is that branch of philosophy concerned with two basic questions: (1) "What is right or good?" and (2) "What should I do?" The moral judgments involved in answering such questions are most highly developed when the process of arriving at them and the reasons for believing in them are clear and convincing. The goal of this chapter is to help consumers of nursing research develop a way of thinking about the complex ethical issues and dilemmas that are often associated with human science.

The ethics of research are the product of recent years, although they rest on long-honored moral traditions. In the not-so-distant past, violations of human rights under the guise of scientific advancement took place with shocking frequency. From 1932 to 1972 more than 400 black Alabama sharecroppers and day laborers were subjects in a government study designed to deliberately withhold treatment for syphilis to study the untreated disease. James H. Jones has recounted this sad tale in his book *Bad Blood: The Tuskegee Syphilis Experiment* (1981). In the early 1960s Timothy Leary and Richard Alpert (a lecturer and an assistant professor at Harvard University) stretched the tolerance of the scientific community with their use of human subjects in studying the effects of psilocybin and LSD. In 1963 a physician injected hospitalized elderly patients at the Jewish Chronic Disease Hospital in Brooklyn with live cancer cells without informing them. Additional accounts of research using the poor and the mentally retarded crowd history books.

This chapter helps you to answer the question "How ethical is a given research project?" It also provides you with a list of characteristics of ethical research. It describes codes formulated to help protect the dignity and rights of individuals and social groups. It also acquaints you with four fundamental rights of human research subjects and the basic procedures used to ensure these rights.

MAKING SCIENCE ETHICAL

Many medical research studies can be conducted with either animal or human subjects. Nursing research, however, tends to focus more consistently on people—their health attitudes, experiences associated with illness, values, coping behaviors, support systems, community networks, and environmental stressors. Being aware of the rights of human subjects is therefore a major part of a nurse's responsibility when planning a research project, assisting in someone else's research, or evaluating a research article.

Characteristics of Ethical Research

Ethical research includes protecting the rights of human subjects but encompasses a broader list of characteristics:

- *Scientific objectivity.* The investigator reports all data points, including those that are unsupportive of hypotheses, is aware of personal values and biases, and does not preconceive a study's outcome or engage in any misconduct, fraud, or acts of bad faith in connection with the research.

- *Cooperation* with duly authorized review groups, agencies, and institutional review boards. The researcher submits the proposed research to the appropriate committee in charge of reviewing provisions for the protection of subjects' rights and is willing to comply with the committee's recommendations. Many journals require that study reports contain a statement that the research was approved from an ethical standpoint by the appropriate institutional committee.

- *Integrity* in representing the research enterprise. The investigator does not withhold information about the study's possible risks, discomforts, or benefits or intentionally deceive study subjects on these matters.

- *Equitability* in acknowledging the contributions of others. Credit is given where credit is due, by listing coauthors in publications or by acknowledging the work of others in speeches and presentations.

- *Nobility* in the application of processes and procedures to protect the rights of human subjects. The investigator works actively to protect subjects from harm, deceit, coercion, and invasions of privacy, even when the study may be inconvenienced.

- *Truthfulness* about a study's purpose, procedure, methods, and findings. The investigator does not attempt to disguise the research or conduct it "under cover."

- *Impeccability* in use of any privileges that may be associated with the researcher's role. Data are kept anonymous and confidential. The researcher is discreet about what he or she learns about people.

- *Forthrightness* about a study's funding sources and sponsorship. The researcher discloses all sources of financial support as well as any special relationship between a study and its sponsors in publications and presentations of research findings.

- *Illumination* of nursing's body of scientific knowledge through publications and presentations of research findings. Research should yield fruitful results.

- *Courage* to publicly clarify any distortions that others make of the researcher's findings.

Codes of Research Ethics

The preceding characteristics of ethical research are reflected in most professional codes of ethics for research. Box 12–1 presents a summary of the American Nurses' Association's Human Rights Guidelines for Nursing in Clinical and Other Research. Conducting research based on such codes helps investigators ensure that their research remains ethical as well as scientific.

Box 12–1 American Nurses' Association Human Rights Guidelines for Nurses in Clinical and Other Research

These guidelines attempt to specify several important entities: (1) the type of activities that are involved, (2) the rights that are to be protected, (3) the persons to be safeguarded, and (4) the mechanisms necessary to ensure that protection is adequate.

Guideline 1: Employment in Settings Where Research Is Conducted

Conditions of employment in settings in which clinical or other research is in progress need to be spelled out in detail for all potential workers. . . . Anyone employed in work that carries the potential of risk to others needs to be advised as to the types of risks involved, the ways of recognizing when risk is present, and the proper actions to take to counteract harmful effects and unnecessary danger.

Guideline 2: Nurses' Responsibilities for Vigilant Protection of Human Subjects' Rights

In all instances the prospective subject must be given all relevant information prior to participation in activities that go beyond established and accepted procedures necessary to meet his or her personal needs. . . . Nurses must be increasingly vigilant in their concern for subjects and patients who by reason of their situation and/or illness are not able to protect themselves effectively from externally imposed threat or injury. They must be sensitive to the tendency toward exploitation of "captive" populations such as students, patients, and inmates in institutions and prisons. All proposals to be used need to be discussed with the prospective subject and with any workers who are expected to participate as a subject or data collector, or both. Special mechanisms must be developed to safeguard the confidentiality of information and protect human dignity.

Guideline 3: Scope of Application

The persons for whom these human rights guidelines apply include all individuals involved in research activities and include the following groups: patients, donors of organs and tissue, informants, normal volunteers including students, and vulnerable populations that are "captive" audiences such as the mentally disordered, mentally retarded, and prisoners.

Guideline 4: Nurses' Responsibility to Support the Accrual of Knowledge

Just as nurses have an obligation to protect the human rights of patients, so do they also have an obligation to support the accrual of knowledge that broadens the scientific underpinnings of nursing practice and the delivery of nursing services.

Guideline 5: Informed Consent

To safeguard the basic rights of self-determination, consent to participate in research or unusual clinical activities must be obtained from the prospective subject or his legal representative. The subject needs to receive:

- a description of any benefit to the subject or to the development of new knowledge that might be expected

Box 12–1 (*continued*)

- an offer to discuss or answer any questionsbout the study

- a clear statement to the subject that he or she is free to discontinue participation at any time he wishes to do so

- full freedom from direct or indirect coercion and deception

Guideline 6: Representation on Human Subjects Committees

There is increasing public support for systematic accountability to ensure that individual rights are not denied human subjects who participate in research studies. In most instances, the protective mechanism takes place through a committee judged competent to review studies and other investigative activities that involve human subjects. The profession of nursing has an obligation to publicly support the inclusion of nurses as regular members of Institutional Review Committees of this kind.

Source: American Nurses' Association, 1975 Adapted and summarized with permission.

THE RIGHTS OF HUMAN RESEARCH SUBJECTS

Protecting the rights of human subjects who are involved in research has become a high priority throughout all the professional and scientific communities. Nurse researchers are often among the most responsible and conscientious investigators when it comes to respecting the rights of subjects. The responsibility for assuring that a study is ethical is no longer exclusively the investigator's. Recent guidelines such as those in Box 12–1 have been established to ensure an unbiased review. They rely on two historical documents: The Nuremberg Code and the Declaration of Helsinki.

The Nuremberg Code

The first internationally accepted effort to set up formal ethical standards governing human research subjects is now known as the Nuremberg Code, or Nuremberg Articles. When the U.S. secretary of state and secretary of war learned that the defense of the Nazi doctors during the trials of war criminals after World War II would center on justifying their atrocities on the ground that the doctors were "engaged in important research," the American Medical Association was asked to appoint a group to develop a code of ethics for research against which sadistic experiments on concentration camp prisoners would be judged.

The code they developed requires informed consent in *all* cases and makes no provision for any special treatment of children, the elderly, or the mentally incompetent. Its definitions of the terms *voluntary, legal capacity, sufficient understanding,* and the *enlightened decision* have been the subjects of numerous court cases and the focus for several presidential commissions

---

Box 12–2 Articles of the Nuremberg Tribunal

1. The voluntary consent of the human subject is absolutely essential. . . .

2. The experiment should be such as to yield fruitful results for the good of society, unprocurable by other means of study, and not random and unnecessary in nature. . . .

3. The experiment should be so designed and based on the results of animal experimentation and knowledge of the natural history of the disease or other problems under study that the anticipated results will justify the performance of the experiment. . . .

4. The experiment should be conducted to avoid all unnecessary physical and mental suffering and injury. . . .

5. No experiment should be conducted where there is a prior reason to believe that death or disabling injury will occur. . . .

6. The degree of risk to be taken should never exceed that determined by the humanitarian importance of the problem to be solved by the experiment. . . .

7. Proper preparations should be made and adequate facilities provided to protect the subject against . . . injury, disability, or death.

8. The experiment should be conducted only by scientifically qualified persons. . . .

9. The human subject should be at liberty to bring the experiment to an end. . . .

10. During the experiment the scientist . . . if he has probable cause to believe that a continuation of the experiment is likely to result in injury, disability, or death to the experimental subject . . . will bring it to a close.

Source: Katz 1972 pp. 289–290.

---

engaged in standard setting. The code itself disallows any research on subjects who are not capable of giving consent. See Box 12–2 for the Articles of the Nuremberg Tribunal.

The Declaration of Helsinki

The Declaration of Helsinki was issued in 1964 by the World Medical Association as a guide for physicians engaged in clinical research. Revised in 1974, the declaration differentiates between two major types of research: (1) that which is essentially therapeutic and (2) that which is essentially directed toward developing scientific knowledge and has no therapeutic value for the subject. The contemporary application of this document in nursing research emphasizes the requirement to inform research subjects when a clinical or nonclinical study will have no personal benefit to them and to avoid any subtle suggestion to the contrary. Both the Nuremberg Code and the Declaration of Helsinki served as the basis for the U.S. policies and regulations issued in 1966.

U.S. Policies and Procedures

The ethical protection of the rights of human subjects in research studies is no longer left solely to the judgment of the individual investigator, nor is the researcher's need to know something or even the benefit of society considered adequate justification for any and all research practices. Previous abuses of human beings in the interest of science have resulted in insistence by the government agencies that support nursing, medical, biological, and social research that ethical standards be followed if a project is to be funded. In fact, the U.S. surgeon general, in 1966, and subsequent secretaries of the Department of Health, Education, and Welfare (1971) issued regulations governing the use of human subjects in research funded by the National Institutes of Health. The rules require that before research proceeds, an **institutional review board** (IRB) functioning in accordance with specifications of the department must review and approve all studies. In 1981 two regulations were added. One excepted several categories of research from the review requirement. The other provided the option of an expedited review in instances where risks were presumed to be minimal, such as use of noninvasive procedures, collection of external secretions, voice recording, and the like.

Four Basic Rights

Balancing the obligation to conduct the most valuable study with the obligation to safeguard the rights of human subjects is not an easy task and embroils researchers and reviewers alike in stormy ethical issues. From a moral point of view, however, four basic rights of research subjects must be protected in all instances.

The Right Not to Be Harmed   The regulations of the Department of Health, Education, and Welfare (now the Department of Health and Human Services) defined risk of harm to a research subject as exposure to the possibility of injury going beyond everyday situations. They included physical, emotional, legal, financial, and social harm. Withholding treatment in order to study the course of a disease is clearly a physiological danger. But risks to human subjects in a nursing study may also be more subtle. For example, parents who are asked to complete a questionnaire, ostensibly dealing with "health issues," after the death of their child may experience undue anxiety and the awakening of guilt if sensitive items are included that could evoke disturbing feelings. The risk is particularly high if no **debriefing** (the process of disclosing to the subject any information that was previously withheld) is conducted afterward and no provision for referral to counseling is included in the study protocol.

   Merely agreeing to be confined for an extended period in a hospital for research purposes exposes a subject to an increased risk of hospital infections, boredom, and missed opportunities. Participating in a randomized treatment study (see chapter 7) places the subject at a 50% risk of receiving care or treatment that may not be as effective as the standard or control treatment with which the experimental treatment is being compared. Simple procedures such as venipuncture performed for research purposes involve risks that range from a small bruise to death.

Other risks associated with nursing research studies include:

- Loss of confidentiality, which could occur if a nursing faculty member required students enrolled in a course to complete a questionnaire about personal experiences with recreational drugs.

- Loss of privacy by becoming a subject in multiple studies because of one's serious illness or condition (for example, a cancer patient who is terminally ill may be willing to agree to anything to sustain hope for recovery).

- Being subject to additional procedures and tests as a consequence of participating in clinical research and then being charged for them. Most institutions require that investigators assume costs for tests done for research purposes.

- Being duped into thinking that participating in a study will positively affect one's care or condition directly, when in fact the advancement of knowledge or the development of a new commercial product may be the only benefit.

- Exploitation by commercial sponsors who ask patients to donate extra blood or endure discomfort or inconvenience so that the firm can develop a new, marketable product.

In summarizing the riskiness of research procedures, Reynolds (1972) identified five categories, in order of increasing risk:

1. No positive or negative effects expected on the research subjects. Such studies include chart reviews and tissue studies. Formal consent procedures and forms may be waived by some review boards in such cases.

2. Temporary discomfort, anxiety, or physical pain. Here the discomfort is no more than would be encountered in day-to-day living and ceases with the termination of the experiment. Simple venipuncture for taking a blood sample would fit into this category.

3. Unusual levels of temporary discomfort that may last beyond the end of the study and that may require a debriefing interview or conference to return a subject's anxiety to normal. An interview or questionnaire that evokes strong feelings or upsets the subjects might fall into this category, as would research in which subjects are not told from the start the authentic question under investigation.

4. Risk of permanent damage, such as might result from the use of an investigational drug or device.

5. Certainty of permanent damage. Examples of this fifth category exist among the abuses of human subjects cited earlier in this chapter—the Tuskegee syphilis study and the like.

Concern for protecting human research subjects has been extended beyond research that threatens bodily harm, such as drug toxicity or discomfort, to include research that threatens a subject's self-esteem, self-worth, values, composure, privacy, and even religious freedom. The risks of anxiety, embarrassment, or other stressors must be weighted against the benefits in any study, and the **risk-benefit ratio** must be clearly disclosed to all research subjects before they agree to participate. Two key considerations that evolve when attempting to apply the right not to be harmed: (1) Certain subjects are vulnerable and may not be able to evaluate risks involved in a study (for example, unconscious patients). (2) The risk-benefit ratio of a research project may not justify exposure of subjects to the risks.

In the first instance, children, fetuses, the mentally disabled, the elderly, captives, the dying, and the sedated or unconscious are **vulnerable groups of subjects.** In such cases a guardian or advocate should be identified to provide special consideration and protection. Even here, however, there seem to be no simple answers, only complicated ones. For example, can a mother who has volunteered for an abortion have the interest of the fetus in mind when evaluating the risks associated with an untested intrauterine fetal research procedure? The fundamental rule here is that the less able a subject is to give informed consent, the greater the burden on the investigator to protect the subject's rights.

The second issue in calculating the risk-benefit ratio requires that risks to research subjects be justified by potential benefit to them (in the case of clinical research) or to society (in the form of knowledge produced). The benefits, in short, should exceed the risks. Even then, the risks to a cancer patient of increased side effects from combining near-toxic levels of multiple chemotherapeutic agents may not always be justified by advancing society's knowledge of cancer treatment. This risk-benefit ratio continues as a primary objective standard by which we can judge the ethics of certain research procedures. Its calculation involves naming the benefits and weighing them as well as considering the following two questions: (1) How important is the research? and (2) How serious are the risks to human subjects? Some critics, however, cite this standard as "typically American" in its pragmatism, in that it judges the morality of research practices by the results produced. Often the benefits of "basic" research (see chapter 1) are difficult to identify. In any case, if harm, be it physiological or psychological, is involved, the investigator must explain how the risks will be minimized. The subjects must be fully aware of the risks, and the nature of the benefits expected from the study must be convincing. *Minimal risk* means that the risks of harm anticipated in the proposed research are not greater than those ordinarily encountered in daily life or during the performance of routine examinations or tests.

The Right to Full Disclosure Full disclosure involves informing subjects about the following aspects of any study:

- the nature, duration, and purposes of the study
- the methods, procedures, and processes by which data will be collected, expressed in straightforward lay terminology (for example, teaspoons or

ounces of blood to be drawn, rather than cc's)—in short, what will happen to them

- the use to which findings will be put and any personal or societal benefits that could derive from the research

- any and all inconveniences, potential harms, or discomforts that might be expected, including becoming a target for inclusion in future studies, risking loss of privacy or confidentiality, and commitment of personal unreimbursed time

- any results or side effects that might follow from participation in a study, including follow-up interviews or questionnaires

- alternatives to participating in the study that are available to the subject

- the right to refuse to participate or to withdraw at any time

- the identities of the investigators and how to contact them

Full disclosure means that deception, either by withholding information about a study in the interest of protecting its validity or by giving a subject false information about the study, is unethical. Examples of deception in research abound: Researchers have taken undercover jobs in mental institutions as nursing aides or attendants while engaging in observational research. Parents have been told that a study was focusing on child development rather than on their own attitudes and behavior toward their battered children. The scientific rationale for deception is that knowing the point of the research would influence either the natural behavior of the subjects or their willingness to consent to participate, or both. Researchers may argue, for example, that informing staff nurses that the amount of time they spend on paperwork as compared with patient care is being studied might alter their usual behavior.

The Right of Self-Determination   Research subjects who have the right of self-determination will feel free from constraint, coercion, or undue influence of any kind. Many research subjects feel pressured to participate in studies if they are in powerless, dependent positions, such as being a patient in a nursing home, or if they feel they must please nurses who are responsible for their treatment and care. To allow these patients self-determination, researchers will avoid coercive or seductive language in introduction letters and consent forms. Instead of referring to a study as the investigation of "a promising new relaxation technique for controlling the pain experienced by cancer patients," for example, investigators will use a more neutral expression, such as "an experimental pain control technique involving meditation." Similarly, any promises of getting special attention or of becoming famous by making a contribution to science, or other such masked inducements, are strictly avoided. For example, a nursing study investigating the effects of injection rates on the intensity of first and second pain of intramuscular injection stated forthrightly that (1) there were no known additional risks from being in the study, other than that the injection a subject received might be more or less painful than an injection given by another method, and (2) there were no personal benefits to the study subjects because the purpose of the study was to learn about intramuscular injection pain.

The Right of Privacy, Anonymity, and Confidentiality   *Privacy* enables a person to behave and think without interference or the possibility that private behavior or thoughts may be used to embarrass or demean the person later. A study is considered truly *anonymous* if even the investigator cannot link a subject with information reported. *Confidentiality* means that any information that a subject divulges will not be made public or available to others.

The use of instruments such as hidden tape recorders, cameras, or one-way mirrors without a subject's knowledge or permission is an invasion of privacy. Personal activities, opinions, attitudes, beliefs, letters, diaries, and records are generally private property and may not be used as sources for research data without a subject's permission. Even certain records such as school or health records are released only with a person's consent. Invasion of privacy occurs when the subject is not aware of the information being elicited and the use to which it will be put.

If private information is to be collected, at a minimum the investigator will:

1. Maintain the anonymity of subjects by avoiding personally identifiable information on data-collection forms, substituting code numbers for names and keeping a master list under lock and key in a separate place.

2. Preserve the confidentiality of data sources by limiting access to the raw data by people other than the principal investigator. If a loss of confidentiality is threatened, all records and links to identity will be destroyed.

The investigator informs research subjects of the measures that will be used to maintain confidentiality and anonymity and to protect their privacy. For example, in a study of stress and role strain in RN baccalaureate nursing students, subjects were told, "There is no identifier attached to the questionnaire, and once the data are pooled, they cannot be used to identify respondents in any way except for school attended."

ENSURING THAT RESEARCH IS ETHICAL

Although it is the responsibility of investigators to examine their own projects with all the conscience and candor they can summon, federal regulations require that institutions, including universities, hospitals, nursing homes, and health agencies, establish review committees on human research subjects, often called **institutional review boards,** or IRBs.

The Institutional Review Board

The activities that fall under the jurisdiction of board review, as succinctly set forth in the 1974 Code of Federal Regulations, include:

> . . . *any research, development, or related activities which depart from the application of those established and accepted methods necessary to meet the subject's needs or which increase the risk of daily life.*

Thus, an established nursing procedure with therapeutic benefit to patients does not fall under board jurisdiction, because it is not research. Yet a federally funded evaluation study of teaching strategies in a nursing course in which students are randomly assigned to one of two types of teaching will require that the investigator obtain informed consent from the student subjects and undergo board review.

Review boards are formed in any institution that receives significant federal funding or that does a significant amount of drug or device research regulated by the Food and Drug Administration (FDA). Many smaller hospitals and institutions have no board per se but have a research advisory committee that could substitute.

Most boards have instructions for researchers that include steps to be taken to receive board approval, forms for a human-subjects protocol, guidelines for writing a standard consent form, and criteria for qualifying for an expedited rather than a full committee review.

Institutional review boards make final decisions on all federally funded research protocols involving human subjects. Their duty is to protect subjects from undue risk and deprivation of personal rights and dignity. This protection is achieved by reviewing the study's protocol to ensure that it meets the major requirements of ethical research, as summarized in Box 12–3.

Informed Consent

Most review boards use the *Code of Federal Regulations* to define the meaning of **informed consent:**

> . . . *the knowing consent of an individual or his/her legally authorized representative, under circumstances that provide the prospective subject or representative sufficient opportunity to consider whether or not to participate without undue inducement or any element of force, fraud, deceit, duress, or other forms of constraint or coercion.* [pp. 9–10]

Documentation that research meets the criterion of informed consent relies heavily on the board's review of a signed consent form for subjects to be involved in research. The wording of this form is a main focus of most board reviews, because the board must verify that it is suitable for promoting the free self-determination of potential subjects; otherwise, it is difficult to actually verify the consent process.

Vulnerable Subjects

A board reviewing a research protocol will exercise special care if the study involves subjects with *diminished capacity* to give free and informed consent. Prisoners, minors, fetuses, unconscious persons, psychiatric patients, the

Box 12–3 Federal Ethics Requirements for Research

In order to approve research covered by these regulations the IRB shall determine that all of the following requirements are satisfied:

1. Risks to subjects are minimized: (i) By using procedures which are consistent with sound research design and which do not unnecessarily expose subjects to risk, and (ii) whenever appropriate, by using procedures already being performed on the subjects for diagnostic purposes.

2. Risks to subjects are reasonable in relation to anticipated benefits, if any, to subjects, and the importance of the knowledge that may reasonably be expected to result. In evaluating risks and benefits, the IRB should consider only those risks and benefits that may result from the research (as distinguished from risks and benefits of therapies subjects would receive even if not participating in research). The IRB should not consider possible long-range effects of applying knowledge gained in the research (for example, the possible effects of the research on public policy) as among those research risks that fall within the purview of its responsibility.

3. Selection of subjects is equitable. In making this assessment the IRB should take into account the purposes of the research and the setting in which the research will be conducted.

4. Informed consent will be sought from each prospective subject or the subject's legally authorized representative, in accordance with [federal guidelines].

5. Informed consent will be appropriately documented, in accordance with, and to the extent required by [federal guidelines].

6. Where appropriate, the research plan makes adequate provision for monitoring the data collected to insure the safety of subjects.

7. Where appropriate, there are adequate provisions to protect the privacy of subjects and to maintain the confidentiality of data.

8. Where some or all of the subjects are likely to be vulnerable to coercion or undue influence, such as persons with acute or severe physical or mental illness, or persons who are economically or educationally disadvantaged, appropriate additional safeguards have been included in the study to protect the rights and welfare of these subjects.

Source: Committee on Human Subjects 1980.

mentally retarded, students, fellows, and employees are all categories of subjects that many boards will not approve if the desired research data can be obtained from the study of other adult or normal subjects. *Prisoners* are vulnerable because (1) no prisoner is truly a free agent, (2) financial compensation that might seem like a modest sum may constitute an excessive inducement in prison, where earning opportunities are minimal, and (3) prisoners may believe that participation in an experiment will shorten their sentence. *Minors, unconscious patients, psychiatric patients,* and *the mentally retarded* may be unable to evaluate the risks involved, and consent will need to be obtained from parents, guardians, or close relatives. *Students* should prefer-ably be recruited from classes other than an instructor's own and must never have their participation, or lack of it, influence their grades or future recom-mendations from the faculty member conducting research. Similarly, *fellows* and *employees* must be clear that their job, promotion, salary, and status are in no way dependent on serving as a research subject.

Some nurse scientists argue that review boards devised to protect the rights of human subjects in research can sometimes obstruct the efforts of nurse researchers who study certain populations. Robb (1983) believes that researchers who strictly adhere to board conditions for obtaining written in-formed consent from the elderly in institutional settings risk losing entire study populations, because many elderly people prefer being interviewed or observed to signing a consent form. She cites a study designed to evaluate per-spiration patches for estimating digoxin levels as an illustration of one that failed to recruit a single participant, despite the fact that of 312 institutional-ized elderly patients, 107 were taking digoxin. She urges researchers to find creative solutions to the burdens of written consent based on the urgent need for research into this population.

Careful ethical reflection requires that Robb's position be reconciled with the duty to protect the rights of vulnerable subjects. Consent should be con-ceived of as an agreement between two parties, investigator and subject, who have different degrees of power. Investigators are responsible for clarifying to a board what their approach to patients will be. The official consent form is only one way of putting the agreement into written form. Letters of agreement or verbal agreements made after reading an information sheet are alternative ways to document it.

Elements of informed consent under federal guidelines are summarized in Box 12–4.

The Standard Consent Form

Most investigators obtain consent through personal discussion. This process allows questions to be answered on the spot. Consent documents, added to oral consent, have two practical benefits: (1) They can aid the investigator by providing a checklist of discussion items. (2) They can aid the subject as a memory tool to be used at a later time; this suggests that a consent form should be readable and even engaging.

A consent form should tell a reasonable person from the proposed popula-tion the information he or she would wish to know in order to make an informed decision, in language that he or she is likely to understand. The sug-gested formats and language that follow are meant to replace previous, often stilted, language. The organization is adaptable; it can be put in narrative, let-ter, or outline form as desired. Short paragraphs with good margins are easy for most people to read. Boxes 12–5 and 12–6 provide examples of different formats.

Box 12–4 Elements of Informed Consent

A. Basic elements of informed consent. . . .

1. A statement that the study involves research, an explanation of the purposes of the research and the expected duration of the subject's participation, a description of the procedures to be followed, and identification of any procedures which are experimental;

2. A description of any reasonably foreseeable risks or discomforts to the subject;

3. A description of any benefits to the subject or to others which may be reasonably expected from the research;

4. A disclosure of appropriate alternative procedures or courses of treatment, if any, that might be advantageous to the subject;

5. A statement describing the extent, if any, to which confidentiality of records identifying the subject will be maintained;

6. For research involving more than minimal risk, an explanation as to whether any compensation and an explanation as to whether any medical treatments are available if injury occurs and, if so, what they consist of, or where further information may be obtained;

7. An explanation of whom to contact for answers to pertinent questions about the research and research subject's rights, and whom to contact in the event of a research-related injury to the subject; and

8. A statement that participation is voluntary, refusal to participate will involve no penalty or loss of benefits to which the subject is otherwise entitled, and the subject may discontinue participation at any time without penalty or loss of benefits to which the subject is otherwise entitled.

B. Additional elements of informed consent. When appropriate, one or more of the following elements of information shall also be provided to each subject:

1. A statement that the particular treatment or procedure may involve risks to the subject (or to the embryo or fetus, if the subject is or may become pregnant) which are currently unforeseeable;

2. Anticipated circumstances under which the subject's participation may be terminated by the investigator without regard to the subject's consent;

3. Any additional costs to the subject that may result from participation in the research;

4. The consequences of a subject's decision to withdraw from the research and procedures for orderly termination of participation of the subject;

5. A statement that significant new findings developed during the course of the research, which may relate to the subject's willingness to continue participation, will be provided to the subject; and

6. The approximate number of subjects involved in the study.

Source: From *Code of Federal Regulations* 1981.

Box 12–5 Sample Consent Form

Consent to Be a Research Subject

Ms. Nightingale is a nurse studying the way a certain blood component, called XYZ, works. To do the study, she needs blood from healthy people and from people with colds. If I agree to be in the study, a technician will draw a maximum of 100 cc's (approximately 3 ounces) of blood from my arm vein. This will be done in her lab at 1842 Clinics. Drawing blood may be uncomfortable and could produce a bruise or, rarely, an infection. There will be no benefit to me, though the study may produce information of use to nurses in the future.

I have had the opportunity to talk with Ms. Nightingale about the study. I may reach her at 123-4567 if I have questions later.

I will be paid $5.00 for this donation of blood. (If I am an employee, I agree not to participate during my work hours.)

I have received a copy of this form and the Experimental Subject's Bill of Rights to keep. I have the right to refuse to participate or to withdraw at any time without any jeopardy to my employment, my grades, or my care at this clinic.

_____   _____
Date   Subject's Signature

_____   _____
Date   Investigator's Signature

Guidelines

1. The title should mention research in some way—for example, "Consent to Be a Research Subject."

2. The form should be consistent in person and verb tense.

3. The date of typing and page number should appear in the lower left corner.

4. Legal language should not be used. There is no reason to use *herewith* or *hereby,* for example. "I understand that . . ." also tends to place words that might not be true in the subject's mouth. A consent form is at most a piece of evidence, not a legal document.

5. The name and phone number of the investigator should be clear and explicit.

Organization

1. *Statement of purpose and introduction.* This section should answer the questions, "What is being studied?" "Why?" "Why me?" "Who are the investigators?" "What is going on that is different from normal?" This part should set the stage for the remainder of the form and provide a quick review.

Box 12–6 Sample Consent Letter

Dear X:

B. Smith, RN, and L. Jones, RN, are educational researchers who are interested in learning about how students choose their nursing career. They have completed an initial study of people who have no idea what they are going to do, and now they wish to compare this group with people who have a very definite idea about their goals. They have asked me to contact a few of my nursing students to see if they would be interested in responding.

If you agree to participate, please return the questionnaire I have enclosed to them at the address listed. There is identifying information on the form. If you would agree to a further interview, please fill that in at the same time. If you would not agree, then leave the information blank to help protect your own privacy.

You might be interested in further information from them before agreeing to participate. You may call them at 123-4567. Of course, no one must participate in any research if he or she does not wish to do so.

Sincerely,

Professor N, RN, Ph.D.

2. *Procedures.* Subjects want to know, "What will happen to me if I participate that would not otherwise happen to me?" Standard or new procedures that would not ordinarily be done to these patients should be discussed. Procedures should be described in terms of the subjects' experience (blood drawing) rather than laboratory terms (CBC). Procedures affecting the selection of care (random allocation) or others that a subject might wish to know about (for example, contacting a relative) are included. The form must be complete enough to allow a subject to make plans (baby-sitting, transportation).

3. *Risks and discomforts.* Subjects should be able to gain a fair idea of the risks they will be taking and of the discomforts they might experience as a result of consenting. These include potential legal, economic, and psychological risks as well as physical risks. In some behavioral or social science studies, the term *disadvantages* might be more useful. A rule of thumb is that a side effect that is "relatively" frequent or that is "relatively" serious or permanent should be included. A side effect a reasonable person would wish to know about (sterility, scarring) should obviously be mentioned.

4. *Benefits.* An unbiased statement should be included discussing personal and societal benefits. It should not be overstated or read like an advertisement. (Note: Most review boards do not consider money paid to subjects to be a benefit.)

5. *Alternatives.* This section describes the therapeutic or treatment alternatives to participation in the study. If the only alternative is simple refusal (for example, to throw away the questionnaire), this section may be omitted.

6. *Questions.* Few subjects comprehend all details immediately or without some discussion. It is essential for them to have a way to contact an investigator for later discussion. If there is a possibility of emergency reactions, a 24-hour number should be supplied.

7. *Bill of rights.* The experimental subject's bill of rights (see Box 12–7) must be used when physically invasive procedures are involved. Studies that do not use a bill of rights ought to include the final paragraph from the bill of rights on any consent form.

8. *Payment.* Money is offered to pay for expenses, inconvenience, time, and trouble. It should not provide "undue influence" or reflect payment for acceptance of risk.

9. *Signatures.* The subject's signature should always be placed first. Other signatures may be requested. When children are involved, they should be asked to sign if they are old enough (over seven) to consider the questions, and their parents should generally be asked to give "permission" for their participation. The investigator's signature should also be included. A witness is not necessary for most studies but may be desired by the investigator or sponsor.

NURSING AND THE ETHICS OF RESEARCH

Advocates for research subjects, the researcher's own conscience, and review committees whose members have no particular investment in a particular study are all means of safeguarding the rights of human subjects. Nurses who are research investigators themselves or who assist in the research projects of others are in a position to assert and maintain the protective values of the profession. A study design that deprives one group of patients of relaxation techniques for labor pain, for example, would be unethical unless provisions were made for alternatively effective care. Projective psychological tests like the Rorschach inkblot test may represent an invasion of privacy if patients do not know that such tests may measure traits that the patients wish to conceal. Furthermore, patients are vulnerable to requests to participate in research when the person approaching them with the request is the nurse whom the patient depends on for care.

As Walker (1983) points out, obtaining approval for clinical investigations can be time-consuming and cumbersome, making it difficult for some nurses to conduct research in hospitals. But it is difficult for *anyone* to conduct clinical research unless he or she has demonstrated scientific rigor, sophistication, political savvy, and concern for the ethics of research on human subjects.

Box 12-7 Sample Experimental Subject's Bill of Rights

The rights below are the rights of every person who is asked to be in a research study.

As an experimental subject I have the following rights:

1. to be told what the study is trying to find out.

2. to be told what will happen to me and whether any of the procedures, drugs, or devices is different from what would be used in standard practice.

3. to be told about the frequent or important risks, side effects, or discomforts of the things that will happen to me for research purposes.

4. to be told if I can expect any benefit from participating, and, if so, what the benefits might be.

5. to be told the other choices I have and how they may be better or worse than being in the study.

6. to be allowed to ask any questions concerning the study both before agreeing to be involved and during the course of the study.

7. to be told what sort of treatment is available if any complications arise.

8. to refuse to participate at all or to change my mind about participation after the study is started. This decision will not affect my right to receive the care I would receive if I were not in the study.

9. to receive a copy of the signed and dated consent form.

10. to be free of pressure when considering whether I wish to agree to be in the study.

If I have other questions, I should ask the researcher or the research assistant. In addition, I may contact the institutional review board, which is concerned with protection of volunteers in research projects. I may reach the board office by calling 123-4567 from 8:00 A.M. to 5:00 P.M., Monday to Friday, or by writing to the Committee on Human Research, State University.

Participation in research is voluntary. I have the right to refuse to participate and the right to withdraw later without any jeopardy to my nursing care [my grades, my employment].

ANNOTATED RESEARCH EXAMPLE

Example of Ethical Issues in Human Research: The Prayer Experiment

In a study titled "Positive Therapeutic Effect of Prayer on an Intensive Care Population," the subjects were unknowingly to be assigned to one of two groups, experimental or control. If they were assigned to the first group, their bed number, diagnosis, and prognosis would be given to a group of Christians who would then pray for them for the entire time they were in the hospital. The purpose of the study was to "evaluate some of the various ways in which prayer helps critically ill patients."

[margin annotation: variable study purpose]

[margin annotation: study problem experimental design treatment or independent]

Discussion of the Prayer Experiment

risks

Risks
risks

Although the study seems simple and innocuous on the surface, the institutional review board of the university hospital where the study was proposed found that it contained myriad problems and issues that needed to be unraveled. These problems were in the areas of protection of patients' autonomy and in the transmission of private information. The review board acknowledged that although many people would be happy to have someone praying for them, others might not feel so positively and might, in fact, have serious objections. The issue for some members was freedom of religion, for others, it was privacy, and for still others, the simple risk of upsetting very ill patients. Upon reading the results, were they to be published in the lay press, some subjects might be quite angry to learn that they had unknowingly participated in such a study. The Belmont Report (U.S. National Commission 1978) identifies "respect for persons" as one key ethical principle used in research. What if a subject were a deeply committed non-Judeo-Christian or an atheist? Treating the intensive-care patients as if they were uninvolved persons with no feelings about whether a group of Christians who had been given private information about them should be praying for them would not be consistent with this principle. Thus, there

no consent
procedure

low benefit

appeared to be no adequate semblance of informed consent. Finally, the board raised questions about the risk-benefit ratio in this study. It noted that benefit to society is often dependent upon the strength of the research design. It is difficult to determine whether one can ever be empirically "proved" right or wrong on the power of prayer. The committee questioned how the investigator would control for confounding variables, such as someone else, in or out of the prayer group, also praying for the control group members. And how would the researcher distinguish spiritual help from physical help?

The prayer experiment ultimately earned approval from the board once a simple consent form with full disclosure about the risks to human subjects became part of the protocol and the hospital chaplain (not the patient's primary nurse) was designated as the person to approach patients about participating in the study. Even then, its endorsement by the full committee was weak.

Guidelines for Critique

Does the research report contain a statement that the study was approved by an ethical review board or similar institutional committee?

Were vulnerable subjects used?

Were subjects deceived in any way?

Were subjects fully informed of all the procedures involved in the study?

Were careful measures taken to protect subjects from harm and invasion of privacy?

Were subjects apprised of the risks, both obvious and subtle, of participating in the study?

Did the benefits resulting from the study outweigh the risks?

Was informed consent obtained from all subjects? In what form?

Did subjects have the right of self-determination (were they coerced in any way)?

Were subjects debriefed?

Have data been kept anonymous and confidential?

Has the researcher been objective in reporting results, as evidenced by inclusion of data that are unsupportive as well as those that are supportive?

Has credit been given to others who contributed to the research?

Has the researcher disclosed any sources of financial support or sponsorship?

Summary of Key Ideas and Terms

Nursing research, because it regularly involves human subjects, has a particular responsibility for conducting ethical yet scientifically sound studies.

Characteristics that make a study ethical are scientific objectivity, cooperation with authorized review boards, integrity in representing the nature of a study, equitability in acknowledging the work of others, nobility in advocating the rights of human subjects, truthfulness, impeccable use of the researcher's role, forthright honesty about a study's funding sources and sponsorship, illumination of the knowledge base of the discipline, and courage in correcting distortions.

Contemporary codes of research ethics are derived from the Nuremberg Code and the Declaration of Helsinki.

Four basic rights of human subjects are (1) the right not to be harmed, (2) the right to full disclosure, (3) the right of self-determination, and (4) the right of privacy, anonymity, and confidentiality.

One way of increasing the likelihood that research will be ethical is acquiring approval from an institutional review board. Review boards protect human subjects by providing an impartial third-party review of the issues and protections for human rights, such as (1) assuring subjects' informed consent and (2) assuring that an appropriate balance exists between the potential benefits of a study and the risks to human subjects.

Particular care must be exercised in gaining informed consent from vulnerable subjects such as prisoners, children, the mentally disabled, and the like.

Consent forms should be in plain language and should include all the information subjects need in order to give informed consent.

References

American Nurses' Association. *Human Rights Guidelines for Nurses in Clinical and Other Research.* Kansas City, Mo: ANA;1975.

Code of Federal Regulations. Title 45, Part 46. Washington, DC, January 26, 1981.

Committee on Human Subjects. *University of California at San Francisco Handbook.* San Francisco: University of California;1980.

Jones JH. *Bad Blood: The Tuskegee Syphilis Experiment.* New York: Free Press;1981.

Katz J. *Experimentation with Human Beings.* New York: Russell Sage Foundation; 1972.

Robb SS. Beware of the informed consent. *Nurs Res.* May/June 1983;32:132.

U.S. Department of Health, Education, and Welfare. *The Institutional Guide to DHEW Policy on Protection of Human Subjects.* Washington, DC: U.S. Government Printing Office;1971.

U.S. National Commission for the Protection of Human Subjects of Biomedical and Behavioral Research. *The Belmont Report: Ethical Principles and Guidelines for the Protection of Human Subjects of Research.* DHEW Publication No. (05) 78-0012. Washington, DC: U.S. Government Printing Office;1978.

Walker M. As I see it . . . Research with patients requires commitment, savvy. *Am Nurse.* July/August 1983:5.

THE

RESEARCH

CRITIQUE

HOLLY SKODOL WILSON

CHAPTER OUTLINE

In This Chapter . . .

CHAPTER OBJECTIVES

After reading this chapter, you should be able to:

■ Recognize the value of critiquing skills to research consumers

■ Distinguish between a research critique and a research review

■ Formulate strategies that contribute to making a critique constructive rather than destructive

■ Comprehend seven basic criteria for critiquing

■ Comprehend the rationale for asking the framework of critiquing questions and interpreting responses to them

■ Apply the critiquing process to research proposals and reports of findings

■ Appreciate the importance of preparing critiques that are concise, readable, rational, sensitive, accurate, and impartial

13

IN THIS CHAPTER . . .

Criticism, in everyday usage, is full of negative connotations. To criticize is "to censure, to blame, to reprove, to flay, to nit-pick, to find fault, and to pan." But in particular literary, artistic, and scientific terms, criticism takes on an entirely different meaning—one associated with analyzing, reviewing, carefully dissecting, evaluating, or judging the merit of a piece of work. In this case, criticism refers to a finely sharpened skill for ascertaining an author or creator's meaning through an unbiased endeavor to examine the characteristics and qualities of his or her contribution to art or science. In fact, criticism as it was first introduced by Aristotle was meant to be a standard for "judging well."

Leaders in nursing all seem to agree that all nurses, regardless of their educational level, should be prepared with the skills that are essential to functioning in the role of research consumer. As Horsley & Crane (1982) summarized it:

> In this role practitioners read research reports of others, determine the scientific merit and clinical utility of the studies and apply findings where appropriate.

The ability to do all this depends ultimately on the nurse's skill in conducting a critique of the scientific merit of research proposals and reports.

The purpose of this chapter is to describe and illustrate the process of critiquing scientific proposals or reports in sufficient detail that students and practitioners can replicate the process themselves with confidence and credibility. A thoughtful critique of a research report requires more than merely knowing about a list of pertinent questions to ask, such as "Is the study question clearly stated?" or "Is the review of the literature sufficiently comprehensive?" Readers need standards against which to make such judgments. Perhaps equally important is a comprehension of the rationale for both asking and attempting to answer such questions when conducting a scientific critique. This chapter presents a framework of fundamental questions and principles that underpin the process of critiquing a research proposal or report. Then it takes you through a sample critiquing experience that focuses on all aspects of a simulated proposal, using the criteria, questions, and logic of scientific criticism.

WHAT IS A RESEARCH CRITIQUE?

According to Leininger (1968), a **research critique** should be distinguished from a **research review.** A critique is "a critical estimate of a piece of research which has been carefully and systematically studied by a critic who has used specific criteria to appraise . . . the general features. . . . A research review on the other hand merely identifies and summarizes the major features and characteristics of a study" (p. 51). A research critique includes a descriptive account of what is in the study, but unlike a book report that merely summarizes the plot, the emphasis is on *making a judgment about the proposal or report's scientific merits and ultimate worth.* As must be evident from reading other chapters in this text, the scientific way of knowing is often far from flawless. Even the most conscientious researcher may have to compromise great ideas and inquiry strategies because of pragmatic and ethical considerations. The critic's challenge is to determine what the researcher has tried to do and to evaluate the strategies selected, given the overall constraints of the study. A critique presents both the criteria and the evidence for the judgments that are made. These must be sufficient to allow another reader to form an opinion based on the critique. The art of scientific criticism can be demonstrated verbally or in a formal written document, but according to Leininger's classic article, "The most distinctive behavior of a research critic is to act in a judiciously critical but kind manner as he (or she) analyzes another person's work" (p. 53).

WHAT IS THE PURPOSE OF A RESEARCH CRITIQUE?

The purpose of a research critique is to help an investigator refine and improve his or her program of inquiry and to help research consumers decide how to use findings from a study, based on a judicious appraisal of its strengths and limitations. Consider the example below.

Responding to health-related questions such as those in the following example is a regular part of a clinical nurse's role. Responding correctly requires that the nurse be skillful in critiquing studies like the one in this example.

Clinical Example of Needing Research Critique Skills

Mr. H., a 65-year-old retired attorney with a history of hypertension and coronary heart disease, appeared for his regular blood pressure check and presented the nurse practitioner with an article he had clipped from his local newspaper. The headline read: "Beer or Jogging: A Hearty Choice." The article reported on a study, published in the Journal of the American Medical Association *and conducted in Houston, which concluded that "drinking three beers a day is about as good as jogging when it comes to producing an effect that may decrease the risk of coronary heart disease." The researchers had found that volunteer runners and joggers registered about the same high-density lipoprotein (HDL), a type of cholesterol associated with heart disease, as did volunteer sedentary men who drank three cans of beer each day for the three-week period of the study. The rationale was that moderate drinking causes the liver to respond by producing the same or similar enzymes that it produces in response to exercise. Mr. H.'s question to the nurse, of course, was whether he could now substitute three beers a day for the daily walking that he'd been encouraged to do, in view of these new scientific findings.*

(handwritten margin notes) Clients seek health information from nurses. Partial reports of health research appear regularly in the popular press.

findings

Are the clients' conclusions from the findings warranted?

Whether the research critique is undertaken so that scholarly colleagues can exchange information or perspectives that will advance a particular line of inquiry, or whether it is done to better inform health care consumers or other clinicians, a competent critique ought to represent a contribution to knowledge and be helpful.

Yet the critic must not confuse helpfulness with a lack of objectivity or be so earnest in his or her wish not to discourage or offend the investigator as to suppress or drastically disguise the critical points. Nurses who have practice in exercising their critical sensibilities on the day-to-day problems of clinical practice can most certainly learn to bring the same inquiring, honest, benevolent mind to bear on the problems of research quality. Encouraging nurses to become involved with research through the role of research critic can help them identify with and gain a sense of belonging to the scientific community in nursing. Furthermore, it can integrate a research perspective into the evolving tapestry of each nurse's clinical interests. Preparing critiques of research proposals and reports that are objective, comprehensive, correct, respectful, and humane can work to the benefit of the nurse scientist, the nurse clinician, and the patients they serve.

Achieving these mutual goals requires that a critic and an investigator be able to differentiate between *constructive* and *destructive criticism.*

> *Constructive criticism is evident when the critic offers thoughtful comments which are given in such a way that they stimulate the researcher to use suggestions and motivate him (or her) to continue work on the study. In contrast, destructive criticism tends to thwart the researcher's interest in his (or her) work [Leininger 1968 p. 55].*

The careful choice of words in a critique is often cited as one of the most important features of artful and sensitive criticism that the researcher being criticized can use rather than become defensive about. A few helpful do's and don'ts in dealing with the interpersonal aspects of critiquing research are summarized in Table 13–1. Research critiques that bear in mind their real purpose and attend to the potentially delicate social psychology of the researcher-critic relationship can provide valuable opportunities for scholarly and intellectual exchanges that can advance both the science and the professional practice of nursing.

WHAT ARE THE CRITERIA FOR GOOD RESEARCH?

Recognizing the importance of upgrading standards of reporting clinical research, Field (1983) and Fleming and Hayter (1974) suggest that a combination of the following criteria be used when evaluating reports of nursing studies:

1.   clarity and relevance of the purpose

Table 13–1 *Do's and Don'ts for Sensitive Critiques*

Do	*Don't*
1. Try to convey a sincere interest in the study you are critiquing.	1. Avoid excessive nit-picking and fault finding on trivial details.
2. Be sure to emphasize the points of excellence that you discover.	2. Never ridicule or demean an investigator personally.
3. Choose clear, concise statements to communicate your observations rather than ambiguous ones.	3. Don't try to include flattery that is designed merely to boost a researcher's self-esteem.
4. When pointing out a study's weaknesses, include explanations that justify your comments about them.	4. Don't base your summary and recommendations about the study on some loose and perhaps biased attitude toward the state of all science in a particular discipline or on a particular topic.
5. Include supportive and encouraging statements where they are warranted.	
6. Be aware of your own negative attitudes toward a particular approach to science or any personal hostilities that could distort your ability to judge a study on its own merits.	5. Don't write your critique in condescending, patronizing, or condemning language.
7. Offer practical suggestions that are not overly esoteric or unrealistic.	6. Don't forget that your purpose is to advise the researcher and to improve the work.
8. Remember that empathy for the researcher is often crucial to being an effective critic.	

2. researchability of the problem
3. adequacy and relevance of the literature review
4. match between the purpose, design, and methods
5. suitability of the sampling procedure and the sample
6. correctness of the analytic procedures
7. clarity of the findings

Clarity and Relevance of the Study's Purpose

All researchers should specifically state the aims of the study being evaluated. The author should clearly explain the reasons for doing the study and indicate why it is of any importance. Finally, the reader should be convinced that conducting the study is indeed worthwhile. A judgment about the potential value of a nursing study is easier to make if you ask three questions about it:

1. Will the study solve a problem relevant to nursing?

2. Will the facts collected be useful to nursing?

3. Will the study contribute to nursing knowledge?

Many authorities believe that in order to be classified as *nursing research,* studies have to make a first-order contribution to testing clinical nursing interventions or patient responses to them. Others argue that contributions to nursing education and nursing administration, although termed *research in nursing,* are equally justifiable. The key point is to be sure that your critique does not condemn a researcher for failing to accomplish something that was not part of his or her purpose in the first place.

Researchability of the Study Problem

If you recall from chapter 3, a well-stated study problem should at least be able:

1. to be answered through the collection of empirical evidence or data

2. to be stated as a question that involves the existence of a relationship between two or more variables

Having established that the two most fundamental criteria are met in a study problem, other questions relevant to critiquing the quality of a study problem are:

3. Is the statement of the problem clearly and specifically articulated *early* in the proposal or report?

4. Have the investigators placed the study problem within the context of existing knowledge and prior work on the topic?

5. Are the hypotheses, or research questions, explicitly stated?

6. Are the concepts or variables operationally defined so that the methods for measuring them could be replicated?

7. Are the limitations and assumptions of the study included, and are they logically justifiable?

8. Does the problem statement accurately reflect the title of the study?

9. Are the study questions, or hypotheses, clear, specific, testable, and consistent with the study title, purpose, and subsequent literature review?

Adequacy and Relevance of the Literature Review

Whether it is called "a review of related literature" or "a theoretical framework" for the study, evidence that the researcher has a mastery of current knowledge on his or her topic of inquiry and has placed the proposed or reported study within its context is a third criterion for judging the scientific merit of research (see chapter 4). As a critic, you must be convinced that:

1. the investigator has selected references that logically pertain to the subject being studied and the methodology being used.

2. the investigator has not merely presented a laundry list of sources but instead has integrated them into a background synthesis that suggests how the present study resolves controversies, fills gaps in knowledge, extends or refutes what is already known, and so on.

3. the literature review section is logically organized.

4. the review does not omit classic or landmark sources (you may need to consult an expert in the substantive field of the investigation on this point if you are not familiar with the body of literature on a certain topic).

5. the investigator has been open-minded enough to include references to prior work that may not be supportive.

6. the literature review or theoretical framework makes sense as a rationale for framing the specific hypotheses or research questions being examined.

7. the review provides justification for operational definitions of concepts or variables that have been advanced.

8. the review supports the choices of data-collection tools and instruments in the present study.

Agreement of Purpose, Design, and Methods

As you recall, the study design is the overall blueprint selected to answer the research question and enhance the study's validity and reliability, and the methodology is a description of the procedures for data collection and analysis to be used in a study (see chapter 7). As a critic you should ask:

1. Does the investigator name and describe the study design, including its strengths and weaknesses for the problem under scrutiny?

2. Is the study design well matched to the task of answering the specified study questions and controlling extraneous variables that could detract from the value of study findings? (See Box 13–1 for sources of error in research studies.)

3. Does the investigator provide evidence from pilot tests or published literature that the data-collection procedures are reliable and valid?

4. Does the investigator include a copy of the data-gathering instrument or other evidence that it is free from ambiguity, bias, or significant omissions?

5. Are the sources for and adaptations of nonoriginal data-collection tools provided?

6. If the data-collection tools are self-developed, are the processes for developing them and reports for establishing their validity and reliability included?

Box 13–1 Potential Sources of Research Error

Data Characteristics

1. inadequate sampling
2. inaccurate measurement
3. unrepresentative data
4. careless observation
5. intentionally distorted data

Analytical Characteristics

1. mathematical errors
2. incorrect choice of formulas
3. comparison of nonanalogous data
4. generalization based on insufficient data
5. failure to acknowledge significant factors
6. confusion of correlation with causation
7. interpretation manipulated to support prejudice or preconception
8. elimination of contrary evidence

---

7. Are the techniques for data collection logical and practical ways of acquiring empirical evidence on study variables?

8. Does the researcher include checks to guard against possible errors in collecting, recording, and tabulating data?

9. If the design was experimental, do you find evidence of control of extraneous variables, manipulation of independent variables, randomization in both sample selection and assignment of sample members to treatment groups, and replicability?

10. What attempts were made to keep research conditions the same for all sample members?

11. Did the investigator try to keep subjects and researchers who were recording outcomes "blind" with regard to which intervention was being administered to whom?

Suitability of the Sampling Procedure and the Sample

When critiquing the study sample, you should be able to determine:

1. Did the investigator choose to use a probability or nonprobability sample? Why one or the other? (See chapter 9.)

2. What strategies were incorporated to avoid collecting a biased sample about which one could not generalize to the target population?

3. Is the sample representative of the population to which findings are to be generalized?

4. Is the sample size large enough to meet the assumptions of any statistical test that may be used in data analysis?

5. Is the sample size large enough to reduce the standard error?

6. What are the descriptive characteristics of the sample, particularly with respect to any variables that might influence study findings, such as age, education, sex, or physical or psychological condition?

7. What criteria were used to enter eligible sample members into a study?

8. How was informed consent obtained and how were the rights of the human research subjects protected? For example, did each subject get a complete and honest explanation of the purpose of the research, what was going to happen to him or her, and the use to which findings would be put?

9. Finally, were subject losses due to lack of follow-up or to dropping out detailed?

Correctness of Analytic Procedures

Data-analysis methods, including both statistical procedures and qualitative methods and appropriate references to them, should be clearly presented. Presentations of summary data should be clear enough to allow the reader to determine whether the statistical methods were the appropriate ones. Mention of the *power* of the test should be made, so that you and other readers can decide whether the study was conducted on a viable number of subjects and whether an increase or decrease in number of subjects could have affected the results and to what extent. Assumptions related to the use of statistics should all be made clear. In the case of qualitative analysis methods, sufficient detail about the analytic approach should be included so that another investigator could replicate the analytic operations. Specific questions that you should ask in the role of research critic include:

1. Does the author specifically name the statistical tests applied, along with the probability associated with significant values?

2. Does the author explain and provide references for analytic strategies for nonnumerical data?

3. Are the statistical tests used appropriate to the level of measurement (nominal, ordinal, interval, or ratio) represented by the data?

4. Is a distinction made between statistical and clinical significance?

5. Is the statistical procedure the right one to answer the specified rese question?

Clarity of Findings

The results section of a research report normally contains a technical report of how the statistical or qualitative analyses turned out with respect to study questions or hypotheses tested. The discussion of results is usually devoted to a nontechnical interpretation of them. In addition to telling us what the results mean, some researchers use the discussion section to explain why they think the results turned out the way they did. Some authors will use the discussion section to suggest ideas for further research. Results themselves will usually appear in the text of the article, in one or more tables, or in graphs (technically called figures). As a research consumer, you must be able to read, understand, and critically evaluate the results in a research report to avoid uncritical acceptance of findings just because they're in print. You don't have to be a whiz in math to get the drift of a results section in a scientific article. Becoming familiar with research terminology and the principles of scientific evidence will enable you to become much more comfortable with this task. Questions that you should ask about reports and discussions of findings include:

1. Are interpretations of results clearly based on the data obtained?

2. Are reasons given for tabulating or presenting data in particular ways?

3. Can you detect error in any computations?

4. Are there any discrepancies between results presented in graphic form and results presented in the text of the report?

5. Do all the tables and graphs have titles?

6. Are the relationships of the variables in tables clear and easy to figure out? (See Box 13–2 for additional characteristics of good tables.)

7. Has the researcher distinguished between actual findings on the one hand and interpretations made by the researcher on the other?

8. Are the findings explicit enough for you, the critic, to decide whether the interpretations are justified? (For example, some authorities agree that conclusions of any kind cannot be drawn from data returns of less than 51% of the sample.)

9. Are minor or secondary findings overemphasized in the report and major or primary findings underplayed?

10. Are the findings clearly and logically organized?

11. Is the presentation of findings impartial and unbiased?

12. Do generalizations or conclusions go beyond the data collected or the population represented by the sample?

13. Are recommendations for further research offered?

14. Does the researcher include unsuccessful efforts and negative outcomes?

15. Are limitations that might have influenced the results noted?

Box 13–2 Hallmarks of Well-Presented Tables

1. *Every table should have a title.* The title should represent a succinct description of its contents and should help make it intelligible without reference to the text. The title should be clear, concise, and adequate and should answer the questions *What? Where?* and *When?* The title should always be placed above the body of the table.

2. Every table should be identified by a number to facilitate easy reference.

3. The captions, or column headings, and the stubs, or row headings, of the table should be clear and brief.

4. Any explanatory footnotes concerning the table itself should be placed directly beneath the table.

5. In order to emphasize the relative importance of certain categories, different kinds of type, spacing, and indentation can be used.

6. It is important that all column figures be properly aligned. Decimal points and plus and minus signs also should be in perfect alignment.

7. Miscellaneous and exceptional items are generally placed in the last row of the table.

8. Abbreviations should be avoided whenever possible, and ditto marks should not be used in a statistical table.

9. Columns and rows that are to be compared with one another should be close together.

When results are summarized visually in a graph or chart, use the following guidelines to critique the visuals:

1. Decide whether the author has picked the right measure of central tendency. It's important for you to evaluate which is the *best* way to describe the central tendency for any study question.

2. Pay attention to the *range* of numbers in charts or graphs. How variable were the findings?

3. Compare figures presented in the text with those in the charts and tables, keeping alert for contradictions or inconsistencies.

4. Read the captions that accompany figures carefully and compare them with the results and discussion presented in the text. Together they will tell you a great deal about any study that you read.

CRITIQUING A SAMPLE PROPOSAL

You will now have an opportunity to practice applying the critiquing criteria presented earlier in this chapter to the hypothetical sample research proposal in Box 13–3. (A proposal is a comprehensive summary of what the researcher intends to do, how it will be done, and why it is important.) For each part of the critique, do your own analysis before reading my sample analysis.

Clarity and Relevance of the Study's Purpose

Reducing postoperative distress is indeed relevant and useful to nursing. Knowing whether a specific training program can achieve it would contribute to nursing knowledge and perhaps even alter and make more effective the nature of "standard" preoperative preparation. Thus, the sample study is both clear and relevant insofar as its purpose and value for nursing are concerned.

Researchability of the Study Problem

The investigator has met many of the standards for a researchable study problem. The problem can be answered by collecting or measuring empirical data. The investigator has explicitly asked the question: "Can training in cognitive coping skills reduce postsurgical distress in adult patients?" Coping-skills training has been identified as the independent variable and has been given an operational definition. Postsurgical distress has been identified as the dependent variable and has been provided with an operational definition. A specific hypothesis to be tested in the study has been stated: that the training will reduce postsurgical distress. And the study question is accurate and consistent with the title, purpose, and literature review.

The investigator includes some of the study's limitations. But—and this is a rather big *but*—*justification* for accepting the study with those limitations is not included. The influence of age could be controlled for, either through sampling techniques that matched comparative groups by age or through using statistical means to account for any differences in findings that could be attributed to age differences rather than to the independent variable. Similarly, strategies to minimize the Hawthorne effect—the likelihood that any significant differences between Groups A and B are due to the fact that Group A got some kind of "special attention" for four extra hours plus homework activities and group support—could have been incorporated into the study design. Four hours of other individual or group interaction could have been provided to the control group (for example, a general discussion group with the nurse, in which the coping skills were *not* taught). Finally, the possibility of biased self-report data could have been decreased by using a mailed, objective self-report form rather than a face-to-face or even telephone conversation with the nurse (particularly if the nurse doing the follow-up interviews was the same one who did the training program).

Adequacy and Relevance of the Literature Review

Again the investigator has met a number of the standards for an acceptable literature review. The references are pertinent to the subject under investigation,

Box 13–3 Sample Study Proposal

Title

Training in Cognitive Coping Skills and the Reduction of Postsurgical Distress

Purpose

Nursing's major goal after a patient experiences surgery is the patient's uncomplicated recovery. Most patients who are admitted to a hospital for surgery experience anxiety and feel helpless. They are surrounded by unfamiliar machinery and subjected to invasive procedures. Yet ample literature supports the conclusion that the events themselves rarely cause patient anxiety but rather the patients' views and information about the events. This study will demonstrate that training in cognitive coping skills can reduce patient anxiety and contribute to a less distressing postsurgical recovery. Implications of this study are that nurses will have empirical support for their role as health educators, and patients will experience surgery as less traumatic because they feel more independent and in control of their experience. In sum, the specific question for this research is whether cognitive-coping-skills training can reduce postsurgical distress in adult patients.

Hypothesis

The specific hypothesis to be tested in this study is: Patients who are trained in the use of cognitive coping skills before surgery experience less postoperative distress than similar patients who do not receive such training.

Review of Related Literature and Conceptual Framework

The conceptual framework for this study is drawn from related literature in the fields of nursing and psychology. Meichenbaum, Golfried, Mahoney and colleagues have demonstrated that an individual's internal dialogue and mental images influence not only feelings related to a situation but also a person's behavior. Langer and associates (1975) trained surgical patients to use cognitive coping skills, including reappraisal and rehearsing positive aspects of a surgical experience, and found that in their sample there was a significant reduction in postsurgical distress. Further clinical evidence of the value of using cognitive coping skills was present in studies by Meichenbaum and Wine (1970). In their research, students who had received training in coping skills began to label physiological arousal like sweating, increased heart and respiratory rate, and the like as coping rather than debilitating. Other studies have likewise reported reductions in test and speech anxiety following similar training (Wine 1971, Sarason 1973, Norman 1974). Based on the literature cited above, it seems reasonable to assume that surgical patients' internal dialogue and images related to their surgical procedures may influence their postsurgical distress. This study addresses the question of whether a surgical patient's postsurgical distress can be reduced by altering his or her views about the surgical experience through coping-skills training.

Definition of Terms

Cognitive-coping-skills training: a process by which a nurse teaches patients to change distress-provoking thoughts and styles of thinking in order to produce thoughts that decrease distress.

Box 13–3 (*continued*)

Postsurgical distress: constitutes the dependent variable in this study and will be measured operationally using the following indicators:

1. length of stay in the recovery room

2. frequency of pain medication requests

3. time required before eating again by mouth

4. length of hospital stay

5. time required to attain normal routine at home

6. self-report of experience after discharge

7. incidence and severity of postoperative complications

The cognitive-coping-skills training program constitutes the independent variable in this study and will be carried out for all sample members according to the following procedure:

I. Educational Phase

The purpose of the first phase is to convey the idea that there is no 1:1 correlation between a situation and a feeling; rather, the individual's style of thinking and mental images are the major influencing factors in distress.

This section will incorporate didactic and experiential examples of the idea above. Discussion involving sample members will be encouraged. Charts and diagrams will be used to aid in understanding the relationship between events and thoughts. Patients will be told that they probably have not been aware of the influence of thoughts on behavior because they were taught to believe that there is a correlation between the two. They will be told that thinking and thinking styles have become routine and automatic, and thus we are not aware of them. Demonstration of this concept of automatic thinking will be carried out.

There will be a homework assignment given to sample members to bring back the following day. The patients will be asked to visualize the situation of their upcoming surgery and to record their thoughts, images, and feelings concerning the surgery.

II. Rehearsal Phase

The next day, we will work with the data provided by each sample member in the following way:

Cognitive Reappraisal   1. Identify with the patients their distressful thoughts (for example, "I am going to die").

2. Teach the patients to identify their assumptions and distinguish them from facts. (Assumptions are neither true nor false but are only probabilities.)

3. Teach the patients to counter their assumptions, using thoughts and images that are incompatible with the original distress-producing thoughts.

A homework assignment will be given to reinforce what the patients have learned.

Box 13–3 (*continued*)

III. Calming Self-Talk

Patients will be taught how a stress situation occurs and how to prepare themselves. Examples will be given.

Stress comes about in stages:

Stages	*Examples of Calming Self-Talk*
1. what we say to ourselves when preparing for surgery	1. "I can develop a plan to deal with this situation."
2. the actual situation (the surgery)	2. "One step at a time. I can handle this situation."
3. coping with being overwhelmed	3. "When fear comes, just pause."
4. reinforcing self-statements	4. "I can be pleased with my progress."

IV. Cognitive Control through Selective Attention

Patients will be shown that selection of a particular focus (regular breathing, repeating a statement) is incompatible with negative thoughts that produce distress.

Data Collection Procedures and Methodology

Settings for this study will be four private and public hospitals in a West Coast urban area. Patients of either sex who are in the age range 30–55, have had no previous surgery, have no clinically documented illness, are scheduled for a cholecystectomy without common duct exploration, are willing to give informed consent, and have their physician's referral will be admitted to the study *sample* until a total *n* of 100 patients is achieved. Patients will be assigned alternately to Group A or Group B. Group A will receive cognitive-coping-skill training, and Group B, the control group, will receive no special preoperative preparation other than standard care.

The training will be done by the same nurse with special skills in this method and will take one hour for each of four days before admission to the hospital for surgery. Patient data will be obtained from the following data sources:

1. the recovery room chart

2. the ward patient chart

3. telephone interviews to obtain self-reports

4. one follow-up home visit conducted one month after discharge

Limitations in the form of uncontrolled *extraneous variables* that are acknowledged consist of the following:

1. Patients at the younger end of the age range may recover more quickly than patients at the older end.

2. Self-report data may be influenced by sample members' attempting to please the interviewer.

Box 13–3 (*continued*)

3. The absence of comparable preoperative intervention for the control group leaves unanswered the question of whether any differences are due to the training per se or just to any form of special attention.

Data Analysis

The following mock tables reflect the data analysis plan. Scores will be constructed for frequencies of behaviors, summarized in Table I, and frequency of negative and positive comments reported in postoperative phone and home-visit interviews, reflected in Table II. Statistical-analysis procedures will include descriptive data summaries that characterize the study sample and specific techniques appropriate for comparing frequencies for significant differences. Expectations are that the hypothesis will be supported and that both statistically and clinically significant differences will be found between Group A and Group B on the dependent variable of postoperative distress.

Table I: Frequency of Postoperative Distress Behaviors

Distress Behavior	Total Frequency *Group A*	Total Frequency *Group B*
1. Length of stay in recovery room (hours)		
2. Number of pain-medication requests		
3. Time required to begin eating by mouth (hours)		
4. Length of hospital stay (hours)		
5. Time required to attain normal routines at home (hours)		
6. Numbers of postoperative complications		

Table II: Self-Report on Postoperative Distress

Number of Negative Comments		Number of Positive Comments	
Group A	*Group B*	*Group A*	*Group B*
Total	Total	Total	Total

are integrated and logically organized, and provide a rationale for the present study. We can also note the following deficiencies, however:

1. The references are dated (not current).

2. We are left unsure about how this particular study will extend prior work.

3. One of the dates is omitted from the references.

4. The literature review does not provide us with the investigator's rationale for measuring the dependent variable of postsurgical distress in the manner chosen.

5. We really don't get much insight into the researcher's awareness of the range of opinion and extent of research findings in the problem area. For example, we don't know whether this is a well-studied area or whether the references incorporated represent the totality of the work previously done on this topic.

Agreement of Purpose, Design, and Methods

Although the study has been designed to try to answer the research question, we must notice that a number of omissions make it difficult to conclude that efforts to increase its validity and reliability will be successful. For example, the investigator does not ever actually discuss the choice of a study design and therefore does not comment on its strengths and weaknesses. Because sample members are not randomly selected or assigned, we can surmise that this is a quasi-experimental design with a comparative group. But we are not assured that the two groups are actually comparable once they have been constructed, because analysis of demographic data is not included in the analysis plan.

We have commented earlier on the ways in which the procedures fail to control for some of the extraneous variables that could affect the study findings. We also have no results of pilot studies or power analyses on which to base any decisions about the reliability and validity of data-collection operations and adequacy of sample size. For example, is it correct to assume that the number of requests for pain medication is necessarily an indicator of postoperative distress? Might cultural or personal preferences about taking medication be a factor here? The investigator also does not provide us with copies of the data-collection and data-recording tools, making it hard to assess exactly how self-report data, in particular, will be obtained and making it impossible to actually replicate the study. Not knowing what tools or instruments will be used makes it impossible for us to know their sources, their tested validity and reliability, or how they were developed—if they were. Finally, although conditions were apparently to be the same for all members of Group A, who experienced the experimental treatment, conditions for Group B were not comparable to those for Group A, and we have no reason to believe that the rater or interviewer was blind when collecting the postoperative data on the dependent variable.

Suitability of the Sampling Procedure and the Sample

The investigator does tell us the size of the intended sample, the fact that it will be collected from four different hospital settings, and the criteria used to enter eligible sample members into the study. What we find missing is the rationale for these choices. Why not a random sample and assignment to groups? On what basis was the sample size of 100 made? Addition of more of the sampling logic and reporting on the characteristics of the two groups in the study's final report both represent areas for improvement.

Correctness of Analytic Procedures

The logic of analysis of data in the study is underdeveloped and incomplete. Why focus exclusively on absolute frequencies? Are they all of equal weight or importance? What, specifically, will be performed statistically to answer the study question and test the hypothesis for significant differences between the two groups? The analysis section is perhaps the weakest single aspect of the study proposal. We are unable to answer any of the questions appropriate for conducting a critique of a study's analytic procedures, even though sample tables are incorporated. For instance, we don't know the name of the statistical tests to be applied, the probability associated with significant values, how any extra qualitative data might be analyzed or if it will be, whether the intended statistical tests are appropriate to the level of measurement and study question, and what the researcher intends to do about clinically significant findings that may not be "statistically" significant.

Clarity of Findings

Because this is a study proposal rather than a study report, there are, of course, no research findings. Instead, review the questions under this criterion and apply them to a report of findings in a current nursing research journal. And remember that it is neither just nor reasonable to criticize a piece of work such as the simulated proposal we have just dissected for failing to be or do something that the author never intended for it. Our sample proposal could, however, be improved by a less abrupt conclusion that would serve as an abstract or summary of the entire study.

CRITIQUING RESEARCH—SOME FINAL TIPS

The preceding criteria, questions, principles, and illustrations are all intended to serve as guidelines in critiquing research proposals or reports of study findings. It is never justifiable to apply them without giving sufficient rationale for your opinion that they are appropriate and your conclusions in relation to them. Try to keep in mind the audience for whom the research was intended, and think about the work as a whole even as you scrutinize it for details like the ones suggested in the questions associated with each of the seven criteria. Remember to avoid nit-picking about trivial details, thereby sacrificing the good in favor of the perfect. How you evaluate a piece of research may influence the decisions of others to replicate it or base their practice on it. Try to consult experts and other resource persons on technical aspects that you may feel uncertain about in order to ensure the accuracy and precision of your interpretation. Be considerate in your language. *Science* magazine advises its reviewers: "If you find you have to devote the last paragraphs of your critique to correcting a false impression [about the quality of the research], reconsider your criticisms of it." This doesn't mean that you should withhold criticism, but the merits of the work (or the lack of them) should emerge as the overriding theme of your critique. Be concise, readable, rational, sensitive, accurate, and impartial. Offer explanation and examples. And practice.

Summary of Key Ideas and Terms

In order to fulfill the role of research consumer, expected of all nurses regardless of their educational preparation, you must acquire skills of critiquing research.

A research critique is a critical estimate of a piece of research that has been carefully and systematically studied by a critic who has used specific criteria to appraise its general features.

A research review identifies and summarizes the major features or characteristics of a study.

The critic's challenges are to determine what a researcher has tried to do, to evaluate the strategies used in light of the realistic constraints of the study, and to present both criteria and evidence for making judgments about the quality of the research.

A competent critique ought to represent a contribution to knowledge and scholarly exchange and be helpful to the author of the research.

A helpful critic uses strategies to differentiate his or her criticism from destructive criticism and trivial nit-picking.

Seven conventional criteria can be used as a basis for conducting a critique of a research proposal or report of study findings. These are: (1) clarity and relevance of the study purpose, (2) researchability of the study problem, (3) adequacy and relevance of the literature review, (4) agreement of purpose, design, and methods, (5) suitability of the sampling procedure and sample size, (6) correctness of the analytic procedure, and (7) clarity of findings.

A high-quality critique can influence others to replicate studies or serve as a basis for practice decisions. It should strive to be concise, readable, rational, sensitive, accurate, and impartial, and it should offer explanations for judgments made.

References

Field WE. Clinical nursing research: A proposal of standards. *Nurs Leadership.* December 1983;6:117–120.

Fleming JW & Hayter J. Reading research reports critically. *Nurs Outlook.* March 1974;22:172–175.

Horsley J & Crane J: *Using Research to Improve Nursing Practice: A Guide.* New York: Grune & Stratton;1982.

Leininger MM. The research critique: Nature, function and art. Pages 20–32 in: *Communication Nursing Research: The Research Critique.* Boulder, Colo: WICHE;1968.

USING RESEARCH IN NURSING PRACTICE

HOLLY SKODOL WILSON

CHAPTER OUTLINE

In This Chapter . . .

- Basing Nursing on Research
    - Past Progress
    - Present Barriers
    - Future Strategies
- Using Research Findings in Practice
    - An Institutional Model
    - A Regional Model: The WICHE Project
    - A State Model: The CURN Project
    - The Sigma Theta Tau Regional Research Conferences
- Shaping Practice through Nursing Studies

CHAPTER OBJECTIVES

After reading this chapter, you should be able to:

- Delineate investigative roles for nurses at all levels of educational preparation

- Describe progress made toward building a scientific base for clinical nursing practice

- Formulate strategies for the future of nursing practice that will promote the use of research findings

- Explain the significance of models for applying research findings to practice

- Realize the value and relevance of research in nursing to the development of the profession and to the quality of patient care

14

IN THIS CHAPTER . . .

This chapter gives you some beginning tools essential to becoming an astute and unintimidated consumer of research findings that can actually shape your future clinical nursing practice. You already have one of these tools: A step-by-step guide for understanding a report of study findings and drawing out their clinical implications was presented in chapter 2. Here you will find support for an investigative role of some kind for all nurses. You will learn about where, as a profession, we've been, where we are, and where we'd like to go—and what this all means for using research in our practice. Finally, you'll see some of the characteristics that foster a research orientation in practice settings and hear some success stories about a project that has advanced the profession's commitment to make research every nurse's business.

BASING NURSING ON RESEARCH

Past Progress

The idea that research findings should be used to improve patient care is accepted among contemporary nurses. For at least ten years, nurses have shared the eagerness, expectation, and hope that nursing is at last about to achieve professional status. The strongest force in that direction has been nurses' growing progress in building a scientific base for nursing practice. In our not-so-distant past the study of research was reserved for the master's, doctoral, and postdoctoral levels. Now it is integrated into almost all basic entry-level programs in some form (see Box 14–1). Similarly, just as some degree of research competence is becoming part of every nurse's educational preparation, nursing research departments are springing up in hospitals and health care agencies. The functions of these departments include:

- providing leadership for nurses interested in designing and participating in a variety of scientific investigations
- providing consultation for nurses in investigative roles
- conducting seminars and workshops to help teach research methods
- devising strategies to increase and intensify research activity within the agency
- participating in establishing guidelines for protection of the rights of human subjects (see chapter 12)
- serving on research committees made up of staff nurses
- motivating nurses to become actively involved in seeking solutions to patient problems through scientific inquiry
- considering methods to share significant research findings
- coordinating research displays at appropriate occasions

Box 14–1 Investigative Functions of a Nurse at Various Educational Levels

Associate Degree in Nursing

1. Demonstrates awareness of the value or relevance of research in nursing
2. Assists in identifying problem areas in nursing practice
3. Assists in collection of data within an established structured format

Baccalaureate in Nursing

1. Reads, interprets, and evaluates research for applicability to nursing practice
2. Identifies nursing problems that need to be investigated and participates in the implementation of scientific studies
3. Uses nursing practice as a means of gathering data for refining and extending practice
4. Applies established findings of nursing and other health-related research to nursing practice
5. Shares research findings with colleagues

Master's Degree in Nursing

1. Analyzes and reformulates nursing practice problems so that scientific knowledge and scientific methods can be used to find solutions
2. Enhances the quality and clinical relevance of nursing research by providing expertise in clinical problems and by providing knowledge about the way in which these clinical services are delivered
3. Facilitates investigations of problems in clinical settings through such activities as contributing to a climate supportive of investigative activities, collaborating with others in investigations, and enhancing nursing's access to clients and data
4. Assists others to apply scientific knowledge in nursing practice

Doctoral Degree in Nursing or a Related Discipline

1. Provides leadership for the integration of scientific knowledge with other sources of knowledge for the advancement of practice
2. Conducts investigations to evaluate the contribution of nursing activities to the well-being of clients
3. Develops methods to monitor the quality of the practice of nursing in a clinical setting and to evaluate contributions of nursing activities to the well-being of clients

Graduate of a Research-Oriented Doctoral Program

1. Develops theoretical explanations of phenomena relevant to nursing by empirical research and analytic processes
2. Uses analytical and empirical methods to discover ways to modify or extend existing scientific knowledge so that it is relevant to nursing
3. Develops methods for scientific inquiry of phenomena relevant to nursing

Source: American Nurses' Association 1989.

- interacting with nurses employed in educational institutions to achieve shared goals
- seeking out available community resources for research

Clinicians are increasingly expected to incorporate research findings into practice, and institutions are making changes to facilitate the use and conduct of research in clinical settings (Funk et al 1991). The quantity and quality of nursing research have improved, and new research journals with an emphasis on application of findings are making research results more easily available to practicing nurses.

Present Barriers

Despite progress that has been made, barriers have been identified that limit clinicians' ability to use research results. In a 1991 study by Funk and colleagues, clinicians identified 28 barriers that characterized the nurse, the setting, the research, or its presentation. The two greatest barriers identified, both associated with setting, were "not feeling like he or she had enough authority to change patient care procedures" and "having insufficient time on the job to implement new ideas." Other setting barriers were lack of cooperation and support from physicians, administration, and other staff, inadequate facilities for implementation of research findings, and insufficient time to read research. Such setting factors were rated as the greatest barriers. The presentation and accessibility of research findings represented the next greatest problem area, with the nurses' research skills rated as less problematic.

Future Strategies

Clinicians in Funk and colleagues' survey identified administrative support and encouragement as the best means to facilitate research-based practice innovation. Making involvement in research a staff member's responsibility and providing time to review research literature, explore ideas, pilot test innovations, and develop protocols and policies are suggestions that echo those made by Cronenwett in 1987. Unit-level committees with shared governance could review research findings, propose clinical trials, and report to other staff members on relevant findings. Research should be reported in clinical and specialty journals emphasizing clinical practice implications. Clinical staff could receive library privileges to nearby health science libraries, units could subscribe to health newsletters and journals, and head nurses, in-service coordinators, and research directors all could have research dissemination as part of their job descriptions. Other strategies include:

- making research reports more user friendly
- providing incentives for research involvement
- establishing a center or department for nursing research
- fostering collaborative relationships with university faculty

- establishing a formal research committee or interest group
- starting journal clubs
- conducting research grand rounds
- offering in-service education programs and conferences that focus on research (Funk et al 1991)

While as a group of scientists we are still exploring models for research utilization, there are clear benefits to be obtained here and now for every nurse who shares in the excitement of nursing research. The rest of this chapter will show some of those benefits.

USING RESEARCH FINDINGS IN PRACTICE

An Institutional Model

As long ago as 1983, Morse and Conrad developed an eight-step process by which hospitals and health agencies could put research into practice on the institutional level. These steps are:

1. Identify a clinical need or problem by checking data sources such as management reports, audit scores, incident reports, and patient charts.

2. Use indices to nursing literature and the help of a reference librarian to locate literature relevant to the problem or need identified in step 1.

3. Evaluate relevant research reports by critiquing them (see the questions in chapter 13).

4. If the research study is relevant and scientifically sound, assess its applicability for achieving clinical objectives related to your original problem or need.

5. Prepare a written plan that includes:
   - a statement of the clinical problem
   - a list of clinical objectives for alleviating the problem
   - a description of the new procedures that will reduce or alleviate the problem
   - a detailed budget of labor and equipment costs
   - anticipation of any effects the change suggested in the research might have on hospital policy or procedure
   - a schedule that will help allocate time devoted to the project

6. Obtain cooperation and permission, which involves "selling" the plan to the hospital administration, the nursing staff, the physicians, and the patients.

7. Carry out the plan in an atmosphere of open communication and support.

8. Evaluate the process according to the four possible outcomes that can follow implementation of an innovative technique:
   - The innovation may actually be harmful and therefore should be stopped.
   - The outcome may be neutral, reflecting no change.
   - The outcome may be a realization of the clinical goals.
   - The outcome may be positive or negative but, in either case, unexpected. For example, a program to teach self wound care to the elderly may be so time-consuming that the stress on staff to complete other assignments may become overwhelming.

Whatever the outcome, the authors of this model urge clinicians who attempt to use it to communicate with the researcher who conducted the original study so that new problems can be identified and addressed. Interaction between clinicians and researchers is essential. Research in the practice setting can bring forth major conflicts in the areas of risk taking, vested interests, the rights of research subjects, and the need to produce both scientific and practical knowledge. But collaboration and negotiation between nursing staff and researchers can make it work.

A Regional Model: The WICHE Project

Under the auspices of WICHE (the Western Interstate Commission for Higher Education), the U.S. Department of Health, Education, and Welfare funded a six-year project that had as its original goal investigating the feasibility of increasing nursing research activities through a regional effort. An underlying assumption of the project was that research is necessary to develop a body of validated nursing knowledge on which to base improvements in the quality of nursing given to the public. Many believed that this project was the first large-scale attempt to link the knowledge producers with the practitioners in practice settings.

Part III of the final report of this project (Krueger et al 1978) was devoted to what its author called "research utilization." During the course of the project the participating nurses had an opportunity to identify problems that needed research-based solutions; this activity was not unlike the first step of the institutional model we just examined. The nurses then developed skills in reading and evaluating research for use in practice, learned more about how to locate usable research findings, and developed detailed plans for introducing change into their settings. Although its authors reported that the project was ultimately effective in helping nurses use research in clinical practice, the major problem at that time was the difficulty experienced in finding valid, reliable nursing studies with clearly written implications for nursing care. The categories of clinical problem for which research findings were sought are summarized in Table 14–1.

The implications of the WICHE project were not only that nurses have the skills for evaluating research for possible application in the clinical area but

Table 14–1   *Categories of Nursing Problems Selected by Nurses in the WICHE Nursing Research Development, Collaboration, and Utilization Project*

Nursing Problem	Percentage of Nurses
Clinical nursing	
Patient teaching	29.0
Patient assessment	21.3
Psychosocial problems	3.2
Primary care	4.9
Other direct care	14.7
Problem-oriented records	16.5
Continuity of care	14.7
Nonclinical nursing	4.9

also that *nurse researchers themselves need to write implications for nursing practice into their reports of findings.* Some responsibility must be taken for putting the research report into a form that can be easily used by nurses in the practice setting.

Project participants offered a number of other recommendations based on their experiences. They expressed a need for a centralized index on nursing research (a research hot line), or "Index Nursicus," that would be similar to *Index Medicus* but specifically targeted to research literature. They agreed that research should be taught as part of all basic nursing education and that it should be followed up through continuing education. They urged researchers, in the meantime, to simplify the language used in research reports and to conduct more clinical studies. Participants and project staff alike concluded that

> the use of research in nursing practice would be greatly accelerated by systematic identification, evaluation, and collation of generalizations in a form that is easily accessible to practitioners. Only then can the major difficulties of research utilization be diminished and valid research findings made available. [Krueger et al 1978 p. 299]

In the final recommendation the following conclusions were drawn:

> Institutions must value and be committed to research in order to develop resources for its conduct. The value is institutionalized through its stated philosophy and goals. It is operationalized through job descriptions, recruitment policies, [and] retention and promotion criteria that reward nurses with research skills. [p. 332]

It seems that the WICHE project's message was that nursing research will move forward only if skilled researchers collaborate with others who have clinical competency and ideas for clinically useful research problems.

A State Model: The CURN Project

The second effort to apply research in practice was the five-year Conduct and Use of Research in Nursing (CURN) project, sponsored by the Michigan State Nurses' Association. This project attempted to stimulate the conduct of research in clinical settings and help nurses learn new ways of using research findings in their practice. It resulted in a set of nine volumes (Horsley 1981–1982), which earned the 1983 Book of the Year Award presented by *The American Journal of Nursing*. The volume titles give a sense of the range of clinical research that was involved:

- *Mutual Goal Setting in Patient Care*
- *Closed Urinary Drainage Systems*
- *Distress Reduction Through Sensory Preparation*
- *Pain*
- *Intravenous Cannula Change*
- *Preventing Decubitus Ulcers*
- *Preoperative Sensory Preparation to Promote Recovery*
- *Reducing Diarrhea in Tube-Fed Patients*
- *Structured Preoperative Teaching*

The project's principal investigator, Jo Anne Horsley, concluded from the project that research will be accepted by practicing nurses if it is relevant to practice and is communicated broadly through journals and conferences.

The Sigma Theta Tau Regional Research Conferences

Yet another prototype to explore the dissemination and utilization of research in nursing practice was the Sigma Theta Tau Regional Research Conferences. The primary goal of these conferences was to promote research-based nursing practice by identifying study findings that were ready to be used in practice. A second goal was to suggest further steps to be taken in research areas where the findings were not yet ready for clinical application.

SHAPING PRACTICE THROUGH NURSING STUDIES

This book, particularly through its many examples from the nursing research literature, has tried to show you that nursing research published to date can indeed shape nursing practice and that you have the tools to make a preliminary assessment of a study's clinical potential. Here is an illustration of the first point:

Example of Nursing Research that Can Change Practice and Decrease Cost

Between 1982 and 1985, Mary Naylor, Dorothy Brooten, Linda Brown, and Lynne Borucki, nurses at the University of Pennsylvania School of Nursing, conducted a randomized clinical trial of early hospital discharge and nurse specialist home follow-up of very-low-birthweight infants (1991). The purpose of the study was to determine the safety, efficacy, and cost savings of early hospital discharge of infants who weighed less than 1,500 grams and who were provided with home follow-up by a nurse clinical specialist. Families in the early discharge group received instruction, counseling, home visits, and daily on-call availability of a hospital-based nurse specialist for 18 months after infant discharge. Infants in the early discharge group were sent home an average of 11 days earlier, weighed 200 grams less, and were 2 weeks younger at discharge than the infants in the control group. Findings from this study, published in the New England Journal of Medicine, *were that the two groups of infants did not differ in the number of rehospitalizations, in acute care visits, or in measures of physical and mental growth. Furthermore, this care model saved $18,560 per infant. Following publication in the* New England Journal of Medicine, *the study results were featured on local and network television and in newspapers across the country, including the* Wall Street Journal, New York Times, Boston Globe, *and* Los Angeles Times. *Findings were also reported in* Medical Economics *and the* London Economist, *attesting to this nursing study's far-reaching impact (1991).*

As far as the second point is concerned, you can begin your assessment of research by noting that good clinical studies, according to Fuller (1982), have the following characteristics in common:

1. They study a problem that occurs frequently in a definable population of patients.
2. The standard way the problem has been dealt with is unsatisfactory.
3. Some index of the problem can be measured.
4. The proposed solution alters patient care.

When you read or hear reports of clinical studies, use the following preliminary set of questions to help you consider their scientific merit and possible utility (Fawcett 1982):

1. Has the original study been replicated?
2. If so, are the findings similar in a variety of situations?
3. Is corroboration of findings in clinical situations done with actual patients who receive nursing care?
4. What were the risks and benefits of the nursing action tested in the study?

5. Does the study focus on a significant problem in clinical practice?

6. Do nurses have clinical control over the study variables?

7. Is it feasible to carry out the nursing action in the real world?

8. What is the cost of implementing the nursing action?

9. What contribution to client health status does the nursing action make?

10. What overall contribution to nursing knowledge does the study make?

Nursing research that meets these criteria will help you improve the quality of life for patients in your care regardless of their health status. From nursing research, for example, we will learn better ways of intervening with the frail elderly, the chronically ill, and the terminally ill. Research done by nurses includes both laboratory and clinical studies and may cut across traditional disciplines and methods. In the past, research-based nursing practice was more a litany being preached than a reality. But you are part of the tension and excitement of a new era for nursing research. In this era all nurses, whether they make research a central part of their career or not, will need the skills to read, understand, and apply the expanding body of findings to their practice, to participate in the clinical studies of others, and to safeguard the rights of human research subjects under their care. If practitioners collaborate in the entire research process, the outcomes will be used. Remember, the clinician and the researcher have an exchange to make and a profit to share.

ANNOTATED RESEARCH EXAMPLE

Study Problem/Purpose

Focus is on a practical clinical problem

The problem addressed in this study was whether a research-based protocol on oral temperature measurement could be developed and used in the practice setting. The first phase proposed to (a) identify research articles related to the subject, (b) evaluate the quality of the research, (c) assess the adequacy of the research base, and (d) select areas for future study.

Methods

Four procedures were used in this study. The first was an intensive literature search to identify research reports related to clinical thermometry. A classification system for the reports was then agreed upon. The second procedure involved designing a thermometry critique form to be used in reading each of the articles. The third procedure was the development of a table for each classification. These tables were reviewed for completeness and clarity. The final procedure involved evaluating the summary tables to determine whether an adequate research base was available in each of the categories.

a systematic attempt to introduce research findings in a clinical setting

Findings

Forty-eight clinical thermometry articles were published between 1969 and 1989. As a result of this review, it was evident that the data base on oxygen by nasal cannula and its relationship to temperature was adequate, but findings on oxygen by mask and its relationship to temperature needed to be clarified. More clinically based studies are needed before a protocol can be designed and tested in clinical practice.

Source: Longman et al 1990.

[handwritten margin note: Directions for future clinical research are identified]

Summary of Key Ideas and Terms

Applying the growing number of findings from clinical nursing research to practice would be easier if (1) the scientific community were further along in bringing some order to the proliferating research literature; (2) all nursing students were better prepared to find, read, understand, and appreciate these findings; and (3) service organizations were structured to foster such applications.

Evidence of progress toward establishing a *scientific basis* for nursing practice includes (1) an agreed-upon consensus about investigative roles for nurses at all levels of educational preparation, (2) the emergence of research departments in service agencies, and (3) the establishment of a national research center to coordinate, support, and disseminate nursing research.

Although research conducted by nurses includes various types of study and cuts across traditional disciplines, in the 1990s priority is given to clinical research directly related to developing the knowledge and information needed for the improvement of nursing practice.

Various models have been developed for using nursing research in practice.

Researchers can benefit nursing practice not just by the findings they discover, but also by the new questions they raise.

Applying research findings to clinical practice requires that investigators make their work more accessible to practitioners, that practitioners develop their skills of critical reading and keep up with research developments, and that service agencies adopt philosophies and strategies that reward putting research findings into practice.

References

American Nurses' Association Committee on Nursing Research. *Guidelines for the Investigative Function of Nurses.* Kansas City, Mo: ANA;1989.

Cronenwett LR. Research utilization in a practice setting. *J Nurs Adm.* 1987; 17(7,8):9–10.

Fawcett J. Utilization of nursing research findings. *Image.* June 1982;14:57–59.

Fuller E. Selecting a clinical nursing problem for research. *Image.* June 1982;14:60–61.

Funk SG, Champagne MT, Wiese RA & Tornquist EM. Barriers to using research findings in practice: The clinician's perspective. *Applied Nurs Res.* May 1991; 4(2):90–95.

Horsley JA. *Using Research to Improve Nursing Practice.* (Series of Clinical Protocols, 9 vols.) New York: Grune and Stratton;1981, 1982.

Krueger J et al. *Nursing Research: Development, Collaboration and Utilization.* Germantown, Md: Aspen Systems;1978.

Longman AJ et al. Research utilization: An evaluation and critique of research related to oral temperature measurement. *Applied Nurs Res.* February 1990;3(1):14–19.

Morse JM & Conrad A. Putting research into practice. *Can Nurs.* September 1983; 79:40–43.

Naylor MD, Brooten D, Brown L, & Borucki LC. Institutional yields on research: A case study. *Nurs Outlook.* July/August 1991;39(4):166–169.

PROPOSAL WRITING RESOURCES

APPENDIX A

- A–1 GUIDELINES FOR WRITING A RESEARCH PROPOSAL
- A–2 SAMPLE PROPOSAL FORMAT

APPENDIX A–1: GUIDELINES FOR WRITING A RESEARCH PROPOSAL

Components of a Research Proposal

1. a title (usually limited to 54 characters)
2. an abstract (or summary)
3. a statement of the study problem, purpose, and specific aims
4. the theoretical background and/or selective review of related research
5. hypotheses to be tested or research questions to be answered
6. the study setting
7. the sampling procedure and characteristics
8. the data-collection strategies or instruments
9. the plans for storing, retrieving, and analyzing data
10. ethical considerations, such as provisions for informed consent and protection of human and animal rights
11. a timetable or work plan for the conduct of the study
12. a budget and statement of resources available or needed
13. a description of the qualifications of the investigator
14. references
15. appendixes

Steps in Writing a Research Proposal

Step 1: The Problem Statement   The statement of the research problem usually begins a proposal. It must not only convince reviewers that the proposed study is important but also reduce the scope of the problem to manageable terms by specifying a study focus. If any specialized or esoteric concepts or terms are used in the problem statement, they must be defined early and prominently so that reviewers don't base their reading on any misconceptions. The art of identifying and articulating a researchable problem was covered in chapter 3; many experts believe that this step is, in fact, the art of research, because it requires creativity, perceptiveness, and imagination. Although the study problem must not be too broad or grandiose, the potential generalizability of the findings related to studying the problem must also be explicitly stated.

Both the general statement of the purpose of the research and the specific study question should be succinctly expressed and even underlined early in the proposal.

The study problem, purpose, and aims

- are stated with precision

- justify the problem as meriting study

- admit of possible solution

- are intelligible to a reader who is generally sophisticated but may be relatively uninformed in the specific area of investigation

- suggest the significance of conducting the study

It's not a bad idea to conclude the problem-statement section of a proposal with a sentence that begins "Therefore, the specific problem for this investigation is . . ."

Remember that the intention of this first section of your proposal is to make the problem area of your study clear to a reader. Many proposal writers accomplish this by first presenting the larger context in which the problem is found and then narrowing down the big picture to the specific study that is being proposed. They demonstrate the relationship between the two and highlight why their study is important. The problem-statement section is often labeled "Introduction" and consists of three subheadings:

- Statement of the Study Problem (including specific hypotheses or study questions and definitions of terms)

- Specific Objectives (or aims) of the Research (a carefully selected, brief list)

- Significance of the Study (along with any limitations that can reasonably be identified)

Although it is possible to reduce this section to a few seemingly simple parts, a good statement of the problem in a research proposal is usually the product of vigorous intellectual effort and utmost clarity.

Step 2: Theoretical Rationale and Review of Related Literature A review of relevant literature is included in a study proposal to accomplish several purposes:

1. It presents the theoretical basis, rational framework, or organizing scheme of which the proposed study is a part.

2. It offers not a mere bibliography but an analytic and critical appraisal of the important and recent substantive and methodological developments in your area of interest and indicates how your proposed study will refine, revise, extend, or transcend what is now known.

3. It informs and lends support to your assumptions, operational definitions, and even methodological procedures by demonstrating to your reader that the proposed study has profited from scholarly and scientific work that has preceded it.

Critics of this section of study proposals report that the single most obvious flaw is that authors tend to cite theory and prior research that have only the most tenuous connection with the study being proposed. As a result, this section has a disjointed quality, because it looks like a mere catalog or listing of marginally related work lacking in thoughtful, well-developed integration. Avoid statements that imply either that nothing has been done in your research area or that so much has been done that it is impossible for you to summarize. Statements of this sort are usually taken as indications that the investigator proposing the study does not really have a command of relevant literature and knowledge in his or her field. Consider organizing this section of your proposal according to the key concepts or constructs in your proposed research.

Step 3: Design, Methods, and Procedure   By this point in your proposal you have presented the problem(s) you intend to study, the objectives your research will accomplish, the importance and exact meaning of both of these, and the theoretical and empirical background of the present study. Now you must tell your readers or reviewers how you are going to bring about your results, that is, what activities you will conduct to accomplish your study objectives or test your study hypotheses.

Label the Design   Begin by labeling the general approach, or design, of your study (historical, survey, experimental, quasi-experimental, field study, case study, and so on). In effect, this general label allows you to communicate quickly your proposed procedure for inquiry and gives you an opportunity to anticipate questions about why you have selected the design that you have. In short, you should not only identify your plan but also substantiate the reasons for choosing it.

Specify Data-Collection Approaches   Following this labeling and accounting, you should state the exact steps you intend to take to answer every question or test every hypothesis proposed in your study. One organizational technique used by proposal writers is to divide a sheet of paper into columns. Label the first column "Objective #1" or "Hypothesis #1," the second column "Method for #1," and the third "Evaluation for #1" or "Analysis for #1." This strategy helps you to be certain that you indeed have a plan for dealing with all aspects of the problem that you have introduced and that you have set up a data-collection and analysis mechanism or procedure to address each of them.

Describe the Study Setting   Your methods or procedures section should also describe your research setting, if setting is a relevant consideration.

Example: The Study Setting

The proposed study will be conducted at a 450-bed community hospital located in the greater Pittsburgh area. It has the only accredited cancer care program in the immediate area, and the investigator is currently the oncology clinical nurse specialist employed by this hospital. Furthermore, she is familiar with referring physicians.

Discuss Your Study Sampling   You should discuss the nature and size of the sample and the rationale behind sampling decisions. The sampling procedure should be identified and explained in adequate detail so that your study can be replicated and so that the extent of generalizability of your findings can be determined. If your sample members must meet specific criteria, these should be listed. For example, one pediatric nurse engaged in a descriptive study of adolescent cancer patients' experience of fatigue proposed the following sampling criteria:

> *Cancer patients (n = 40) will consist of adolescent leukemia patients admitted to any of three city hospital inpatient units or seen in these institutions' outpatient clinics. Furthermore, they must be able to read, write, and speak English as a primary language, be able to complete data-collection instruments, and be willing to maintain daily diary recordings. Finally, they must have confirmation of their cancer diagnosis. Exclusion criteria include patients who are (1) under psychiatric care; (2) taking antidepressants, sedatives, or thyroid medications; and (3) diagnosed as having diabetes, anemia, or thyroid disease.*

Discuss Confounding Variables   Confounding variables that might plague your study need to be addressed in your procedures section. You may eliminate some of them by using random sample selection and random assignment to comparative groups. Some may be addressed by your sample size or exclusion criteria. Others may be controlled for with certain statistical operations. But still others may be beyond any of these attempts to reduce their influence and must be identified as limitations of your study or constraints on the generalizability of your findings. Most authorities agree that it is preferable for you to acknowledge problems, errors in design, or limitations rather than to attempt to ignore or disguise them. It is important to indicate that whatever compromises you have made with regard to the control of extraneous variables were given careful thought, that you are definitely aware of which variables need to be controlled in order to preserve the integrity of your study, that you have chosen not to control some, and why you believed it was not possible to do so.

Most reviewers of research proposals are experienced scientists and scholars themselves, although they may not be experts on your specific study problem. They will recognize weaknesses and flaws in a study design such as lack of control or comparative groups, a Hawthorne effect, a regression effect, pretest effects, and a biased sample. Your design discussion ought to show how you have attempted to make your study as precise as is practical to do.

Present Data-Collection Tools or Instruments   You must also enumerate and discuss the data-collection instruments you propose to use. If you expect to use published and previously tested tools for data collection, you need tell your readers why you selected them and how they are appropriate t sure the variables that are important to your study question. The dis this relationship often appears in connection with the operatio of each of your study variables. The measures that you elect not only be consistent with the variable's operational definitio empirical evidence attesting to their validity, reliability, and objec

Assistance in evaluating certain instruments can be found in annual test reviews and compendia such as Oscar Buros's *Mental Measurement Yearbooks* (1938–present) and others available in your library. If no instruments exist or are available to investigate the variables of interest to you, it is probably better to propose a methodological study to develop tools rather than to argue that instrument plans will be forthcoming. If "homemade" or "self-developed" instruments are to be used, be sure to justify them in terms of their fit with the operational definition of your study variables. Discuss the procedures you plan to use to develop them, and then establish their reliability and validity.

Present Your Analytic Procedures   Finally, the methods or procedures section should present a method of analysis that is consistent with your study questions and levels of measurement. The assumptions of the statistics should fit the data that will be obtained. Most authorities seem to agree that it is not always possible to anticipate every analysis procedure that will be used. It is to your advantage, however, to expose your readers and reviewers to evidence that you have thought through each step that you will need to take to test every hypothesis or respond to every question in your study problem. Many advisers will encourage you to generate mock tables that will organize your data before you collect any, so that others know what you have in mind when it comes to analysis. For many proposal writers, this is an appropriate point at which to consult a computer programmer or statistician who can make suggestions for your analysis plan or even your data-collection procedures.

A careful plan and procedures section of your proposal need not prohibit discovery of serendipitous findings or inhibit your creativity. Instead, it must support your contention that you know how to answer the research question and possess the attributes of a serious scholar, at least with regard to using an approach that is consistent with systematic inquiry.

Step 4: Timetable or Work Plan   A timetable or work plan accomplishes two main aims:

1. It clarifies for the reader the overall flow of research-related activities. (This point is particularly important when the research project is complex.)

2. It constitutes evidence that you have carefully and realistically considered exactly what you intend to do to carry out the proposed study.

The timetable or work plan can be presented in a number of different formats, but in all cases, it must provide a clear, sequential statement of the operations that will be carried out in your study and must be consistent with the descriptive sections of your written proposal. Whether a table, graph, flowchart, PERT diagram, or path analysis is used, the following information should be included:

1. the tasks or project activities

2. an estimate of the amount of time required for each, and scheduled dates

3. personnel requirements for each activity

The simplest way to portray a timetable or work plan in a research proposal is simply to list research activities and associated dates or blocks of time.

Step 5: Sections on Personnel, Budget, Facilities, and Resources

Personnel   This section of your proposal tells reviewers about the people who will be needed to conduct your study. It is, of course, crucial that the principal investigator, project director, or codirectors be identified and that their qualifications be convincingly presented. Educational preparation, both formal and informal, professional experience, prior research positions in the field, and previous publications related to the proposed study all strengthen one's case. Although it may be expedient to opt for including a "canned" biographic sketch that is already available in your files, reviewers are more likely to be impressed by a presentation of project personnel, their "job descriptions," and background information that has been carefully selected to highlight particular competencies relevant to this study.

Budget   The budget section of a proposal states your project in monetary or financial terms. The total dollar amount is usually determined by the nature of the study you are proposing. The goal in preparing a budget is to make it realistic. If you have underbudgeted, you may not have sufficient resources to carry out your proposed plan of activities. A written budget narrative should accompany the actual list of costs, in order to explain the reasons for requesting certain items and to link up the budget details with the project activities.

Facilities and Other Resources   You should indicate the special facilities that are available to you in carrying out your proposed study. One customarily mentions the libraries (and their holdings), computer resources, special equipment or laboratories, office space, and secretarial support services.

If your study requires you to collect data in organizations or institutions other than your own setting, evidence of their willingness to cooperate with you, in the form of letters of agreement or contracts, should be attached. Many funding sources view an institution's willingness to allow you to use their facilities as added support for your proposal.

Step 6: Abstract and Title   Most proposals begin with a short (approximately 300-word) abstract, or summary. Even though it usually appears at the beginning of the document, most researchers write it last. The purpose of an abstract is to convey the essence of your proposed study to the reviewers. It not only introduces your study's importance to reviewers but may also be used as the basis for subsequent press releases or publications and may be used as the basis for entering your project into a computerized record-keeping system. It goes without saying, then, that your abstract should be composed carefully, accurately, and clearly. An abstract should include the most important points that you wish to stress about your proposed research and should provide the maximum amount of pertinent information as concisely as possible. A well-written abstract not only presents the central idea of the study but also convinces the reader or reviewer that it is both interesting and important. It should whet the appetite and prepare the reader for the body of the proposal.

The title serves similar purposes but in an even more abbreviated way. Try to avoid jargon and clichés in study titles. Instead, use key terms that will orient a reader to the nature of your study and *make sense.*

General Hints on Preparing a Proposal

Consider Your Audience, and Write for Strangers   Although *you* have no doubt devoted what might seem like an astounding amount of time to thinking through both your research topic and the approach you intend to take to it, remember that the readers and reviewers of your proposal may not be as well informed in your area of interest as you are. *Explain everything clearly and logically.* Avoid using jargon or abbreviations that may be commonplace in your nursing specialty area but "Greek" to others.

Flaws in structure and internal consistency will be easily identified by readers who are unfamiliar with your subject. Develop a chain of logic throughout your proposal that hangs together and has no weak links. For instance, objectives of the research must logically flow from the problem statement, and each hypothesis or objective must have a corresponding data-collection and data-analysis procedure that addresses it. Choices of descriptive or inferential statistical methods must be consistent with the purpose of your study and the level of inquiry you are proposing. Check your proposal to be certain that objectives are not dropped along the way or that certain data-collection plans are not advanced without a corresponding plan for analyzing them. If your study uses a naturalistic and/or interpretive approach, stay clear and precise on the qualitative method you are employing. For example, don't use phenomenology to "generate a grounded theory."

Good writing, like good speaking, uses visual aids. Make use of headings and subheadings, underlining, diagrams, flowcharts, tables, and other strategies that signal to the reader what the critical parts of your proposal are without requiring him or her to plow through endless pages of undifferentiated prose. Most standard proposal forms have 10-, 20-, or 25-page limits.

Package Your Proposal So That It Is Attractive   In addition to not being well informed about your research interest, your reviewers and readers may also be less enthusiastic about the value or importance of your study than you are. It's up to you to convey not only what your project hopes to find out but also why doing it is important to the world, to nursing, or to the funding agency.

Conveying a sense of enthusiasm for your project does not require Madison Avenue techniques. But making your proposal physically attractive is an effective strategy for increasing its appeal. You should definitely do the following:

- Put your proposal aside, and then reread it with some critical distance.

- Make revisions where necessary.

- Be sure to correct errors in spelling, grammar, and referencing. (The care you give to such details in your proposal often conveys something about your attention to the details of your research.)

- Check your proposal for consistent use of the future tense. (After all, you are proposing to do something in the future.)

- Type your proposal, or have it typed (using letter-quality or double-strike type if it's done on a word processor and printer).

- Number the pages.

- Proofread your proposal, and proofread it again.

Balance Detail and Flexibility   A proposal should reflect a balance between sufficient detail, so that reviewers are convinced that the study is worthwhile, and the investigator has the ability to conduct it, and sufficient flexibility. Writing such a plan is a craft that must be finely honed. The issue of length comes up here, and two general guidelines coexist: (1) When in doubt about including or excluding some piece of relevant information bearing on your proposed project, *it's better to include rather than to exclude it.* (2) Page limitations are set for a purpose and should be respected. The solution to these seemingly incompatible guidelines is to *use appendixes to provide auxiliary information* and try not to crowd details into the main body of the proposal. Appendixes can give reviewers the benefit of the findings of a pilot study. They can also locate the proposed study within the context of a broader program of research. And they can incorporate the qualifications of the investigator. All these additional pieces of information may assist a reviewer in making a decision about your proposal without unduly burdening someone who may because of limited time be reading a mass of proposals according to the "skip and skim" approach.

Evaluation of Your Proposal

Readers and reviewers can use a number of criteria to evaluate your proposal. To get an idea of what these criteria encompass, you can examine the various checklists in Box A–1 that are used by funding agencies in evaluating research proposals.

Box A–1 Evaluation Checklists

I. National Institutes of Health (checklist of deficiencies)

A. *The Problem*
- The problem is not of sufficient importance or is unlikely to produce any new or useful information.
- The proposed research is based on a hypothesis that rests on insufficient evidence, is doubtful, or is unsound.
- The problem is more complex than the investigator appears to realize.
- The problem has only local significance, is one of production or control, or otherwise fails to fall sufficiently clearly within the general field of interest to the prospective sponsor.
- The problem is scientifically premature and warrants, at most, only pilot study.
- The research as proposed is overly involved, with too many elements under simultaneous investigation.
- The description of the nature of the research and of its significance leaves the proposal nebulous and diffuse without clear research aim.

B. *The Approach*
- The proposed tests, methods, or scientific procedures are unsuited to the stated objective.
- The description of the approach is too nebulous, diffuse, and lacking in clarity to permit adequate evaluation.
- The overall design of the study has not been carefully thought out.
- The statistical aspects of the approach have not been given sufficient consideration.
- The approach lacks scientific imagination.
- Controls are either inadequately conceived or inadequately described.
- The material the investigator proposes to use is unsuited to the objectives of the study or is difficult to obtain.
- The number of observations is unsuitable.
- The equipment contemplated is outmoded or otherwise unsuitable.

II. U.S. Office of Education (list of shortcomings)

A. *Problem*
- Limited significance
- Local significance only
- Incomprehensible; not spelled out
- Not appropriate to this granting agency
- Overly ambitious objectives

B. *Procedures*
- Insufficient detail; vague
- Evaluation procedures inadequate
- Selection of subjects unclear, undefined, and/or unrealistic
- Research design inadequate
- Variables uncontrolled
- Discrepancy between objectives and procedures
- No theoretical construct or rationale

Box A–1 (*continued*)

- Research design overly complex; too many research components
- Statistical procedures unspecified
- Pilot study necessary
- Time schedule inappropriate

C. *Personnel and Facilities*
- Inadequate training and/or experience
- Time commitment inadequate or unspecified
- Consultants needed
- Personnel not specified
- Duties not specified
- Personnel specified but insufficient information provided

D. *Economic Efficiency*
- Budget too high for expected result
- Request for operational or support money

III. National Science Foundation

A review of the evaluation instructions provided to outside reviewers of National Science Foundation (NSF) research proposals reveals concern about the same general areas noted for the U.S. Office of Education and the National Institutes of Health. The instructional letter for one program area asks the review to comment on such points as the scientific merit of the research that is proposed and the qualifications of the applicant. It also requests a response to the following questions:
- Is the research well planned?
- Is the research important?
- Is the applicant aware of recent developments in the field?
- Is the applicant adequately trained to undertake the project?
- Is the support requested appropriate for the project?

The definitions of rating terms used by another NSF program may provide further insight into the criteria employed:

Excellent — The problem is very important and well defined in the proposal. The investigators are highly competent and fully capable of doing the job. Strongly deserves support.

Very Good — The problem is important and adequately defined in the proposal. The investigators are competent and the research will contribute to their growth. Deserves support.

Good — The problem may be important, but the research is not well defined. The approach is routine, but might contribute to graduate education or developing the potential of the principal investigator. The proposal is marginal in its present form.

Fair — The problem is probably unimportant or not well enough defined in the proposal to allow evaluation. The approach is questionable. The proposal is not deserving of support in its present form.

Poor — The problem is unimportant, subprofessional, or has been solved by others.

Source: Sonoma State University Academic Foundation.

APPENDIX A–2: SAMPLE PROPOSAL FORMAT

Center for Research
Research Prospectus to Develop Proposal

To: Center for Research Coordinating Committee

From: _____
              (Name of unit/organization)

    through _____
              (contact person)

Section A—Complete the following section relating responses to the proposed project.

1. Objective (overall or long-term goal of proposed research)

    _____

    _____

    _____

2. Rationale (behind investigator's initiation of this prospectus)

    _____

    _____

    _____

3. Significance to the Profession

    _____

    _____

    _____

4. Summary of all Center for Research Staff and Other Resources Requested

    _____

    _____

    _____

Section B—Complete the following section relating responses to proposal development.

1. Time Frame (include time frame for proposal development and for proposed study)

    _____

_____

_____

_____

_____

2. Staff Needed to Develop Full Proposal (include consultants)

_____

_____

_____

_____

_____

_____

3. Budget for Proposal Development (only)

_____

_____

_____

_____

_____

Section C—Complete the following section relating responses to the proposed project (be as specific as possible with information available).

1. Specific Aims or Research Questions (measurable objectives of proposed project)

_____

_____

_____

2. Methods of Procedure (give general outline for research plan including nature and accessibility of subjects and sampling procedures; list instruments to be used or developed, kinds of data expected, data-collection procedures, and procedures for data analysis and interpretation)

_____

_____

_____

_____

_____

_____

_____

3. Time Frame (include time frame for proposal development and for proposed study)

_____

_____

_____

_____

4. Staff, Facilities, and Resources Needed to Conduct Project

_____

_____

_____

_____

5. Total Budget and Identification of Potential Funding Sources

_____

_____

_____

_____

HUMAN SUBJECTS REVIEW RESOURCES

APPENDIX B

APPENDIX B–1: SAMPLE EXPEDITED
HUMAN SUBJECTS PROTOCOL

Submission date _____ 10/13/82 _____

Principal Investigator   *University*   Nursing–Mental
(UCSF Faculty) ___ Professor Holly Wilson ___   *Title* _Professor_ *Dept.* ____ Health ____

Co-Investigator   Sandra L. Scheetz,   *Is principal investigator*
and Title _____ M.S., R.N., Doct. Cand. ____   *the sponsor/adviser only? Yes* _X_ *No* __

Mailing Address
(campus if possible) _____ N511E School of Nursing _____ *Phone* _____ 476-3903 _____

Project
Title _The Influence of Social Network Characteristics on the Performance of Self-Care_

____ by the Chronically Mentally Ill in the Community ____

(A) *The point of this project is (explain background, rationale, basic design, etc.):*

To investigate the influence of the characteristics of social network on the performance of self-care by the chronically mentally ill (CMI) in the community.
    Much recent research has focused on the individual's primary group and
the relationship to psychiatric epidemiology. More specific information is
needed about the person's ability to function on a day-to-day basis, which is
one aspect of the psychiatric disability. This is important because chronic
mental illness is a major health problem today, and because one of the primary problems with this group is self-care. The proposed descriptive, longitudinal study would be an attempt to describe the social network of the CMI
over time and the relationship of network characteristics to the performance
of self-care in this population.

(B) *The subject population(s) will be selected (or excluded) on the following
criteria (consider how access will be gained as well as any problems relevant
to special subject populations such as children, prisoners, etc.):*

One hundred twenty subjects who will be residing in the community will be
solicited from inpatient psychiatric units. Criteria for inclusion are (1) adults
ages 18–45; (2) voluntary admission to hospital; (3) English speaking; (4) diagnosis at discharge of schizophrenia, affective disorder, or borderline personality; (5) on, or approved for, Supplemental Security Income (SSI); (6) hospitalized one time in the past 5 years for at least 6 months OR hospitalized two or
more times in the past 12 months; (7) must agree to participate in the study.
Exclusion criteria are (1) physical deformities, physical injuries, and serious
or chronic physical conditions; (2) organic psychoses; (3) primary diagnosis of
substance abuse. Subjects will be asked to involve a friend or relative in a
home-visit follow-up.

(C) *The following procedures involving humans will be done for purposes of*

the study (if known, the expedited review category number from Consent
Forum, *issue 5, is* 9) *(if applicable, include interview themes and questionnaires if not commonly known):*

1. Charts will be reviewed by agency staff to determine eligibility.

2. Information Sheet (attached) will be given to potential subjects by agency
    staff.

3. Those interested in participating will be given the Informed Consent (at-
    tached) and the opportunity to discuss it with the investigator. They will
    be asked to sign the Consent.

4. Relative or friend named by subject will be contacted by investigator and
    invited to participate in follow-up (Time 1 & Time 2). Informed Consent
    for Relative or Friend will be signed prior to administration of question-
    naires at follow-up.

5. Consenting subject (pts) will be given the following:
    a. Demographic Data Sheet—at Baseline.
    b. Modified Norbeck Support Questionnaire (Norbeck, Lindsey & Carrieri
       1981)—at Baseline, Time 1, & Time 2.
    c. Social Relationship Scale (McFarlane 1980)—at Baseline, Time 1, &
       Time 2.

6. Level of Rehabilitation Scale (Carey & Posavac 1978)—rated by nurse at
    Baseline; rated by investigator questioning relative or friend at Time 1 &
    Time 2.

7. Katz Adjustment Scale (Katz & Lyerly 1963) Forms S2 & S3 Subject and
    R2, R3 Relative, all completed at Time 1 & Time 2.

8. Consent to participate at Time 2 will be reviewed at Time 1 with subject
    and relative/friend.

(D) *The risks involved in these procedures and the methods of minimizing
the risks, inconveniences, or discomforts are (include any potential for loss of
privacy):*

It is possible that subjects will become frustrated or anxious while responding
to the questionnaires. If the investigator or the subject determines that this is
occurring, another appointment will be set up to complete the questionnaires.

The privacy of prospective subjects will be maintained by having agency
staff do the initial screening for eligibility. Only the names of those who
would like to participate will be given to the investigator. Subjects will be
given a code number, and all identifying information will be separated from
the responses. The code number will be retraceable only by the investigator
for purposes of follow-up. Complete confidentiality of all information will be
maintained.

Subjects' right to refuse to continue in the study or to withdraw at any
time will be respected. It will be concluded that those who miss three follow-
up appointments are "withdrawing" and will be dropped from the study.

All questionnaires will be filled out, and all appointments will be made at the subjects' convenience as to time and place.

(E) *Describe the anticipated benefits, if any, to subjects, and the importance of the knowledge that may reasonably be expected to result:*

There will be no immediate or direct benefit to subjects. This study has the potential to extend our theoretical knowledge about the network characteristics of the specific subpopulation of the chronically mentally ill over time, and knowing more about the relationship between network characteristics and performance of self-care by the chronically mentally ill is of clinical significance.

(F) *Describe the consent process and attach all consent documents. If waiver from use of written consent is requested, give the justification:*

Patients will be screened initially by agency staff. Those who meet the inclusion criteria will be given an Information Sheet for Prospective Participants (attached), which explains the study. Those who wish to participate will be given the Informed Consent (attached) and the opportunity to discuss the study with the investigator. The Informed Consent also includes a choice for the subject to participate in the 12-month follow-up. This aspect of the Consent will be reviewed with the subject at the 1-month visit should the subject not wish to continue. Potential subjects will be asked to sign the Consent Form. Those who agree to participate will be given a copy of the Consent and the Information Sheet to keep.

Source: Used with permission of Sandra Scheetz, RN, MS, DNS

APPENDIX B–2: INFORMATION SHEET FOR PROSPECTIVE PARTICIPANTS IN A RESEARCH STUDY

Sandra Scheetz is a nurse and a doctoral student at the University of California, San Francisco. She is conducting a research study of persons, like yourself, who will be discharged from the psychiatric unit to return to the community to live. You are invited to participate in this study.

The following are answers to questions that people ask most often about the study.

1. What is the purpose of the study?

The main purpose of this community follow-up study is to help nurses and other mental health professionals learn more about how patients get along on a day-to-day basis after they leave the hospital.

2. What would be required of *me?*

Prior to leaving the hospital, you will be asked to fill out one personal information sheet and two paper-and-pencil questionnaires. These are *not* tests.

Also before discharge an appointment will be made to see you approximately 4–6 weeks after you leave the hospital. The follow-up visit will be either at your home or at the hospital, whichever is more convenient for you.

At the follow-up visit, you would be asked again to fill out three paper-and-pencil questionnaires.

You will also be asked to have a relative or close friend, someone you see on a daily basis, participate in the study by being present at the follow-up visit. You will choose this person to participate. This friend or relative will also be asked to fill out two short questionnaires and to answer some questions about how you are getting along.

3. What good will the study do *me?*

There will be no direct benefit to you. Perhaps you will get some satisfaction from knowing that, by answering the questionnaires, you have provided information that may help other patients returning to the community.

4. What will be done with the information I give about myself?

You are one of 120 people who are being studied in the community follow-up. All of the people are former patients like yourself. The information will be carefully studied by the researcher, who will write a report on the results of the study. These results may also be published in the professional journals where they can be read by other mental health professionals. Therefore, in the long run, the information you provide will be helpful for many people who are hospitalized, as you were, and helpful to the many professionals who give care to those patients.

Your name will not be used anywhere in the reports. Your answers will be given a special number to be used instead of your name. The information you provide will *not* be a part of your chart or treatment records and will not be shared with the professionals who give you care.

5. Will filling out the questionnaires take a long time?

No. The average time for each set of questionnaires is 1 hour, once in the hospital and once at the follow-up visit, for a total of 2 hours. Some people may finish in 30 minutes, and others may take more than 1 hour. The time needed for your friend or relative to fill out the questionnaires and to answer questions is approximately 30 minutes.

6. What if I am unable to keep my follow-up appointment?

Please call Sandra Scheetz at 123-4567 or 890-1234 to let her know. If you need to call long distance, please call Mrs. Scheetz at 890-1234 and she will accept a collect phone call. She will be glad to schedule another time for you that is more convenient.

7. How will I remember my follow-up appointment time?

About 1 week before the appointment time, you will receive a postcard in the mail to remind you.

8. Who will be present at the follow-up visit?

You and your relative or friend will be seen only by Sandra Scheetz or her research assistant.

9. Why do I have to ask a relative or friend to take part in the study?

Your relatives or friends who see you every day are the people who know most about how you are getting along. Of course you, yourself, will provide the most information, but another person will often notice things that you overlook. Research has already shown that a relative's report is a very useful source of information, even when the patient's own report about him- or herself is also available.

10. What if I have other questions that haven't been answered here?

Please feel free to call Sandra Scheetz at 123-4567 (or leave a message). Or tell your nurse that you would like to speak to Mrs. Scheetz, and she will contact you on the unit the next time she is there.

What next?

If you would be willing to participate in this study, please fill in the information below, detach it, and give it to your nurse or to the research assistant on the unit. You will then be asked to sign a "Consent to Be a Research Subject" before filling out any questionnaires.

You may keep this information sheet for yourself and to share with your relative or friend.

Thank you for taking the time to read this!

Source: Used with permission of Sandra Scheetz, RN, MS, DNS

APPENDIX B–3: CONSENT TO BE A RESEARCH SUBJECT

Sandra Scheetz is a doctoral student in nursing studying psychiatric patients who return to live in the community and how they get along on a day-to-day basis after they leave the hospital.

If I agree to be in the study, I will fill out two questionnaires and a personal information sheet prior to leaving the hospital. I will also meet with Sandra Scheetz or her research assistant at my home or at the hospital approximately 1 month after discharge to fill out three additional questionnaires. I have agreed to have a relative or friend of my choosing participate in the home visit to answer additional questionnaires and additional questions.

I (AGREE) (DO NOT AGREE) (circle one) to be a participant in the 12-month follow-up study. Participating in this follow-up would require a second home visit with Sandra Scheetz or her research assistant. This second home visit would be like the first one and would be approximately 12 months after my discharge from the hospital.

Filling out the questionnaires may be an inconvenience to me and may take as long as 2 hours total. However, I may fill out the questionnaires at my convenience before leaving the hospital, and may also make the follow-up appointment at a time and place convenient to me. If I agree to participate in the 12-month follow-up, I will be contacted by phone or mail several times over the intervening 11-month period in order to find out if my address has changed and to make arrangements for the final home visit. This may be an intrusion on my privacy.

There will be no medical benefit to me, and I will not be paid for my participation. The study may produce information of use to medical health professionals in the future.

I have had the opportunity to talk with Sandra Scheetz or her research assistant about the study. If I have further questions, I may reach her at 123-4567 (or leave a message). If I have any comments about participating in this study, I should first talk with Mrs. Scheetz. If for some reason I don't want to do this, I may contact the Committee on Human Research, which is concerned with protection of volunteers in research projects. I may reach the committee between 8 A.M. and 5 P.M., Monday through Friday, by calling 800-0000.

I have been offered a copy of this form and an Information Sheet to keep.

I have the right to refuse to participate or withdraw from the study at any time. Refusing to participate will in no way affect my care at this medical center at any time.

Subject Signature

Date

Source: Used with permission of Sandra Scheetz, RN, MS, DNS

SELECTED STATISTICAL INFORMATION

APPENDIX C

APPENDIX C–1: TABLE OF RANDOM NUMBERS

71,510	68,311	48,214	99,929	64,650	13,229
36,921	58,733	13,459	93,488	21,949	30,920
23,288	89,515	58,503	46,185	00,368	82,604
02,668	37,444	50,640	54,968	11,409	36,148
82,091	87,298	41,397	71,112	00,076	60,029
47,837	76,717	09,653	54,466	87,988	82,363
17,934	52,793	17,641	19,502	31,735	36,901
92,296	19,293	57,583	86,043	69,502	12,601
00,535	82,698	04,174	32,342	66,533	07,875
54,446	08,795	63,563	42,296	74,647	73,120
96,981	68,729	21,154	56,182	71,840	66,135
52,397	89,724	96,436	17,871	21,823	04,027
76,403	04,655	87,277	32,593	17,097	06,913
05,136	05,115	25,922	07,123	31,485	52,166
07,645	85,123	20,945	06,370	70,255	22,806
32,530	98,883	19,105	01,769	20,276	59,402
60,427	03,316	41,439	22,012	00,159	08,461
51,811	14,651	45,119	97,921	08,063	70,820
01,832	53,295	66,575	21,384	75,357	55,888
83,430	96,917	73,978	87,884	13,249	28,870
00,995	28,829	15,048	49,573	65,278	61,493
44,032	88,720	73,058	66,010	55,115	79,227
27,929	23,392	06,432	50,201	39,055	15,529
53,484	33,973	10,614	25,190	52,647	62,580
51,184	31,339	60,009	66,595	64,358	14,985
31,359	77,470	58,126	59,192	23,371	25,190
37,842	44,387	92,421	42,965	09,736	51,873
94,596	61,368	82,091	63,835	86,859	10,678
58,210	59,820	24,710	23,225	45,788	21,426
63,354	29,875	51,058	29,958	61,221	61,200
79,958	67,599	74,103	49,824	39,306	15,069
56,328	26,905	34,454	53,965	66,617	22,137
72,806	64,421	58,711	68,436	60,301	28,620
91,920	96,081	01,413	27,281	19,397	36,231
05,010	42,003	99,866	20,924	76,152	54,090
88,239	80,732	20,778	45,726	41,481	48,277
45,705	96,458	13,918	52,375	57,457	87,884
64,274	26,236	61,096	01,309	48,632	00,431
63,731	18,917	21,614	06,412	71,008	20,255
39,891	75,337	89,452	88,092	61,012	38,072
26,466	03,735	39,891	26,362	86,817	48,193
33,492	70,485	77,323	01,016	97,315	03,944
04,509	46,144	88,909	55,261	73,434	62,538
63,187	57,352	91,208	33,555	75,943	41,669
64,651	38,741	86,190	38,197	99,113	59,694
46,792	78,975	01,999	78,892	16,177	95,747
78,076	75,002	51,309	18,791	34,162	32,258
05,345	79,268	75,608	29,916	37,005	09,213
10,991	50,452	02,376	40,372	45,077	73,706

APPENDIX C–2: THE STANDARD NORMAL (z) DISTRIBUTION

z	.00	.01	.02	.03	.04	.05	.06	.07	.08	.09
0.0	.0000	.0040	.0080	.0120	.0160	.0199	.0239	.0279	.0319	.0359
0.1	.0398	.0438	.0478	.0517	.0557	.0596	.0636	.0675	.0714	.0753
0.2	.0793	.0832	.0871	.0910	.0948	.0987	.1026	.1064	.1103	.1141
0.3	.1179	.1217	.1255	.1293	.1331	.1368	.1406	.1443	.1480	.1517
0.4	.1554	.1591	.1628	.1664	.1700	.1736	.1772	.1808	.1844	.1879
0.5	.1915	.1950	.1985	.2019	.2054	.2088	.2123	.2157	.2190	.2224
0.6	.2257	.2291	.2324	.2357	.2389	.2422	.2454	.2486	.2517	.2549
0.7	.2580	.2611	.2642	.2673	.2704	.2734	.2764	.2794	.2823	.2852
0.8	.2881	.2910	.2939	.2967	.2995	.3023	.3051	.3078	.3106	.3133
0.9	.3159	.3186	.3212	.3238	.3264	.3289	.3315	.3340	.3365	.3389
1.0	.3413	.3438	.3461	.3485	.3508	.3531	.3554	.3577	.3599	.3621
1.1	.3643	.3665	.3686	.3708	.3729	.3749	.3770	.3790	.3810	.3830
1.2	.3849	.3869	.3888	.3907	.3925	.3944	.3962	.3980	.3997	.4015
1.3	.4032	.4049	.4066	.4082	.4099	.4115	.4131	.4147	.4162	.4177
1.4	.4192	.4207	.4222	.4236	.4251	.4265	.4279	.4292	.4306	.4319
1.5	.4332	.4345	.4357	.4370	.4382	.4394	.4406	.4418	.4429	.4441
1.6	.4452	.4463	.4474	.4484	.4495	.4505	.4515	.4525	.4535	.4545
1.7	.4554	.4564	.4573	.4582	.4591	.4599	.4608	.4616	.4625	.4633
1.8	.4641	.4649	.4656	.4664	.4671	.4678	.4686	.4693	.4699	.4706
1.9	.4713	.4719	.4726	.4732	.4738	.4744	.4750	.4756	.4761	.4767
2.0	.4772	.4778	.4783	.4788	.4793	.4798	.4803	.4808	.4812	.4817
2.1	.4821	.4826	.4830	.4834	.4838	.4842	.4846	.4850	.4854	.4857
2.2	.4861	.4864	.4868	.4871	.4875	.4878	.4881	.4884	.4887	.4890
2.3	.4893	.4896	.4898	.4901	.4904	.4906	.4909	.4911	.4913	.4916
2.4	.4918	.4920	.4922	.4925	.4927	.4929	.4931	.4932	.4934	.4936
2.5	.4938	.4940	.4941	.4943	.4945	.4946	.4948	.4949	.4951	.4952
2.6	.4953	.4955	.4956	.4957	.4959	.4960	.4961	.4962	.4963	.4964
2.7	.4965	.4966	.4967	.4968	.4969	.4970	.4971	.4972	.4973	.4974
2.8	.4974	.4975	.4976	.4977	.4977	.4978	.4979	.4979	.4980	.4981
2.9	.4981	.4982	.4982	.4983	.4984	.4984	.4985	.4985	.4986	.4986
3.0	.4987	.4987	.4987	.4988	.4988	.4989	.4989	.4989	.4990	.4990

Source: Mosteller, F & Rourke, R. *Study Statistics.* Table A1, Reading, Mass: Addison-Wesley; 1973. Reprinted with permission.

APPENDIX C–3: *t* DISTRIBUTION

α

Degrees of freedom	.005 (one tail) .01 (two tails)	.01 (one tail) .02 (two tails)	.025 (one tail) .05 (two tails)	.05 (one tail) .10 (two tails)	.10 (one tail) .20 (two tails)	.25 (one tail) .50 (two tails)
1	63.657	31.821	12.706	6.314	3.078	1.000
2	9.925	6.965	4.303	2.920	1.886	.816
3	5.841	4.541	3.182	2.353	1.638	.765
4	4.604	3.747	2.776	2.132	1.533	.741
5	4.032	3.365	2.571	2.015	1.476	.727
6	3.707	3.143	2.447	1.943	1.440	.718
7	3.500	2.998	2.365	1.895	1.415	.711
8	3.355	2.896	2.306	1.860	1.397	.706
9	3.250	2.821	2.262	1.833	1.383	.703
10	3.169	2.764	2.228	1.812	1.372	.700
11	3.106	2.718	2.201	1.796	1.363	.697
12	3.054	2.681	2.179	1.782	1.356	.696
13	3.012	2.650	2.160	1.771	1.350	.694
14	2.977	2.625	2.145	1.761	1.345	.692
15	2.947	2.602	2.132	1.753	1.341	.691
16	2.921	2.584	2.120	1.746	1.337	.690
17	2.898	2.567	2.110	1.740	1.333	.689
18	2.878	2.552	2.101	1.734	1.330	.688
19	2.861	2.540	2.093	1.729	1.328	.688
20	2.845	2.528	2.086	1.725	1.325	.687
21	2.831	2.518	2.080	1.721	1.323	.686
22	2.819	2.508	2.074	1.717	1.321	.686
23	2.807	2.500	2.069	1.714	1.320	.685
24	2.797	2.492	2.064	1.711	1.318	.685
25	2.787	2.485	2.060	1.708	1.316	.684
26	2.779	2.479	2.056	1.706	1.315	.684
27	2.771	2.473	2.052	1.703	1.314	.684
28	2.763	2.467	2.048	1.701	1.313	.683
29	2.756	2.462	2.045	1.699	1.311	.683
Large	2.575	2.327	1.960	1.645	1.282	.675

APPENDIX C–4: CRITICAL VALUES OF
THE CHI-SQUARE (χ^2) DISTRIBUTION

α

Degrees of freedom	0.995	0.99	0.975	0.95	0.90	0.10	0.05	0.025	0.01	0.005
1	—	—	0.001	0.004	0.016	2.706	3.841	5.024	6.635	7.879
2	0.010	0.020	0.051	0.103	0.211	4.605	5.991	7.378	9.210	10.597
3	0.072	0.115	0.216	0.352	0.584	6.251	7.815	9.348	11.345	12.838
4	0.207	0.297	0.484	0.711	1.064	7.779	9.488	11.143	13.277	14.860
5	0.412	0.554	0.831	1.145	1.610	9.236	11.071	12.833	15.086	16.750
6	0.676	0.872	1.237	1.635	2.204	10.645	12.592	14.449	16.812	18.548
7	0.989	1.239	1.690	2.167	2.833	12.017	14.067	16.013	18.475	20.278
8	1.344	1.646	2.180	2.733	3.490	13.362	15.507	17.535	20.090	21.955
9	1.735	2.088	2.700	3.325	4.168	14.684	16.919	19.023	21.666	23.589
10	2.156	2.558	3.247	3.940	4.865	15.987	18.307	20.483	23.209	25.188
11	2.603	3.053	3.816	4.575	5.578	17.275	19.675	21.920	24.725	26.757
12	3.074	3.571	4.404	5.226	6.304	18.549	21.026	23.337	26.217	28.299
13	3.565	4.107	5.009	5.892	7.042	19.812	22.362	24.736	27.688	29.819
14	4.075	4.660	5.629	6.571	7.790	21.064	23.685	26.119	29.141	31.319
15	4.601	5.229	6.262	7.261	8.547	22.307	24.996	27.488	30.578	32.801
16	5.142	5.812	6.908	7.962	9.312	23.542	26.296	28.845	32.000	34.267
17	5.697	6.408	7.564	8.672	10.085	24.769	27.587	30.191	33.409	35.718
18	6.265	7.015	8.231	9.390	10.865	25.989	28.869	31.526	34.805	37.156
19	6.844	7.633	8.907	10.117	11.651	27.204	30.144	32.852	36.191	38.582
20	7.434	8.260	9.591	10.851	12.443	28.412	31.410	34.170	37.566	39.997
21	8.034	8.897	10.283	11.591	13.240	29.615	32.671	35.479	38.932	41.401
22	8.643	9.542	10.982	12.338	14.042	30.813	33.924	36.781	40.289	42.796
23	9.260	10.196	11.689	13.091	14.848	32.007	35.172	38.076	41.638	44.181
24	9.886	10.856	12.401	13.848	15.659	33.196	36.415	39.364	42.980	45.559
25	10.520	11.524	13.120	14.611	16.473	34.382	37.652	40.646	44.314	46.928
26	11.160	12.198	13.844	15.379	17.292	35.563	38.885	41.923	45.642	48.290
27	11.808	12.879	14.573	16.151	18.114	36.741	40.113	43.194	46.963	49.645
28	12.461	13.565	15.308	16.928	18.939	37.916	41.337	44.461	48.278	50.993
29	13.121	14.257	16.047	17.708	19.768	39.087	42.557	45.722	49.588	52.336
30	13.787	14.954	16.791	18.493	20.599	40.256	43.773	46.979	50.892	53.672
40	20.707	22.164	24.433	26.509	29.051	51.805	55.758	59.342	63.691	66.766
50	27.991	29.707	32.357	34.764	37.689	63.167	67.505	71.420	76.154	79.490
60	35.534	37.485	40.482	43.188	46.459	74.397	79.082	83.298	88.379	91.952
70	43.275	45.442	48.758	51.739	55.329	85.527	90.531	95.023	100.425	104.215
80	51.172	53.540	57.153	60.391	64.278	96.578	101.879	106.629	112.329	116.321
90	59.196	61.754	65.647	69.126	73.291	107.565	113.145	118.136	124.116	128.299
100	67.328	70.065	74.222	77.929	82.358	118.498	124.342	129.561	135.807	140.169

Source: Owen D. *Handbook of Statistical Tables*. Attached tables. Reading, Mass: Addison-Wesley, 1962. Reprinted with permission.

APPENDIX C–5: STATISTICS SYMBOLS

x	value of a single score	r	linear correlation coefficient
f	frequency with which a value occurs	r^2	coefficient of determination
Σ	summation	r_s	Spearman's rank correlation coefficient
n	number of scores in a sample	m	slope of the straight line with equation $y = mx + b$
$n!$	factorial		
N	number of scores in a finite population	b	y intercept of the straight line with equation $y = mx + b$
$\bar{x}$	mean of the scores in a sample		
μ	mean of all scores in a population	y'	predicted value of y
s	standard deviation of a set of sample values	d	difference between two paired scores
		$\bar{d}$	mean of the differences d found from paired sample data
σ	standard deviation of all values in a population	s_d	standard deviation of the differences d found from paired sample data
s^2	variance of a set of sample values		
σ^2	variance of all values in a population	s_c	standard error of estimate
z	standard score	T	rank sum used in Wilcoxon signed-rank test
$z(\alpha/2)$	critical value of z		
t	t distribution	H	Kruskal-Wallis test statistic
$t(\alpha/2)$	critical value of t	R	sum of the ranks for a sample; used in the Wilcoxon rank-sum test
df	number of degrees of freedom		
F	F distribution	μ_R	expected mean rank; used in the Wilcoxon rank-sum test
χ^2	chi-square distribution		
χ^2_R	right-tailed critical value of chi-square	σ_R	expected standard deviation of ranks; used in the Wilcoxon rank-sum test
χ^2_L	left-tailed critical value of chi-square		
p	probability of an event *or* the population proportion	G	number of runs in runs test for randomness
q	probability or proportion equal to $1 - p$	μ_G	expected mean number of runs; used in runs test for randomness
p_s	sample proportion		
q_s	sample proportion equal to $1 - p_s$	σ_G	expected standard deviation for the number of runs; used in runs test for randomness
$\bar{p}$	proportion obtained by pooling two samples		
$\bar{q}$	proportion or probability equal to $1 - \bar{p}$	$\mu_{\bar{x}}$	mean of the population of all possible sample means $\bar{x}$
$P(A)$	probability of event A		
$P(A/B)$	probability of event A assuming event B has occurred	$\sigma_{\bar{x}}$	standard deviation of the population of all possible sample means $\bar{x}$
$\bar{A}$	complement of event A	E	maximum error of the estimate of a population parameter *or* expected value
H_0	null hypothesis		
H_1	alternative hypothesis	Q_1, Q_2, Q_3	quartiles
α	probability of a type I error *or* the area of the critical region	$D_1, D_2, \ldots, D_9$	deciles
		$P_1, P_2, \ldots, P_{99}$	percentiles
β	probability of a type II error		

GLOSSARY

Abstract A statement located at the beginning of a research article that summarizes the work as briefly as possible.

Accessible Population The feasible population from which the sample is drawn.

After-only/posttest-only design The simplest quasi-experimental design wherein data from the experimental and control groups are collected only at the end of treatment or after exposure to the independent variable.

Agency for Health Care Policy Research (AHCPR) A federal agency that is responsible for implementing a program to improve health services nationwide and that includes funds for studies of clinical nursing practice.

Alternative Hypothesis A statement that there is a difference between two populations with respect to a measure or variable. Also called a *research hypothesis.*

Analysis of Variance (ANOVA) An inferential statistical procedure that compares the mean scores of two groups on a measure or variable of interest.

Analytic Induction A method of qualitative analysis that searches for concepts and propositions in the data rather than attempting to quantify categories.

Applied Research Research directed toward solving practical problems.

Basic Research Research conducted to develop theories.

Basic social process (BSP) Patterns or core variables that account for most of the variation in interaction in a grounded theory study.

Before-after design A study design in which subjects are measured on the same variable before and after the experimental treatment.

Biased Sample A sample that is not representative of the population it aspires to represent.

Bimodal Distribution A distribution or set of scores with two modes.

Case Study   An in-depth analysis of an individual, a family, a social setting, or a group conducted under natural conditions.

Census   A study based on an entire population.

Central Tendency   A measure of a central value or trend in a set of numbers. The three measures of central tendency are the mode, the median, and the mean.

Chi-Square   A nonparametric statistic that measures the relationship between two variables.

Clinical Trial   A study aimed at developing and evaluating a new program, product, method, or procedure.

Cluster Sampling   A type of probability sampling in which the study population is divided into groups or clusters and elements are randomly selected from each cluster.

Comparative Group   Another term for a control group.

Complex Hypothesis   A statement that predicts the relationship between two or more independent variables and two or more dependent variables.

Concept   The building block of theory that allows one to categorize and organize observations.

Conceptual Framework   Background of existing literature that may not contain a specific theory but that does synthesize sensitizing concepts.

Concurrent Validity   A type of criterion-related validity that assesses the relationship or consistency between a score on a current test and a score or rating on a different test that measures a similar construct.

Confounding Variable   A variable other than or in addition to the study's independent variable that may have an effect on the dependent variable. Also called an *uncontrolled* or *extraneous variable.*

Construct   (1) Abstract concepts constructed or derived from existing theory. (2) A concept used in a theory to account for a relationship in observable events.

Construct Validity   An estimate of how well a particular instrument measures a theoretical construct.

Content Analysis   A procedure for analyzing qualitative data by establishing categories.

Content Validity   An assessment of the content of an instrument to ensure that it adequately represents or includes the entire content area or domain it purports to measure.

Continuous Variable   A variable with a range of variability.

Control Group   Subjects in an experiment who do not receive the experimental treatment or intervention and whose scores provide a comparison against which the scores of the experimental group can be interpreted.

Convenience Sampling   A type of nonprobability sampling that allows the use of available or accessible research subjects.

Correlation   A measure of the association or relationship between two interval or ratio-level variables.

Correlation Coefficient   A measure of the association or relationship between two variable values, ranging from +1 to −1. A correlation of .0 indicates no relationship between the variables, and values approaching ±1 indicate a strong relationship.

Criterion-Related Validity   A measure of the validity of a psychosocial instrument. There are two types of criterion-related validity: predictive and concurrent. Predictive validity assesses how well a score on a current test can predict future performance. Concurrent validity indicates an individual's current standing on a criterion measure related to the construct of interest.

Critical Value   The value of a statistic that needs to be exceeded in order for the null hypothesis to be rejected.

Data   The information the investigator collects from subjects in a study. Data may be either quantitative or qualitative.

Data Cleaning   A systematic process of checking a data set for errors.

Debriefing   The process of disclosing to a research subject any information that may have been withheld previously.

Deductive Approach   An approach to theory building that begins with existing theory and tests hypotheses deduced from that theory; moves from general to specific.

Delphi Technique   A type of expert sampling where several rounds of questionnaires focusing on a specific topic are sent to experts with the aim of eliciting their opinions and determining group consensus.

Dependent Variable (DV)   The effect or outcome variable that depends on the independent variable; usually symbolized as y.

Description (analytic)   A qualitative analysis method that generates new classes or categories by an active inspection of data.

Description (straight)   A qualitative analysis method that uses a classification scheme from existing literature.

Descriptive Analysis   A range of possible statistical procedures for summarizing data.

Dichotomous Variable   A variable with only two categories.

Direct Measure   A variable that can be directly measured, such as age or income.

Directional Hypothesis   A statement that specifies the direction of the relationship between variables.

Distribution   A visual display of a set of scores characterized by shape. The shape of a distribution can be either symmetrical or skewed.

Ecological Validity   A measure of a study's procedures to determine if they are clear, explicit, and consistent enough to be replicated by another investigator.

Empirical Data   Evidence gathered by the senses.

Empiricism   *See* **Positivism.**

Ethics   A branch of philosophy concerned with what is right or good and what one should do.

Exemplar   A short story or vignette that captures similar meanings in phenomenologic research.

Experiment   A study design in which investigators randomly select a sample, randomly assign sample members to control and experimental groups, and manipulate at least one independent variable; can be used to determine cause and effect.

Expert Sampling   A type of nonprobability, purposive sampling that involves choosing experts based on their knowledge concerning an area relevant to the study.

Ex post Facto Study   A study that investigates something after the fact.

External Criticism   The examination of historical data sources for their validity, genuineness, or authenticity.

External Validity   The generalizability of a study's results or findings.

Extraneous Variables See **Confounding variables**

F-Value   A ratio used in analysis of variance procedures calculated by dividing the between-group variance by the within-group variance. A large F-value leads to a rejection of the null hypothesis, and a small F-value leads to acceptance of the null hypothesis.

Face Validity   Subjective judgments by experts or respondents about the degree to which a test appears to measure the relevant construct.

Factor-Isolating Question   A researchable question that asks "What is this?"; a question that isolates, describes, categorizes, or names factors or situations.

Factor-Relating Question   A researchable question that asks "What is happening here?"; a question that asks how factors relate to one another.

Factorial Design   A design that involves matching on a nominal variable that can't be rank ordered but is assumed to have an effect on the dependent variable or to interact with the independent variable; results in increased numbers of cells and the need for larger samples.

Field Research   A term that encompasses the various methods of qualitative data collection.

Fieldwork   A mode of scientific inquiry that immerses the researcher in processes of day-to-day life. Also called *naturalistic inquiry.*

Frequency Distribution   A method of organizing and presenting data in which numerical values are arranged with the number of corresponding cases for those values from lowest to highest or from highest to lowest.

Frequency Polygon   A method of graphing and visually displaying frequency data.

Grand Theory   An explanation of how something occurs under a great variety of conditions. Also called *formal theory.*

Grounded Theory Methodology   One of the most carefully systematized methods for generating categories, propositions, and theoretical explanations based on qualitative data.

Hawthorne Effect   The effect on a dependent variable that might be attributed to participation in a study.

Hermeneutics   The study of human meanings and practices emphasizing the interpretation of lived experience and behaviors from narrative text or stories of informants; from the Greek word meaning "to interpret." Also called *phenomenology*.

Histogram   A type of bar graph used to visually display frequency data.

Historical Study Design   A study design used to learn about the past based on data that already exist.

Hypothesis   A statement about predicted relationships between variables.

Independent Variable (IV)   A variable that the investigator manipulates; the cause, condition, treatment, or input variable; usually symbolized as x.

Inductive Approach   An approach to theory building that generates hypotheses and explanatory schema from data; moves from specific to general.

Inferential Statistics   Statistic techniques used to generalize from the sample to the larger, unmeasured population.

Informed Consent   The knowing consent of an individual or his or her legally authorized representative to participate in research without undue inducements or any form of fraud, deceit, duress, or other constraint or coercion.

Institutional Review Board (IRB)   A committee established to review ethical issues related to human research.

Internal Consistency Reliability   A measure of how well all the items in a particular instrument relate to one another.

Internal Criticism   A determination of the accuracy of statements contained within historical data sources.

Internal Validity   Whether or not the manipulation of a study's independent variable made the difference on the dependent variable.

Interrater Reliability   An assessment of the consistency of an instrument or measure despite different raters or users.

Interval Estimate   A range of numbers calculated from the sample and used to infer or estimate the population parameter.

Interval Scale   Ordered measurement categories or numbers with equal distances between successive values.

Level 1 Question   A question in exploratory and descriptive research used when little knowledge is available about a topic that asks, "What is it?"

Level 2 Question   A question that looks for relationships between variables.

Level 3 Question   A question that assumes a relationship between variables and asks "Why" or "How."

Level of Significance   Expressed as a numerical value or decimal point; the likelihood of making a Type I, or alpha, error. Also called the *p value.*

Likert Scale   An ordinal scale commonly used in psychosocial research that measures the level of a subject's agreement or disagreement with a statement.

Materials   The measurement devices used to collect data from subjects.

Mean   A measure of central tendency that is calculated by summing a set of scores and dividing the sum by the total number of subjects; commonly referred to as the "average."

Measurement   The process of assigning numerical values to the concepts under investigation.

Median   A measure of central tendency that represents the middle score in a set of data or scores. The median lies at the midpoint of the distribution and divides the set of scores into halves.

Methodological Note (MN)   The type of field note that the researcher uses to give instructions to him- or herself; a critique of tactics or reminder about what might be useful.

Methodological Study   A study designed to develop, validate, or evaluate research tools or techniques.

Mode   The most frequent or most common score in a set of data; a measure of central tendency that is used most often with nominal-level data.

Multimodal Distribution   A distribution or set of scores with two or more modes.

National Center for Nursing Research (NCNR)   A center established as part of the National Institutes of Health by congressional mandate to fund nursing research training.

National Nursing Research Agenda (NNRA)   A concentrated effort to set priorities for nursing research.

Naturalistic (also called interpretive)   Philosophy of science borrowed from social sciences that focuses on understanding meaning under natural conditions; associated with qualitative methodologies.

Naturalistic/Interpretive Study Design   A study design that uses qualitative methodologies to discover meaning and understanding under natural conditions.

Necessary Condition   A condition that must occur if an effect is to occur.

Negative Case   Datum that runs counter to the researchers' propositions.

Nominal Scale   A scale used to collect categorical or labeled data; arbitrarily assigns a numerical value to represent a category or name.

Nominal Distribution   A bell-shaped distribution that is symmetrical and unimodal.

Nondirectional Hypothesis   A statement that predicts there is a relationship between variables without specifying direction.

Nonparametric Test   A statistical test that does not require a normal distribution of a variable.

Nonprobability Sampling   A nonrandom sampling technique in which not all elements in the population have equal chances of being selected for inclusion in the sample.

Null Hypothesis   (1) A statement that no difference exists between the populations being compared. (2) A statement that there are no significant differences in a study outcome variable (the dependent variable) other than what can be attributed to chance. (3) A statement that there is no relationship between study variables. Also called a *statistical hypothesis*.

Nursing Research   Research on the problems, or outcomes, of nursing care.

Objectivity   An attempt to distance the research process as much as possible from the scientist's personal beliefs, values, and attitudes.

Observational Note (ON)   The type of field note that describes the who, what, where, when, and how of a situation, event, or interaction with as little interpretation as possible.

Operational Definition   Specification of how a study variable will be measured.

Ordinal Scale   A scale used to collect ordinal, or "ordered," data. Ordinal data is numbered or ranked from low to high values; the distance between these values is not necessarily equal.

Outlier   An extreme score in a set of data.

Paired Comparison   A data-collection or measurement technique in which respondents are asked to choose between two objects or stimuli based on a specific property or dimension.

Paradigm Case   A whole case that stands out, vividly revealing patterns of meaning in phenomenologic research.

Parametric Test   A statistical test that requires that specific assumptions about the sampling distribution are met. The sampling distribution of the statistics must be close to normal distributions or the sample large enough (usually 20 or more) that the sampling distribution is approximately normal.

Personal Note (PNs)   The type of field note that researchers use to keep track of personal reactions, reflections, and experiences.

Pilot Study   A small-scale practice run.

Point Estimate   A single number from a sample used to infer or estimate the population value.

Population   The larger group of subjects from which a sample is drawn. The sample is meant to represent the distribution of scores in the wider population. The total possible membership of the group under study; the group to whom study results will be generalized.

Population Parameter   A numerical description of a variable or measure in a population. Population parameters are generally estimated with data from a smaller subgroup or sample of the population.

Population Validity   Measurement of whether the findings can be generalized from the sample to the total population of interest to the investigator.

Positivism   A philosophy of science that attempts to measure phenomena objectively; associated with quantitative methodologies. Also called *empiricism*.

Power   The probability that an inferential statistical test will reject the null hypothesis and support the research hypothesis; related to both sample size and effect size.

Predictive Validity   A type of criterion-related validity that assesses how well a score on a current test can predict future performance.

Preexperimental Design   A posttest-only study design with no control group.

Primary Source   Firsthand information in historical studies.

Probability Sampling   A sampling technique in which each element in the population has an equal and random chance of being selected for inclusion in the study.

Proxy Measure   A measure or value of something that cannot be measured directly.

Pure-Applied Continuum   Stages of a study's nursing practice relevance ranging from highly theoretical to highly pragmatic.

Pure Research *See* **Basic Research**

Purpose   Specifies the overall goal of a study; what will be accomplished.

Purposive Sampling   A type of nonprobability sampling in which the researcher selects a particular group or groups chosen on certain relevant criteria.

Qualitative Analysis   The nonnumerical organization and interpretation of data for the discovery of patterns, themes, forms, and qualities from textual data.

Quantitative Data   Numerical data collected from the subjects in a study.

Quasi-experimental Design   A design used when it is not possible to implement all the characteristics of an experimental design such as random assignment to experimental and control groups.

Quota Sampling   A type of nonprobability sampling in which the researcher decides the best, most relevant groups or strata to be included in the study. A quota of each of these strata is sampled.

Randomized Block Posttest Design   A variation on the after-only design that involves assigning subjects to experimental and control groups after they have been ranked with respect to some variable that is important to the dependent variable.

Range   A measure of the dispersion of a set of scores.

Ranking Technique   A data-collection or measurement technique in which respondents are asked to reorder a set of objects or stimuli based on a specific property.

Ratio Scale   A scale consisting of ordered measurement points with equal distances between successive values and an absolute zero point.

Reliability   The consistency, accuracy, and precision of a measure.

Representative Sample   A sample that is similar to the larger population from which it was drawn with regard to the distribution of major characteristics.

Research Critique   A critical estimate of the scientific merit of a piece of research that has been carefully and systematically studied.

Research Design   A set of procedures that tell an investigator how data should be collected and analyzed to answer a study question; a blueprint for the conduct of the research.

Research Hypothesis   A statement of the anticipated relationship between variables.

Research in Nursing   The broad study of the nursing profession, including historical, ethical, policy, and educational studies.

Research Problem   A statement or question that can be addressed through empirical evidence that provides the basis and direction for a study; a problem that can be investigated using the process of scientific inquiry.

Research Process   The tool of science.

Research Review   A summary of the major features and characteristics of a study.

Response Bias   A potential bias in the data collected when there is a low response rate in a study.

Response Set   A tendency to respond to items in a similar manner based on irrelevant criterion.

Reverse-scored Item   A test item worded in the opposite way from the majority of items in order to avoid response bias.

Risk-Benefit Ratio   The balance between the risks of participating in a study and the scientific benefits expected.

Sample   (1) A subgroup of the larger population under study; used to make inferences and estimates about the larger, unmeasured population. (2) Those elements of a population from whom data will be collected and from whom generalizations will be made.

Sample Survey   A study based on a sample of the total population.

Sampling Error   The fluctuation of a statistic from one sample to another drawn from the same population.

Sampling Frame   All the subjects in the population.

Sampling Interval   The distance between elements or subjects selected in a sample.

Scatter Plot   A visual presentation of the relationship between two variables.

Scientific Inquiry   A process in which observable, verifiable data are collected to describe, explain, and/or predict events.

Secondary Source   An account other than a firsthand account used as data in historical studies.

Semantic Differential Scale   A psychosocial scale designed to quantify concepts in terms of their word meanings or semantic properties.

Semistructured Interview   An interview that begins with an outline of topics but in which the interviewer and the subject are free to deviate from the agenda as the conversation unfolds. Focused interviews require that all predetermined topics or questions be covered in some form by the end of the interview. Also called a focused interview.

Simple Hypothesis   A statement that predicts the relationship between one independent variable and one dependent variable.

Situation-Producing Question   A researchable question that asks "How can I make it happen?"; a question that establishes goals for nursing actions.

Situation-Relating Question   A researchable question that asks, "What would happen if . . . ?"; a question in which the investigator manipulates variables to see what will happen.

Skewed Distribution   A distribution of a set of scores that is not symmetrical about the mean. Skewed distributions are off-center relative to the mean and have longer tails in one direction than in the other. Positively skewed distributions have longer tails to the right, and negatively skewed distributions have longer tails to the left.

Snowball Sampling   A kind of nonprobability sampling in which subjects suggest other potential subjects to the researcher.

Sorting Technique   A data-collection or measurement technique in which subjects are given a stack of cards with one item per card and asked to sort them into piles based on a specific dimension such as level of difficulty or alternativeness.

Split-Half Reliability   An indicator of the internal consistency of an instrument.

Standard Deviation   A measure of the variability of a set of scores; the distance a "typical" score varies from the mean.

Standard Error of the Mean   The standard deviation of a distribution of means of samples. The smaller the standard error of the mean, the more accurately a sample mean reflects a population mean.

Standard Score   A score that indicates how many standard deviations away from the mean a particular score is. Represented by z.

Standardized Instrument   An instrument that has been developed, tested, and refined and is commonly used to measure a particular variable or construct.

Statistic   A numerical description of a sample. There are two kinds of statistics: descriptive and inferential.

Statistical Analysis System (SAS)   A computer program that can perform a number of statistical calculations on data.

Statistical Hypothesis See **Null hypothesis 3.**

Stratum   A homogeneous subpopulation.

Subscale   One of several specific measures that contribute to a broader measure or scale.

Substantive Theory   An explanation of a process or phenomenon under a specific set of conditions; a middle-range theory.

Sufficient Condition   A condition that is always followed by an effect.

Survey Research Design   A study design in which information is collected from a sample of subjects who resemble the total population on characteristics important to the researcher; used to describe characteristics, opinions, attitudes, and so on, as they exist.

Symmetrical Distribution   The distribution of a set of scores that is symmetrical about the mean and can be divided into two even halves.

Systematic Sampling   A type of probability sampling in which every element is drawn from a population.

T-Test   A statistical test used to determine whether two groups are significantly different from each other.

Test of Knowledge   A test used to assess knowledge in a given area or areas.

Test-Retest Reliability   A measure of the stability of an instrument over repeated periods of use.

Thematic Analysis   A strategy in phenomenological research that involves recognizing common themes in textual data.

Theoretical Framework   An essay in which an investigator summarizes existing concepts, theories, methods, and findings and relates them to his or her study.

Theory   An explanation of the world; a vision or view on truth or reality; a set of interrelated constructs, concepts, and propositions that present a systematic view of phenomena by specifying relationships for the purpose of describing, explaining, and predicting.

Time Series Design   A design used when the investigator can study only one group but uses before measures to establish a baseline against which to compare posttreatment measures of the dependent variable.

Triangulation   (1) The acquisition of different slices of data in the same study, for example, interviews and observations. (2) The combination of qualitative and quantitative methods in the same study. (3) The obtainment of different perspectives on the same issue or question.

Type I Error   A rejection of the null hypothesis when it is really true. Also called *Alpha Error*; the researcher concludes that a relationship exists when it does not.

Type II Error   An acceptance of the null hypothesis when it is really false. Also called *Beta Error*; the researcher concludes that *no* relationship exists when it does.

Uncontrolled Variable *See* **Confounding Variable.**

Unimodal Distribution   A distribution or set of scores with only one mode.

Unstructured Interview   An interview, either scheduled or spontaneous, in which the respondent is free to talk about anything of relevance to the research.

Validity   The relevance of a measure. A valid instrument measures the concept or construct it claims to measure.

Variability   The dispersion of a set of scores or how a set of scores is spread out.

Variable   Any factor that varies.

Vulnerable Group   A group of research subjects such as the elderly, captives, the unconscious, infants, the mentally disabled, and others for whom obtaining informed consent is difficult.

INDEX